SUPER
FOODS
COOKBOOK

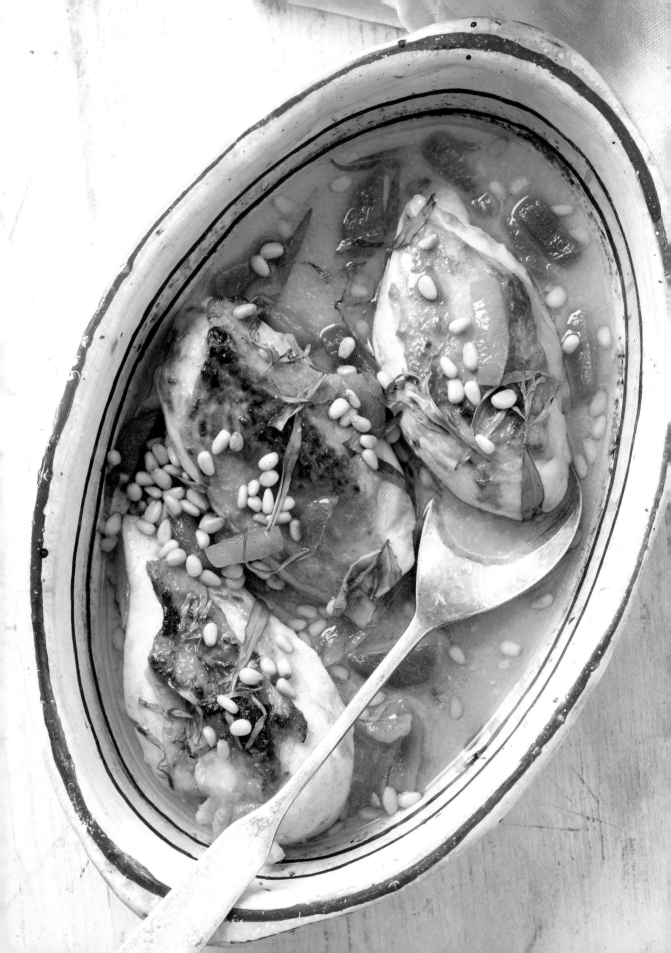

SUPER FOODS
COOKBOOK

184 Super Easy Recipes to Boost Your Health

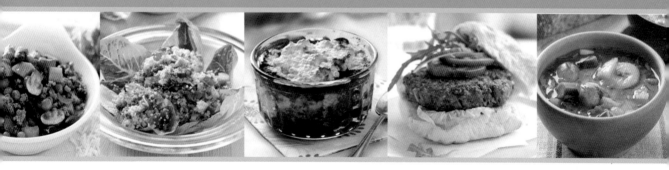

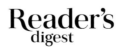

Reader's digest

The Reader's Digest Association, Inc.
New York, NY / Montreal

A READER'S DIGEST BOOK

This edition first published 2014.

This book is adapted from *Super Foods Super Easy*, produced in the United Kingdom in 2012 by Vivat Direct Limited (t/a Reader's Digest), using the services of Creative Plus Publishing Limited, for The Reader's Digest Association, Inc.

Library of Congress Cataloging-In-Publication Data
Super foods cookbook : 184 easy recipes to boost your health / editors of Reader's digest.
    pages cm
  Includes index.
  Summary: "Eat your way to optimum health with 184 recipes that pack a nutritional punch. Each recipe contains at least one superfood designed to boost energy, promote health and well-being, and protect against disease. Discover the exceptional nutritional content and disease-fighting qualities of super foods like broccoli, blueberries, and salmon and delicious, healthful ways to prepare them. By including super foods as part of a balanced diet, you can protect your heart, immune system, digestive system, skin, and bones, and even reduce the risk of developing certain medical conditions later in life. In Super Foods Cookbook you'll find 184 health-boosting recipes, all of which include at least one super food. Each recipe offers clear step-by-step cooking instructions, ingredient information, and invaluable tips. These recipes and foods are proven to prevent, fight, and beat problems big and small."– Provided by publisher.
  ISBN 978-1-62145-197-6 (paperback) – ISBN 978-1-62145-198-3 (epub) 1. Cooking. 2. Natural foods. 3. Functional foods. 4. Health. I. Reader's Digest Association. II. Reader's digest. III. Title: Superfoods cookbook.
  TX714.S868 2014
  641.3'02–dc23
                    2014026105

Picture credits
All photography David Munns, copyright The Reader's Digest Association, except for the following:
8 top left Elizabeth Watt; 12 all Shutterstock; 18 iStockphoto; 38 iStockphoto; 56 Shutterstock; 64 all Shutterstock; 76 Shutterstock; 90 iStockphoto; 98 all Shutterstock; 110 Jodi Pudge/Gettyimages; 126 Paul Debois/GAP Photos; 134 all Shutterstock; 144 iStockphoto; 146 Shutterstock; 164 all Shutterstock; 174 Shutterstock; 188 Shutterstock; 196 all Shutterstock; 206 Graham Strong/GAP Photos; 229 iStockphoto; 238 Andrea Jones/GAP Photos; 244 all Shutterstock; 256 David Dixon/GAP Photos; 272 Jim Franco Photography/ Gettyimages. Illustrations: Shutterstock

We are committed to both the quality of our products and the service we provide to our customers. We value your comments, so please feel free to contact us.

The Reader's Digest Association, Inc.
Adult Trade Publishing
44 South Broadway
White Plains, NY 10601

For more Reader's Digest products and information, visit our website:
        www.rd.com
        www.readersdigest.ca

Printed in China

1 3 5 7 9 10 8 6 4 2

NOTE TO READERS
The information in this book should not be substituted for, or used to alter, medical therapy without your doctor's advice. For a specific health problem, consult your physician for guidance.

While the creators of this work have made every effort to be as accurate and up to date as possible, medical and pharmacological knowledge is constantly changing. The writers, researchers, editors and publishers of this work cannot be held liable for any errors and omissions, or actions that may be taken as a consequence of information contained within this work.

Please note that measurements were converted from metric to imperial measurements. Nutritional data is generally correct and should be used as a general guide in determining your nutrient requirements.

CONTENTS

Welcome to the NEXT STAGE OF the healthy food revolution

Put down your health books, take up your knife and fork, and discover how to eat your way to a healthier lifestyle, easily, quickly, and deliciously. Savor our recipes and move into the super food nutritional fast lane.

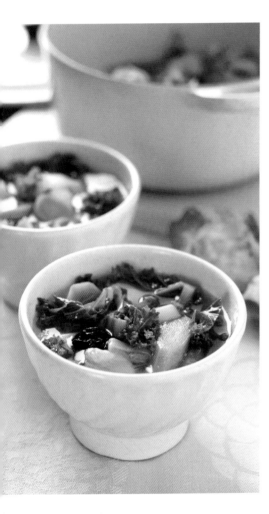

Super Foods Cookbook is a cookbook with a difference—a fantastic selection of tasty, contemporary, easy recipes for everyday living, each of them packed with foods that have been demonstrated to promote long-term health, aid healing, and even help to fight some diseases. And all this can be done without fuss, complicated preparation, or lengthy cooking time—and with supermarket staples.

WHAT IS A SUPER FOOD?

Super foods, such as broccoli, blueberries, and salmon, contain natural ingredients with exceptional nutritional values or protective qualities. They contain natural chemicals, compounds, and nutrients that, for example, may help to protect against the impact of diseases such as cancer and type 2 diabetes, as well as fight the effects of aging, help to lower cholesterol levels, and improve mental alertness.

Here are five top reasons for including more super foods in your daily diet:

● Super foods will help you to meet the seven-a-day fruit and vegetable target that health professionals recommend as a minimum daily amount to protect your body and maintain well-being.

● Many super foods such as lentils and oats have a low glycemic index (GI) value, which means that their carbohydrates are absorbed slowly into the bloodstream. Such foods stave off hunger and keep you feeling full longer which helps with weight control.

● Many super foods such as whole-wheat pasta and carrots are a good source of fiber. This helps your digestive system to work effectively, and some forms of fiber can help to lower cholesterol.

● All super foods are low in, or free from 'bad' fats, such as saturated fats and trans fats, which can increase the risk of heart disease.

● Super foods naturally provide high levels of the essential vitamins and minerals that your body needs for a healthy nervous system, a fully functioning brain, and other key body processes, such as the regulation of blood clotting and the efficient working of your cells and organs.

Turn to the Super Food Benefits Chart (see pages 10–11) for a list of the main super foods featured in our recipes and the conditions they can help to reduce and possibly even prevent, as well as their positive health benefits in the body.

MAKING YOURS A **BALANCED DIET**

Super foods should form a large part of a healthy, well-balanced diet. Follow this checklist of what food types to include regularly to keep your mind and body performing at their best.

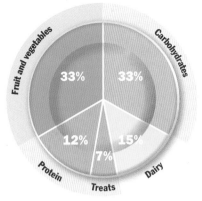

Protein
Essential for building and maintaining muscles and internal organs, protein is also needed to build new cells and repair damaged tissue in your body. High-protein foods include lean meat, poultry, fish, seafood, low-fat dairy foods, eggs, and legumes.

Carbohydrate
The staple of most diets, carbohydrates provide energy for your body throughout the day and as you sleep. About 50 percent of your daily energy should come mainly from whole-grain foods, such as brown rice, whole-wheat pasta, and whole-grain bread. Within this total, no more than 10 percent should come from sugary foods. The best type of sugar is found naturally in fruit and vegetables, not added.

Fat
Providing your body with energy and fat-soluble vitamins, and protecting your vital organs, are among the many roles fat has to play. Eating too much fat, though, especially saturated fat, can lead to weight problems and heart disease. The good fats are unsaturated fats, such as olive oil or canola oil. Other healthy fats include omega-3s, found in oily fish, nuts, and seeds.

Vitamins and minerals
Vitamins A, the B group, C, D, E and K are the essential nutrients for keeping your body in good working order. Major minerals (those found in relatively large amounts in the body) are iron, calcium, zinc, selenium, magnesium, and potassium. Vitamins and minerals appear in small quantities in lots of different foods, so a varied diet is the best way to obtain them all.

Dietary fiber
You need about 30 g of fiber per day to keep your digestive system in good working order. Some types of fiber also help to lower cholesterol levels, which is vital if you want to maintain a healthy heart. Unrefined (unprocessed) plant-based foods contain the highest amounts of fiber. Good examples include whole grains, legumes such as lentils and beans, dried fruit, and fresh fruit and vegetables.

Fluids
Water is vital for physical well-being. An average adult needs to drink almost 2 quarts of fluids every day. Water is the best thirst quencher, but tea, coffee, and low-fat milk are also included. Food can also supply some of your fluid requirements—many fruit and salad ingredients have a high water content.

EATING WELL

Build your food intake around the main food groups for healthy living. The optimum amount of nutrients needed to maintain health varies from person to person—depending on sex, age, height, weight, and activity levels—but as a rule of thumb, about one-third of the food you eat should come from high-fiber carbohydrates such as whole grains, legumes, and potatoes, another third from fruit and vegetables, with the rest made up from fish, poultry, lean meat, and low-fat dairy foods, with only limited amounts of processed fatty or sugary foods.

A NOTE ON SEASONING

Salt Avoid adding salt to your cooking and when serving—too much can lead to high blood pressure. Choose low-sodium stock, or make your own stock. Salt is not added to the cooking water of vegetables, rice, and pasta in our recipes. We have not overseasoned the recipes.
Herbs Use herbs and spices to boost flavor—many have their own health properties. Fresh is best, but use dried if you prefer or if it's more convenient.
Sugar Replace processed sugar with natural sweetness from fresh and dried fruit whenever you can.

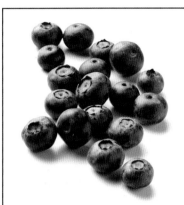

FREEZING SUPER FOODS

Using a freezer to store food ready to use at any time is a great idea—vegetables, fruit, meat, poultry, fish, and even some fresh herbs and spices retain their nutritional value when frozen.

Freeze meat, poultry, and fish on the day of purchase and do not store them for longer than 3 months. Never refreeze meat, fish, or poultry.

Frozen vegetables are very handy—either when store-bought or fresh from the garden. If freezing your own produce, always freeze as soon as possible after picking to avoid losing essential vitamins and minerals. Wash and chop the vegetables ready for freezing, then blanch in a saucepan of boiling water for 2–3 minutes. Lift out with a slotted spoon, refresh under cold water, drain, and pack into labelled containers. Once opened, reseal bags of frozen vegetables securely. Salad vegetables cannot be frozen.

Always defrost food thoroughly in the refrigerator before cooking. Do not cook raw poultry or meat from frozen as it may not cook completely. Some seafood and fish can be cooked from frozen—follow the recipe instructions.

SUPER EASY **PLANNING** AND **SHOPPING**

Healthy cooking does not mean costly lists of little-known ingredients. Much of it is about making a few easy changes to your usual routine and planning ahead, such as making best use of your freezer (see left).

A WELL-STOCKED PANTRY

Stock up on super-food pantry staples and you will always be able to make delicious, healthy food even if you forget to plan ahead. These are the staples that should always be on your shelves:
- grain products such as brown rice, rolled oats, bulgur, couscous, quinoa, a few different whole-wheat pasta shapes, noodles, and flour
- dried and canned legumes, including lentils, cannellini beans, kidney beans, and chickpeas
- a variety of unsalted nuts and seeds
- oils for cooking and salads—canola oil and olive oil are best
- natural sweeteners such as agave syrup, honey, and maple syrup
- whole and ground spices, plus a selection of seasonings, such as low-salt soy sauce, stock cubes, herbs, and pepper.

THE SAVVY SHOPPER

All the ingredients in our recipes are easy to find in supermarkets. If your local store has a fish or meat counter, ask the fishmonger or butcher to prepare the food fresh for you. You are likely to end up with less waste—and even save money.

Also try specialty shops either at shopping centers or online, and make use of local farmers' markets for top-quality produce that is locally and ethically farmed. Choose organic ingredients whenever possible as they should be free from pesticides and artificial additives.

Fish When buying fish, look for sustainable sources—try to avoid endangered bluefin tuna, orange roughy (ocean perch) and shark, and use more abundant varieties such as snapper, haddock, and flounder.

Poultry Choose free-range chicken and turkey where possible. They are slightly more expensive than cage-raised and may have a better flavor.

Meat Beef, pork, and lamb are sold ready cubed, sliced, or ground, which will save on preparation time. Steaks, chops, and tenderloin are best for quick cooking. Always choose lean ground meat. Choose grass-fed or wild meat where available.

Fruit and vegetables Fresh is best, but ready-prepared packs will save you time.

LET'S GET **COOKING**

Super Foods Cookbook contains 184 health-boosting recipes, and all include at least one super food. Each recipe page offers clear step-by-step cooking instructions, ingredient information, and invaluable tips.

● **Ingredients** Each ingredient is listed on the page in the order that it is needed in the recipe, with exact quantities given, either in weight or numbers. Unless otherwise stated, all ingredients such as eggs, fruit, and vegetables are medium in size.

● **Alternative ingredients** The majority of recipes in this book include different ingredient suggestions so you can include the foods you prefer—or adapt the recipe to what you have available.

● **Nutritional values** If you're keeping an eye on your calories or your intake of fat, protein, and fiber, these values are available to give you guidance at a glance.

● **Cook's tips** Expert practical advice is provided so you can get the most from our recipes—from how to remove seeds from a cardamom pod to the best cut of lamb to choose for a stir-fry.

● **Super food information** Every recipe page tells you about the health benefits of one super food ingredient. Refer to the Glossary (right) if there are any terms that are unfamiliar to you. Also, special features on 14 major super foods appear throughout the book. Each provides information on the food's health-promoting benefits and includes five simple mouth-watering recipes.

CONVERSION CHART

Weight		Volume	
Imperial	**Metric**	**Metric**	**Imperial**
1 oz	25 g	1 fl oz	30 mL
2 oz	50 g	2 fl oz	50 mL
3 oz	75 g	5 fl oz	150 mL
4 oz (¼ lb)	125 g	10 fl oz	300 mL
6 oz	175 g	1 pint	500 mL
8 oz (½ lb)	250 g	1 qt	1 L
10 oz (⅔ lb)	275 g	1 gal	4 L
12 oz (¾ lb)	350 g	¼ cup	50 mL
16 oz (1 lb)	500 g	⅓ cup	75 mL
2 lb	1 kg	½ cup	125 mL
		⅔ cup	150 mL
		¾ cup	175 mL
		1 cup	250 mL

GLOSSARY

anthocyanin: a type of plant pigment that may help to protect the body against heart disease (see also flavonoid).

antioxidant: a substance that helps to protect against and destroys harmful free radicals that can damage the body's cells.

beta-carotene: part of a family of natural antioxidants found in many fruit and vegetables. It can be converted to vitamin A in the body.

cholesterol: fatty substance made predominantly by the body from saturated fat in the diet. Too much cholesterol in the blood can increase the risk of heart disease.

ellagic acid: a plant chemical that may have anti-cancer properties.

flavonoid: a plant pigment with beneficial antioxidant properties.

folate: form of B vitamin folic acid that occurs naturally in food. Folate helps to produce and maintain new red blood cells in the body.

glycemic index (GI): a ranking of carbohydrate foods based on the rate at which they raise blood glucose levels after eating. A low GI rating means only a gradual rise in blood glucose levels, which may help with weight control and reduce the risk of heart disease and diabetes.

immune system: the body's defense system, composed of cells, tissues, and organs, which protects the body against infection.

monounsaturated fat: can help to lower harmful cholesterol in the blood and keep the heart healthy.

phytochemical: describes a wide variety of compounds produced by plants that may help to reduce the risk of cancer.

polyunsaturated fat: heart-healthy fats that lower harmful cholesterol in the bloodstream. They provide essential fatty acids.

saturated fat: can raise harmful cholesterol in the blood, increasing the risk of heart disease.

vitamin: a substance found in food that is essential to maintain a healthy body.

SUPER FOODS BENEFITS CHART

	Aging (skin)	Cancer	Cholesterol lowering	Depression	Diabetes (type 2)	Digestive health	Eye health	Fatigue	Heart health	Immune function	Menopause	Mental alertness	Osteoporosis	Rheumatoid arthritis	Stroke prevention	Weight control
Apples	•	•	•	•	•	•	•		•	•	•	•		•	•	•
Apricots	•	•	•	•	•	•	•		•	•	•	•	•	•	•	•
Avocados	•	•	•	•	•	•	•		•	•	•	•	•	•	•	
Bananas	•	•	•	•	•	•		•	•	•	•	•	•	•	•	•
Beans		•	•					•	•	•	•	•				•
Beef (lean)	•			•				•	•							•
Beets	•	•	•	•	•	•	•		•	•	•	•			•	•
Bell Peppers	•	•	•	•	•	•	•		•	•	•	•	•	•	•	•
Berries	•	•	•	•	•	•	•		•	•	•	•	•	•	•	•
Broccoli	•	•	•	•	•	•	•		•	•	•	•	•	•	•	•
Butternut squash	•	•	•	•	•	•	•	•	•	•	•	•		•	•	•
Cabbage	•	•	•	•	•	•			•	•	•	•	•	•	•	•
Carrots	•	•	•	•	•	•	•		•	•	•	•	•	•	•	•
Cauliflower	•	•	•	•	•	•			•	•	•	•		•	•	•
Cherries	•	•	•	•	•	•			•	•	•	•	•	•	•	•
Chicken		•		•	•		•	•	•			•				•
Chicken livers		•		•	•		•	•	•				•	•	•	•
Citrus	•	•	•	•	•	•	•		•	•	•	•	•	•	•	•
Dried fruit	•	•	•	•	•	•		•	•	•	•	•	•	•	•	•
Eggplant	•	•	•	•	•	•			•	•	•	•			•	•
Eggs		•		•			•	•	•	•	•		•	•		•
Garlic		•	•		•	•			•						•	•
Grains		•	•	•	•	•		•	•	•	•	•		•	•	•
Grapes	•	•	•	•	•	•			•	•	•	•		•	•	•

The chart below lists top super foods and shows you where they may be particularly beneficial when eaten as part of a balanced diet for the health issues, diseases, and conditions indicated in the headings. Use this chart as a guide only—always talk to your doctor if you have any concerns about your health.

	Aging (skin)	Cancer	Cholesterol lowering	Depression	Diabetes (type 2)	Digestive health	Eye health	Fatigue	Heart health	Immune function	Menopause	Mental alertness	Osteoporosis	Rheumatoid arthritis	Stroke prevention	Weight control
Lentils		•	•	•	•	•		•	•	•	•	•	•		•	•
Low-fat dairy	•	•		•	•	•		•	•	•	•	•	•	•	•	•
Mangoes	•	•	•	•	•	•	•		•	•	•	•	•	•	•	•
Mushrooms	•	•	•	•	•	•	•	•			•	•		•	•	•
Nuts	•	•	•	•	•		•		•	•	•	•	•	•	•	•
Oats		•	•	•	•			•	•	•	•	•			•	•
Oily fish	•	•	•	•	•				•	•	•	•		•	•	•
Olive oil	•	•	•		•				•	•		•	•	•	•	
Onion		•	•		•	•			•	•	•	•			•	•
Pears	•	•	•	•	•	•			•	•		•			•	•
Peas	•	•	•	•	•	•	•	•	•	•	•	•	•	•	•	•
Pineapples	•	•	•	•	•	•			•	•	•	•			•	•
Pomegranates	•	•	•	•	•	•	•		•	•	•	•	•	•	•	•
Seafood	•	•	•	•	•		•	•	•	•	•	•	•	•	•	•
Seeds	•	•	•	•	•	•	•	•	•	•	•	•	•	•	•	•
Soybeans	•	•	•	•	•	•		•	•	•	•	•	•	•	•	•
Spinach	•	•	•	•	•	•	•	•	•	•	•	•	•	•	•	•
Sweet potatoes		•	•	•	•	•	•	•	•	•	•	•		•	•	•
Tomatoes	•	•	•	•	•	•	•		•	•	•	•	•	•	•	•
Turkey		•	•	•	•		•	•	•	•		•	•	•	•	•
White fish		•	•	•	•				•	•	•		•	•		•
Whole-grain bread		•	•	•	•	•		•	•	•	•	•	•	•	•	•
Whole-grain rice		•	•	•	•	•		•	•	•	•	•	•	•	•	•
Zucchini	•	•	•	•	•	•			•	•	•	•		•	•	•

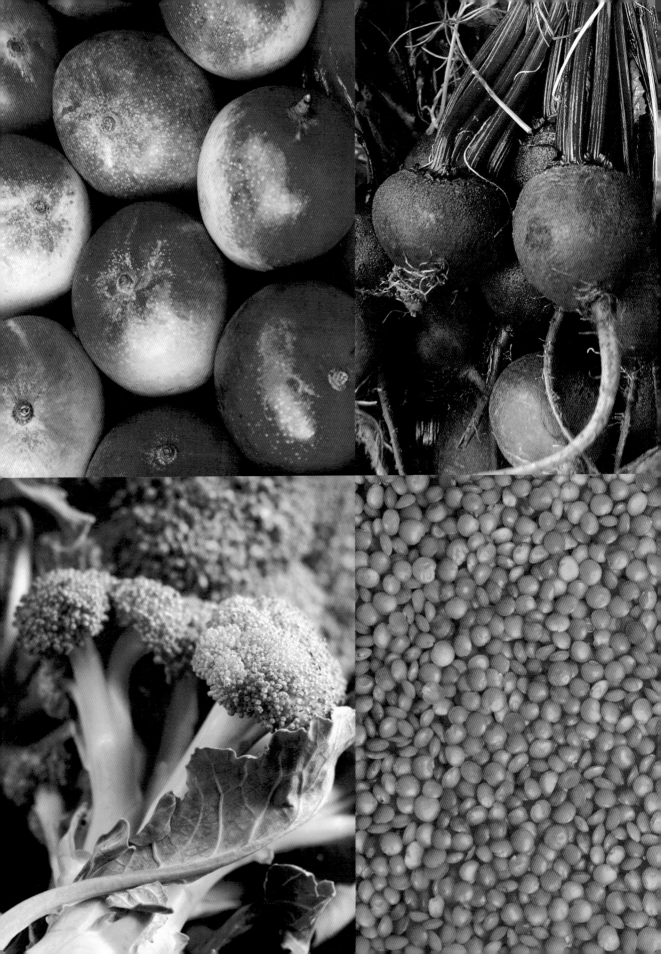

SOUPS, STARTERS *and* SNACKS

CHUNKY **VEGETABLE** SOUP WITH **PASTA**

A real Italian-inspired meal in a bowl—nutritious whole-wheat spaghetti in a rich minestrone-style soup full of tender vegetables. Serve with warmed olive focaccia for a comforting meal.

Serves 4
Preparation 10 minutes
Cooking 30 minutes

1 onion
1 carrot
1 celery stalk
1 yellow bell pepper
1 parsnip
⅓ cup mushrooms
2 tablespoons olive oil
1 bay leaf
1 clove garlic, crushed
1 can (14½ ounces) chopped
   tomatoes
2 cups hot chicken or vegetable stock
3 ounces whole-wheat spaghetti
½ cup grated parmesan, to serve

Each serving provides
• 270 calories • 13 g fat • 4 g
saturated fat • 29 g carbohydrates
• 11 g protein • 7 g fiber

ALTERNATIVE INGREDIENTS
• For a meaty version of this soup,
sauté ¼ cup diced smoked bacon,
chorizo or pancetta in a dry frying pan
for 1 minute before starting step 1.
• Leave out the parsnip and add
⅔ cup fresh or frozen green beans or
fava beans with the pasta.

1 Finely chop the onion. Dice the carrot, celery, pepper, and parsnip, and chop the mushrooms. Heat the oil in a large saucepan over high heat. Add the bay leaf, onion, carrot, celery, and garlic, reduce the heat to low, then cover and cook for 2 minutes.

2 Stir in the pepper and mushrooms, cover, and cook for another 2 minutes. Add the parsnip and tomatoes, then pour in the hot stock and return to a boil. Reduce the heat and simmer, covered, for 20 minutes, or until the vegetables are tender.

3 Break the spaghetti into 1½-inch pieces and stir them into the soup. Return to a boil, reduce the heat, and simmer for 5 minutes, or until the pasta is tender. Ladle the soup into four bowls and sprinkle with parmesan.

COOK'S TIP
● Frozen vegetables are great for everyday meals, saving time on shopping and preparation. There is a wide variety of mixtures, some with bell peppers, celery, and mushrooms as well as the usual carrots, peas, and beans. Use fresh onion and garlic, then add frozen mixed vegetables in step 2 in place of the fresh ingredients. Reduce the cooking time by 5 minutes.

SUPER FOOD

WHOLE-WHEAT PASTA
Most of the goodness of whole grains is concentrated in the outer bran layer. Whole-wheat pasta retains that bran so it contains up to 75 percent more nutrients than pasta made from refined grains. Regularly eating whole-wheat pasta protects against heart disease and may lower the risk of some forms of cancer of the digestive tract.

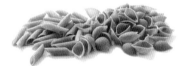

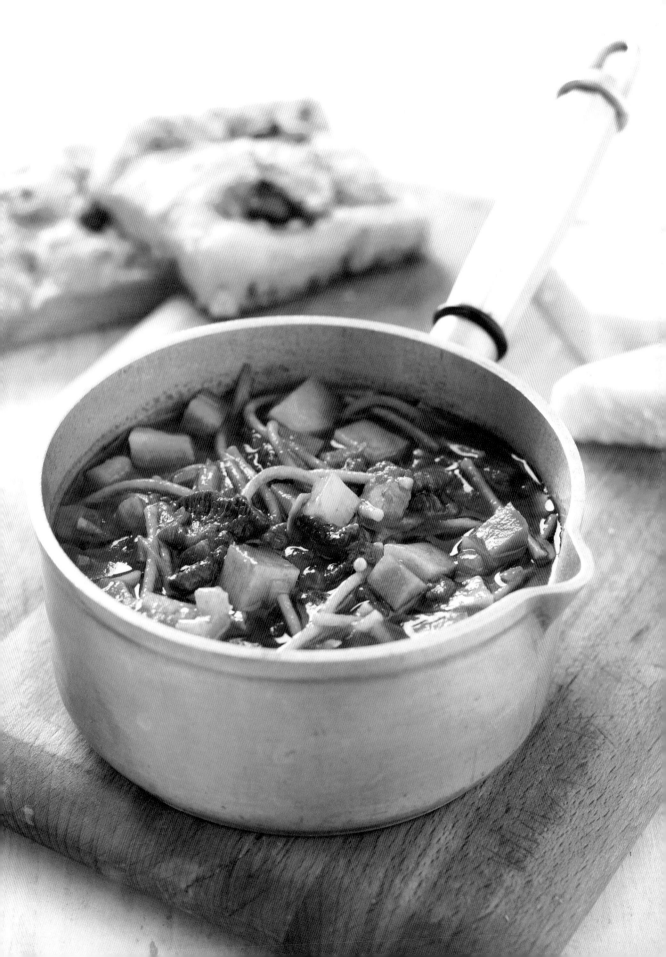

CHILLED **CARROT** AND **ORANGE** SOUP

For a refreshing and healthy cold soup, try this fusion of yogurt, herbs, and two juices whose vibrant orange color is the product of the cancer-fighting pigment beta-carotene.

Serves 4
Preparation 10 minutes
Cooking 2 minutes

2¾ cups carrot juice, chilled
⅔ cup plain yogurt
grated zest of ½ orange and juice
  of 1 orange, about ⅓ cup
4 tablespoons snipped fresh chives
2 tablespoons chopped fresh
  tarragon
1 tablespoon olive oil
4 slices whole-grain bread

Each serving provides
• 181 calories • 6 g fat • 1 g
saturated fat • 26 g carbohydrates
• 7 g protein • 3 g fiber

ALTERNATIVE INGREDIENTS
• For a slightly thicker soup
with a 'nutty' flavor, cut crusts
off 3 extra slices of whole-grain
bread, and process the bread in
a blender with the carrot juice,
yogurt, and chives.
• Fresh cilantro works well
instead of tarragon.
• Try tomato juice in place of
carrot juice and add a dash
of hot sauce for a piquant
tomato soup.

1 Preheat the broiler to high. Pour the carrot juice into a large bowl and whisk in the yogurt until smooth. Add the orange zest, juice, and chives, then whisk again. Ladle into four soup bowls.

2 Mix the tarragon with the oil. Toast the bread for 1 minute on one side under the broiler, then turn and lightly brush the untoasted side with the tarragon oil. Toast for another 1 minute until golden and crisp. Season the soup with freshly ground black pepper to taste and serve.

COOK'S TIPS
● You can make this soup in advance and chill for several hours in the fridge before serving. Add chopped tarragon to the oil well in advance to infuse it with the herb flavor, and then store it in an airtight jar in the fridge until needed.
● If you can't get carrot juice from your supermarket, make it with an electric juicer or in a blender. For this recipe, you will need 2 pounds of peeled or scrubbed carrots. Juice the carrots according to the juicer directions or purée them in a blender. Add a little water if the mixture becomes too dry or the blades stick. Pour the carrot juice into a container and add 2 cups water. Let stand for 30 minutes, then strain through a fine-meshed sieve.

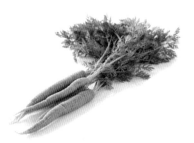

SUPER FOOD

CARROTS
Beta-carotene, found in abundance in carrots and other brightly colored fruits and vegetables, has strong antioxidant properties and may help to protect against cancer. It is converted in the body to vitamin A, which helps to promote healthy skin and improve vision in dim light.

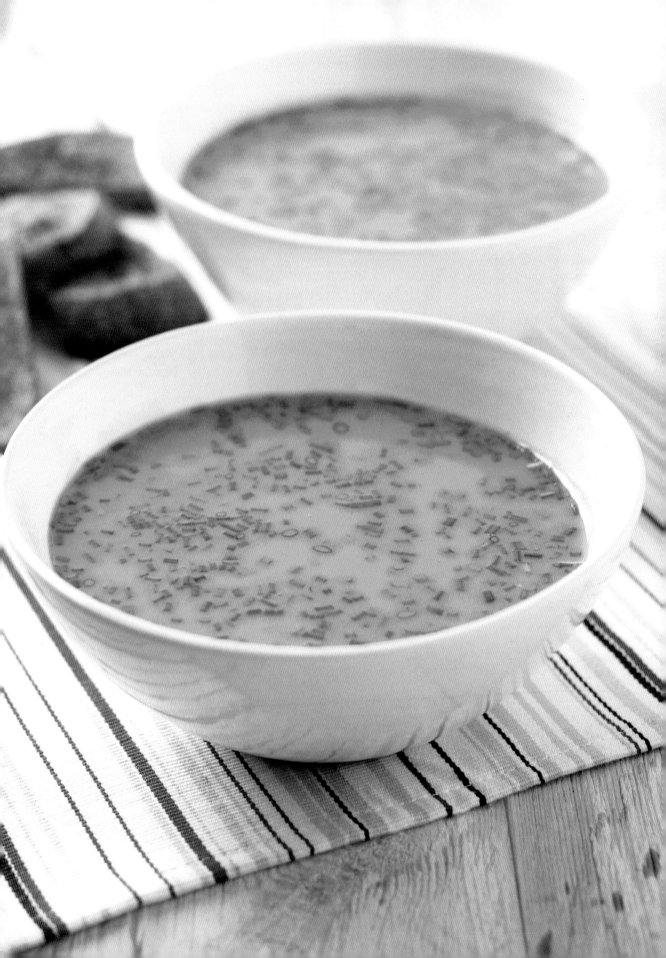

CARROTS

It is no myth that carrots help you to see in the dark, thanks to their high level of beta-carotene, which the body converts to vision-enhancing vitamin A. Yet carrots offer much more – cell-protecting properties for great-looking skin, plenty of fiber to aid digestion, and because they are low in fat and calories, they make a perfect healthy anytime snack.

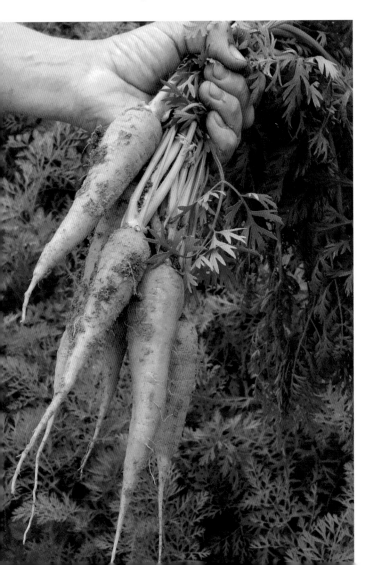

HERBED CARROT AND CORIANDER SOUP

Serves 4
Preparation 10 minutes Cooking 45 minutes

Each serving provides • 112 calories • 5 g fat • 1 g saturated fat • 16 g carbohydrates • 2 g protein • 4 g fiber

Heat **1 tablespoon olive oil or canola oil** in a saucepan over a medium-low heat and then add **5 chopped carrots** and **1 large chopped onion**. Sauté for 5 minutes, or until softened. Add **2 crushed cloves garlic** and **1 teaspoon ground coriander**, and stir occasionally for 1 minute. Pour in **4 cups hot vegetable stock** and bring to a simmer. Cover and cook for 30 minutes. Remove from the heat, let cool a little, then purée in a blender or in the pan with a stick blender until smooth. Stir in the **juice of ½ lemon**, and season to taste. Gently reheat the soup but do not boil. Just before serving, stir in **4 tablespoons chopped fresh cilantro**. Ladle into four bowls and drizzle **1 teaspoon plain yogurt** over each one before serving.

COOK'S TIP
● Give the soup a slightly different flavor by using ground cumin instead of ground coriander.

LAYERED VEGETABLE CASSEROLE

Serves 4
Preparation 15 minutes Cooking 60 minutes

Each serving provides • 381 calories • 8 g fat • 2 g saturated fat • 62 g carbohydrates • 13 g protein • 3 g fiber

Heat **1 tablespoon olive oil** in a flameproof casserole dish and cook **1 large thinly sliced onion** over medium-low heat for 5 minutes to soften, stirring occasionally. Add **1 tablespoon chopped fresh parsley, 1 tablespoon snipped fresh chives**, and **2 crushed cloves garlic**, and stir into the onions. Remove the onion mixture from the casserole dish with a slotted spoon. Cover the bottom of the dish with **1 pound thickly sliced potatoes** then layer over **¼ cup dried split peas**, and a third of the onion mixture. Add the next layer of **5 sliced carrots** and cover with **¼ cup dried split peas**, and one-third of the onion mixture. Top with a layer of **2 sliced parsnips** then **¼ cup dried split peas**, and the remaining third of the onion mixture. Pour in **4 cups hot vegetable stock** and bring to a boil. Reduce the heat, cover and simmer for

30 minutes. Remove the lid and cook for another 20 minutes, or until the vegetables are tender and the sauce has thickened. Top each portion with **1 tablespoon sour cream**.

COOK'S TIPS

● The dried split peas cook in the casserole stock, so there is no need to pre-soak or pre-cook them.

● Serve the casserole with a steamed green vegetable such as broccoli, spinach, or savoy cabbage.

HONEY-BRAISED CARROTS WITH BABY PEAS

Serves 4
Preparation 5 minutes Cooking 12 minutes

Each serving provides • 137 calories • 8 g fat
• 3 g saturated fat • 15 g carbohydrates • 3 g protein
• 5 g fiber

Place **1 pound whole baby carrots** in a saucepan and add **1 tablespoon butter, 1 tablespoon olive oil, 3 tablespoons hot vegetable stock, ½ teaspoon grated nutmeg**, and **1½ tablespoons honey**. Bring to a simmer, cover, and cook for 8 minutes, or until carrots are just tender. Add **1 cup frozen baby peas** to the pan and heat through for 1–2 minutes. Serve the carrots garnished with **1 tablespoon snipped fresh chives**.

COOK'S TIPS

● If baby carrots are not available, use large ones and cut them in half widthwise and lengthwise.

● Serve as a side dish with roast beef or venison to complement their rich meat flavors.

BROWN RICE, LENTIL, AND CARROT SALAD

Serves 4
Preparation 10 minutes Cooking 35 minutes

Each serving provides • 377 calories • 21 g fat
• 3 g saturated fat • 38 g carbohydrates • 9 g protein
• 6 g fiber

Cook ⅔ **cup brown rice** in a saucepan with **1¼ cups hot vegetable stock** and boil, covered, for 30 minutes, or until tender and the stock is absorbed. Cut **3 carrots** into ½ to 1-inch chunks and boil with **1 cup broccoli florets** for 10 minutes, or until tender. Remove the rice from the heat and add ⅔ **cup canned green lentils** to the rice. Stir in gently and allow to cool. Stir the cooked vegetables into the rice with

1 tablespoon finely chopped sun-dried tomatoes. Make a dressing with **2 tablespoons olive oil, 2 tablespoons sesame oil, 1 tablespoon balsamic vinegar, 2 teaspoons finely grated fresh ginger**, and a dash of **store-bought hot pepper sauce**. Stir the dressing and **2 tablespoons chopped parsley** into the rice mixture. Sprinkle **1 tablespoon sesame seeds** over the salad and serve.

COOK'S TIPS

● If you want to use dried lentils, put ⅔ cup green lentils in boiling water and simmer for 25 minutes until tender. Drain before adding to the rice.

● If the rice is not cooked through by the time the stock is absorbed, add a little more hot stock or boiling water and continue cooking until tender. Rice varies in cooking time according to the age and variety of the grains.

● Handy for a buffet, this salad can be stored overnight in the fridge. It will taste even better when the flavors have infused and returned to room temperature.

SWEET AND SOUR NOODLES

Serves 4
Preparation 10 minutes Cooking 10 minutes

Each serving provides • 334 calories • 12 g fat
• 2 g saturated fat • 52 g carbohydrates • 7 g protein
• 5 g fiber

Cook **1 cup medium egg noodles** for 4 minutes, or according to the package directions. In another pan, heat **2 tablespoons olive oil or canola oil** over high heat and add **3 thinly sliced carrots** and **1 sliced leek**. Cook for 3 minutes. Diagonally slice **6 scallions** and add to the pan with **2 chopped cloves garlic** and **1 chopped mild green chile**. Cook for 1 minute. Add **1 teaspoon ground cumin, 1 tablespoon light soy sauce**, and **2 teaspoons honey**, and stir for another minute. Add the noodles and stir gently to heat through. Add **1 teaspoon whole cumin seeds** before serving.

COOK'S TIPS

● Adjust the level of chile heat to your preference with mild, medium, or hot chilies.

● For a heartier meal, add leftover cooked meat, or thin slices of pork or chicken fillet sautéed in 1 tablespoon olive oil or canola oil, when adding the noodles.

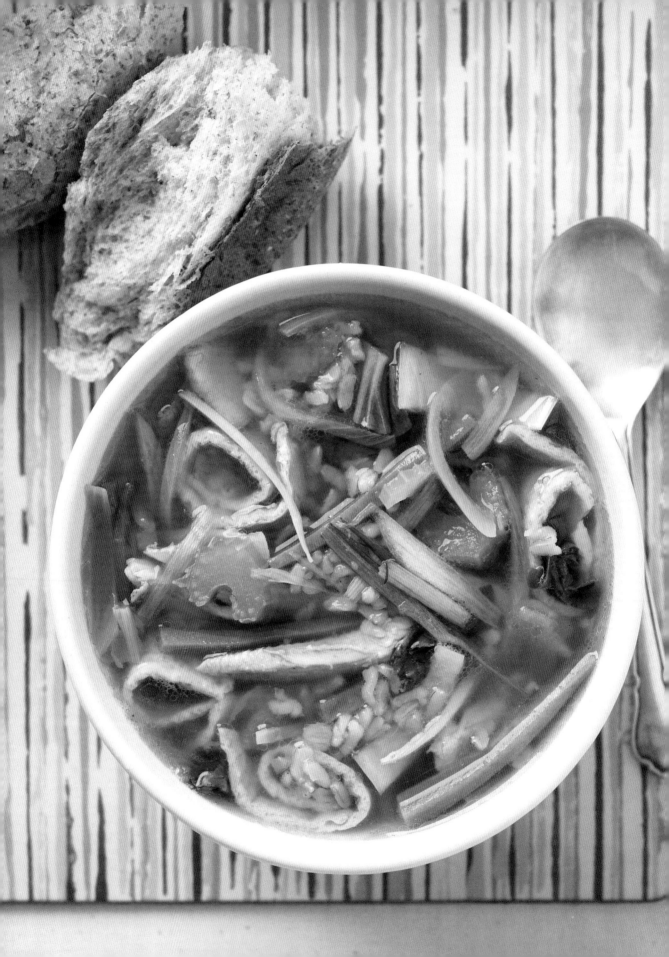

CHICKEN AND RICE BROTH WITH SHREDDED OMELET

Sesame oil, juicy chicken, and vitamin-rich bok choy are just three of the good-for-you ingredients in this delectable soup. Laced with strips of protein-packed omelet, it makes a perfect light meal.

Serves 4
Preparation 15 minutes
Cooking 35 minutes

1 small onion
2 sticks celery
2 carrots
2 tablespoons olive oil or canola oil
1 tablespoon sesame oil
½ pound precooked chicken fingers
⅓ cup brown rice
2 cloves garlic, crushed
4¾ cups hot chicken stock
2 eggs
1 medium bok choy
2 scallions

Each serving provides
• 315 calories • 16 g fat • 3 g saturated fat • 22 g carbohydrates • 22 g protein • 2 g fiber

ALTERNATIVE INGREDIENTS
• Precooked chicken strips are now available in the refrigerated deli case at most supermarkets. If you can't find them, use precooked chicken breast and cut it into thin slices.
• Choy sum, or mustard greens, is a good substitute for bok choy. Alternatively, replace with purple broccoli and allow an extra 1 minute cooking time in step 4.

1 Thinly slice the onion and chop the celery into ½-inch chunks. Cut the carrots into ¼-inch sticks. Heat 1 tablespoon of the olive oil or canola oil and the sesame oil in a large saucepan. Add the chicken and cook over high heat for 1 minute. Stir in the rice, garlic, onion, celery, and carrots. Cook for another minute.

2 Add the hot stock and return to a boil, then reduce the heat. Cover and simmer for 30 minutes, or until the chicken and vegetables are cooked and the rice is tender.

3 Meanwhile, heat the remaining 1 tablespoon of olive oil or canola oil in a frying pan over high heat. Beat the eggs together and pour them into the pan. Cook over high heat for 1 minute, tilting the pan and lifting the edges of the omelet as the egg sets. Remove from the pan, roll up the omelet and slice into ½-inch-wide strips.

4 Slice the bok choy and shred the scallions. When the soup is cooked, add the bok choy and scallions, return to a simmer, and cook for another minute. Season to taste, add the omelet rolls, and ladle into four bowls to serve.

COOK'S TIP
● To wash and prepare bok choy, swish the head in a bowl of water. Rinse between the leaves with running water then shake well. This keeps the head intact and makes slicing easy. Trim off the base and slice as required.

SUPER FOOD

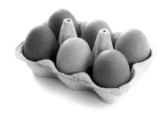

EGGS
Two medium eggs will provide 100 percent of your recommended daily amount of vitamin B_{12}. Researchers believe this vitamin may help to retain mental alertness and protect against Alzheimer's disease. Eggs are also rich in protein and other key nutrients.

BEET AND CRANBERRY BORSCHT

Cranberry juice brings sweetness and fruity goodness to red cabbage and purple beets in a soup that is full of vitamins and antioxidants. Whole-grain bread makes a tasty accompaniment.

Serves 4
Preparation 5 minutes
Cooking 15 minutes

1 onion
2 sticks celery
1 tablespoon olive oil
2 cloves garlic, crushed
pinch of ground nutmeg
⅔ pound red cabbage
1 pound cooked beets
2½ cups hot low-sodium
   chicken stock
2½ cups cranberry juice drink
1 teaspoon red wine vinegar
   or cider vinegar
4 tablespoons low-fat plain yogurt
2 tablespoons snipped chives

Each serving provides
225 calories • 5 g fat • 1 g saturated fat • 37 g carbohydrates • 8 g protein • 7 g fiber

ALTERNATIVE INGREDIENTS
• Use fresh beets instead of cooked. Wash, trim, peel, and dice 1 pound fresh beets and add them to the onion mixture instead of the cabbage in step 2. Add the stock and water, bring to a boil, then reduce the heat, cover, and simmer for 10 minutes. Add the cabbage and cranberry juice drink and continue from step 2.
• Try pomegranate juice drink instead of cranberry for a stronger sweet-sour soup. Increase the quantity of vinegar to 2–3 teaspoons, tasting as you add, to balance the sweeter fruit juice.

1 Chop the onion and dice the celery. Heat the olive oil in a large saucepan over high heat and add the onion, celery, garlic, and nutmeg. Stir the vegetables and reduce the heat to medium, cover, and cook for 4 minutes, or until the vegetables begin to soften.

2 Finely shred the red cabbage and dice the beets. Add the cabbage to the pan and cook, stirring, for 1 minute. Add the hot stock and the cranberry juice drink. Stir in the beets and bring to a boil. Reduce heat to low, so that the soup simmers steadily. Cover and cook for 10 minutes.

3 Stir in the vinegar, season to taste, and ladle the soup into four bowls. Top each serving with 1 tablespoon yogurt and sprinkle with chives.

COOK'S TIPS
● Cut red cabbage into short fine shreds by slicing it into slim wedges and then finely slicing the wedges—the cabbage should then fall apart.
● Vacuum-packed cooked beets, available from some specialty food stores, are a brilliant pantry ingredient with a long shelf life. They work well in this recipe—just make sure they are not the kind preserved with vinegar or acetic acid. Otherwise, boil or bake unpeeled beets until tender, rub off the skins, and use as directed in the recipe.

SUPER FOOD

RED CABBAGE
Cabbage belongs to the brassica family, along with brussels sprouts, broccoli, and watercress. It is bursting with antioxidant nutrients, and also provides vitamin C and B vitamins, such as folate. There is some evidence to link brassicas with a reduced risk of getting cancer, especially cancer of the digestive tract.

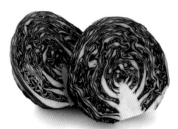

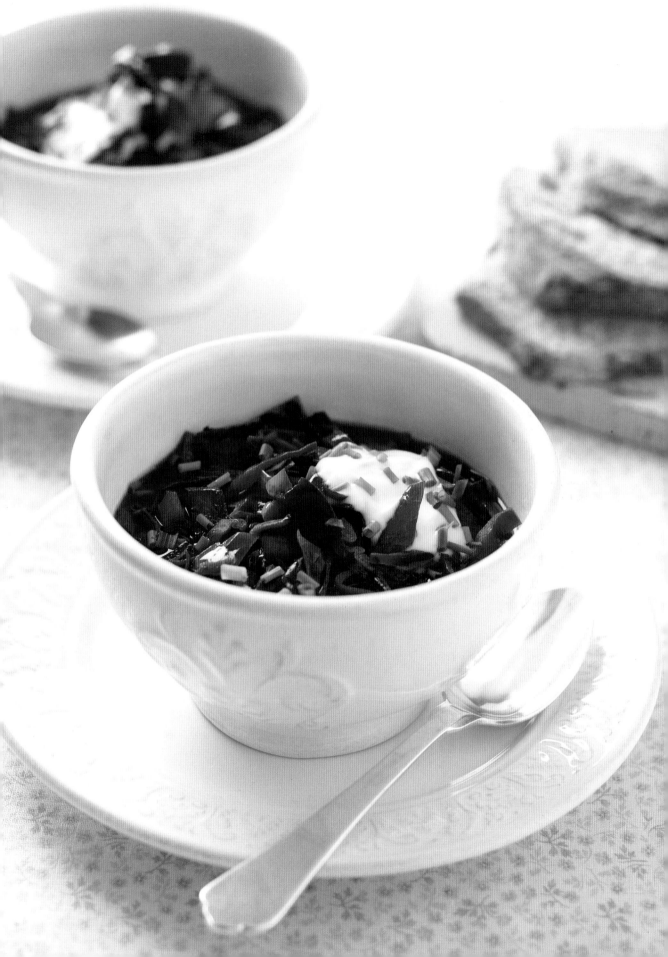

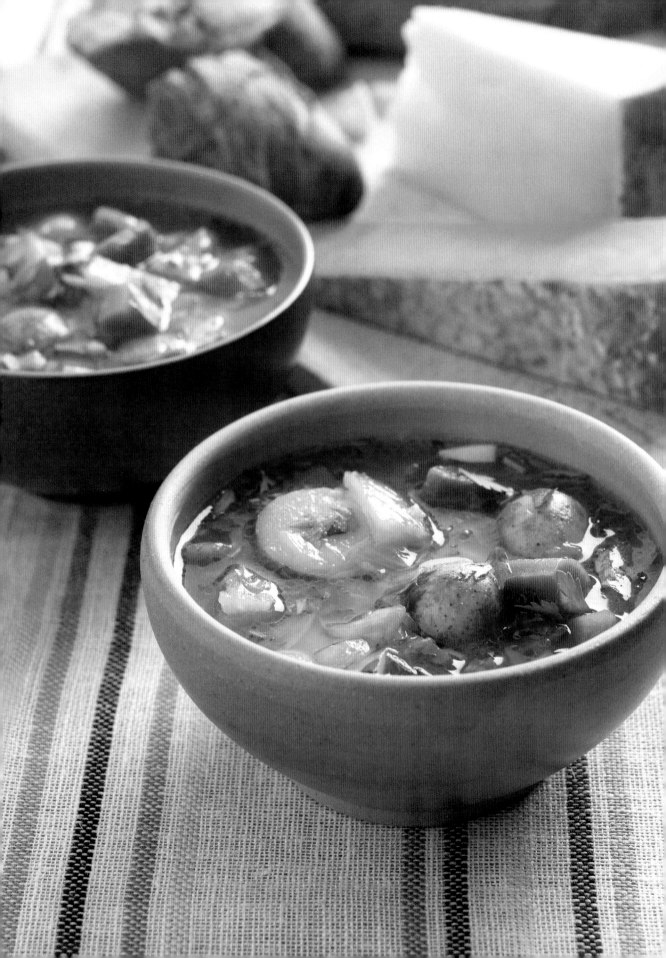

SPRING **VEGETABLE** SOUP

The mild anise flavor of fennel, the firm texture of new potatoes, and a kick of fresh parsley merge temptingly in a hearty soup inspired by a Polish recipe. Serve with bread and cheese.

Serves 4
Preparation 15 minutes
Cooking 25 minutes

1 bulb fennel
2 large onions
2 carrots
1 tablespoon olive oil
1 small sprig rosemary
3 cloves garlic, crushed
1 pound small new potatoes
3¾ cups hot vegetable stock
4 tablespoons chopped fresh parsley

Each serving provides
• 202 calories • 5 g fat • 1 g saturated fat • 36 g carbohydrates
• 5 g protein • 6 g fiber

ALTERNATIVE INGREDIENTS
• Add 4–6 diced celery stalks instead of the fennel for a milder anise flavor.
• If new potatoes are not available, use regular potatoes recommended for boiling, such as russets. Peel them and cut into bite-sized chunks.
• For extra color, add the tips of ½ pound broccolini to the soup for the final 5 minutes of cooking. Return the soup to a simmer before covering the pan so the broccolini cooks.
• Boost the flavor of the soup by adding ¼ pound diced bacon or pancetta in step 2.

1 Trim and chop the stalk and feathery leaves of the fennel and set aside. Cut the bulb into slim wedges, remove the core from the base and thinly slice the wedges into bite-sized pieces.

2 Chop the onions and coarsely dice the carrots. Add the oil, fennel stalk and leaves, rosemary, onions, carrots, and garlic to a large saucepan and cook, stirring occasionally, over high heat for about 3 minutes. Stir in the diced fennel bulb, cover, and reduce heat to low. Cook for another 5 minutes, or until the vegetables have softened, stirring once.

3 Scrub the potatoes, cut them in half, add to the pan, and add the hot stock. Return to a boil and adjust the heat so that the soup simmers steadily. Cover and cook for 10–15 minutes, or until the potatoes are tender. Season to taste and stir in the parsley just before serving.

COOK'S TIPS
● Use good-quality cubed, powdered, or packaged stocks for the best flavor when making soup.
● To make your own vegetable stock, simply simmer together onion, celery, carrot, garlic, parsley, thyme, and bay leaves (and/or any other vegetables and fresh herbs you have on hand) in 2 quarts of water for about 30 minutes.

SUPER FOOD

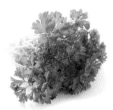

PARSLEY
Though usually served and eaten only in small amounts, parsley is highly nutritious. It contains fiber for a healthy digestive system, the antioxidant vitamin C for cancer prevention, and folate (a B vitamin) for heart health.

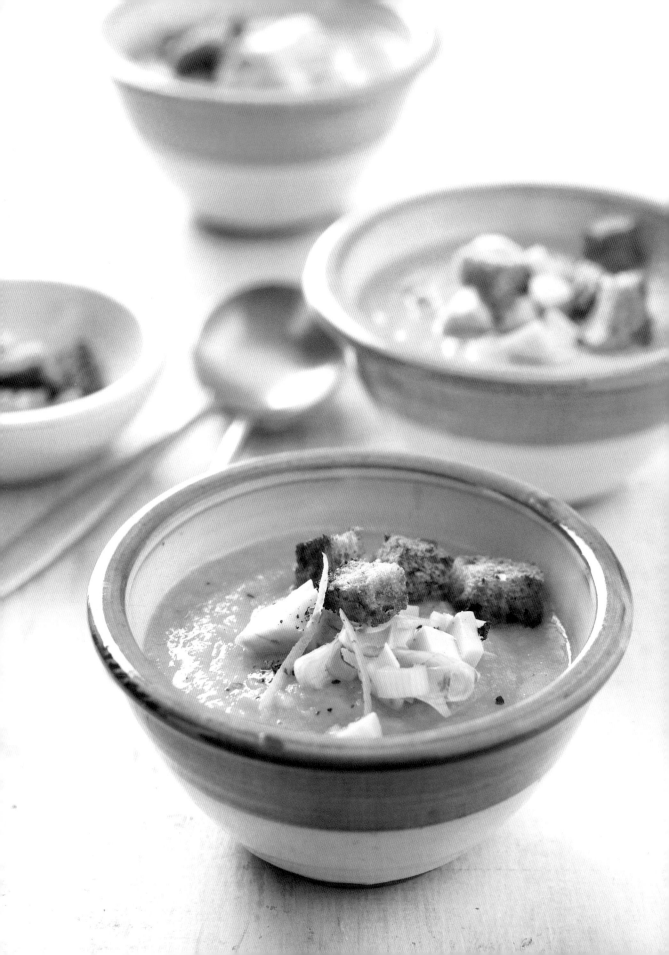

CREAMY **LENTIL** SOUP WITH **CROUTONS**

Perk up the rich flavors of hearty lentil soup with an unexpected zingy topping of avocado, scallions, and lemon zest. Crisp whole-grain croutons add crunch appeal.

Serves 4
Preparation 15 minutes
Cooking 22 minutes

Each serving provides
• 340 calories • 22 g fat • 4 g saturated fat • 25 g carbohydrates • 13 g protein • 8 g fiber

1 onion
2 celery stalks
1 large carrot
1 large rutabaga, about ½ pound
1 tablespoon olive oil
1 clove garlic, crushed
½ cup red lentils
1 bay leaf
2 sprigs fresh thyme
1 tablespoon tomato paste
3¾ cups hot low-sodium chicken
  or vegetable stock

Croutons
2 slices whole-grain bread
1 tablespoon olive oil

1 avocado or 1 cooked potato, peeled
1 scallion
finely grated zest of 1 lemon

ALTERNATIVE INGREDIENTS
• As a change from red lentils, use ⅔ cup green (puy) or brown lentils and increase the amount of stock to 4¾ cups. Simmer the soup for 30–35 minutes, or until the lentils are tender. Do not blend, but serve as a chunky soup.
• Add 1 large diced parsnip instead of the rutabaga for a sweeter flavor.

1 Chop the onion and dice the celery, carrot, and rutabaga into 1-inch pieces. Heat the oil in a large saucepan over high heat. Add the onion, celery, carrot, rutabaga, and garlic. Reduce heat to low, cover, and cook for 2 minutes.

2 Rinse the lentils in a sieve under cold running water. Add the lentils, bay leaf, thyme, and tomato paste to the pan. Add the hot stock, stir, and return to a boil. Reduce the heat, cover, and simmer for 20 minutes, or until the lentils have disintegrated.

3 Meanwhile, make the croutons. Preheat the broiler to high. Brush one side of the bread slices with ½ tablespoon of the olive oil and broil for 1 minute or until golden. Turn them over, brush with the remaining oil, and broil for another minute. Cut toast into 1-inch croutons.

4 Dice the avocado or potato and place in a bowl. Finely chop the scallion and add it to the avocado or potato. Stir in the lemon zest. Remove the thyme and bay leaf from the soup. Purée the soup in a blender, or in the pan with a stick blender until smooth. Season to taste and ladle the soup into four bowls. Top with the croutons and avocado or potato mixture.

COOK'S TIPS
● If using a blender, return the soup to the pan after blending and reheat for 1–2 minutes to make sure that it is piping hot when served.
● Use a grater or zester to remove the lemon zest. Be sure to remove only the yellow skin and not the white pith, as it tastes bitter.

SUPER FOOD

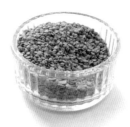

LENTILS
Rich in starchy carbohydrates, lentils have a low glycemic index (GI), so are great for keeping hunger at bay. Their high fiber content is good news for the digestive system, and with iron, B vitamins, and immunity-boosting zinc, lentils are an all-round healthy choice.

SPINACH AND PEA SOUP WITH MINTY YOGURT

This beautiful, garden-fresh soup is just bursting with the flavors of energy-boosting spinach and peas. It is quick to make, too—simply add a refreshing yogurt swirl and then serve.

Serves 4
Preparation 10 minutes
Cooking 18 minutes

1 onion
1 large potato
1 scallion
1 cup low-fat plain yogurt
2 tablespoons chopped fresh mint
1 tablespoon olive oil
1 clove garlic, crushed
2½ cups hot low-sodium chicken stock
1½ cups frozen peas or baby peas
8 ounces fresh spinach

Each serving provides
• 170 calories • 5 g fat • 1 g saturated fat • 17 g carbohydrates
• 13 g protein • 3 g fiber

ALTERNATIVE INGREDIENTS
• Swiss chard, napa cabbage, or lettuce would work well in this recipe instead of the spinach.
• Use a peeled and diced whole cucumber instead of the spinach.
• As a change from the yogurt topping, dice the flesh from 2 ripe avocados, toss them with 2 tablespoons chopped fresh cilantro, and the grated zest and juice of ½ lime. Spoon over the soup just before serving.

1 Chop the onion and dice the potato into 1-inch cubes. Finely chop the scallion. Spoon the yogurt into a bowl and add the scallion and mint. Heat the oil, garlic, onion, and potato in a large saucepan over medium heat. Cook for 2 minutes, or until the onion softens slightly, stirring occasionally. Add the hot stock, stir, return the contents of the pan to a boil, then cover and simmer for 10 minutes.

2 Add the frozen peas, return to a boil, cover and simmer for 2 minutes. Stir in the spinach, cover, and cook for another 3 minutes.

3 Remove the pan from the heat and let the soup cool slightly for 1 minute. Purée using a blender. Reheat for 1–2 minutes, if necessary. Pour the soup into four bowls and serve with generous helpings of the mint yogurt.

COOK'S TIP
● This soup freezes well, without the yogurt topping, for up to 3 months. Make twice the quantity and store half immediately in a lidded container. Thaw completely, then reheat to boiling, stirring frequently, before serving with the yogurt swirl.

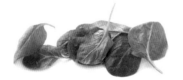

SUPER FOOD

SPINACH
Rich in nutrients, spinach is an excellent source of folate—a vitamin needed for good blood circulation and a healthy pregnancy. The vegetable also contains fiber to promote digestive health and iron to help to prevent anemia.

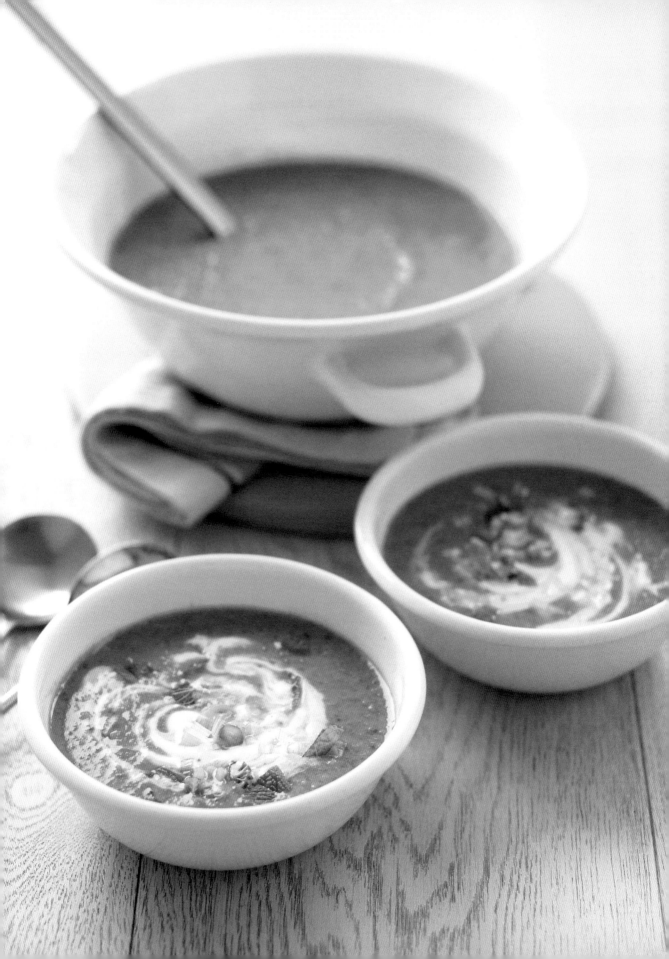

COCK-A-LEEKIE SOUP WITH KALE

Cock-a-leekie soup is a traditional Scottish dish made with leeks and chicken stock, and often thickened with rice or barley and garnished with prunes. This version leaves out the rice or barley and instead includes chunks of tender chicken and sweet kale to keep you energized throughout the day. Serve with a crusty baguette for a light but filling lunch.

Serves 4
Preparation 15 minutes
Cooking 20 minutes

1 pound boneless, skinless
  chicken breast
¾ pound leeks
1 tablespoon olive oil or canola oil
2 large carrots
4¾ cups hot chicken stock
1 bunch kale, about ¾ pound
⅓ cup pitted prunes, quartered

Each serving provides
• 240 calories • 7 g fat • 1 g
saturated fat • 15 g carbohydrates
• 24 g protein • 7 g fiber

ALTERNATIVE INGREDIENTS
• Fresh savoy cabbage or baby collard greens make good alternatives to kale.

1 Cut the chicken breast fillets into 1½-inch cubes. Trim, slice, and rinse the leeks. Heat the oil in a large saucepan over high heat. Add the chicken and leeks, and cook for 5 minutes, reducing heat to medium after the first 1–2 minutes. Stir occasionally.

2 Slice the carrots. Pour the hot stock into the pan. Add the carrots and bring to a boil over high heat, stirring, and reduce heat to low. Cover and simmer for 10 minutes, or until the carrots are tender.

3 Finely shred the kale and stir into the pan. Return to a boil then reduce the heat, cover, and simmer for 4 minutes. Add the prunes and stir them into the soup. Simmer for 1 minute, season to taste and ladle into four bowls to serve.

COOK'S TIPS
● To shred leafy green vegetables such as kale, tightly roll up a few leaves together and slice them thinly with a sharp knife. For short shreds, cut the slices in half. Alternatively, ready-to-cook vegetables, especially frozen, are a labor-saving option for everyday cooking.
● Organic chicken stock is a good choice as it has a light flavor and is not too high in salt.
● If fresh vegetables are not available, use mixed frozen broccoli and cauliflower instead of kale. Add the florets with the prunes in step 3 so that they remain crunchy.

SUPER FOOD

LEEKS
Among a leek's many phytochemicals is a rich amount of carotenoids, especially beta-carotene, a natural antioxidant. With potassium to help to regulate blood pressure, and B vitamins, including folate, leeks are good for heart and digestive health.

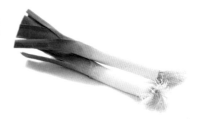

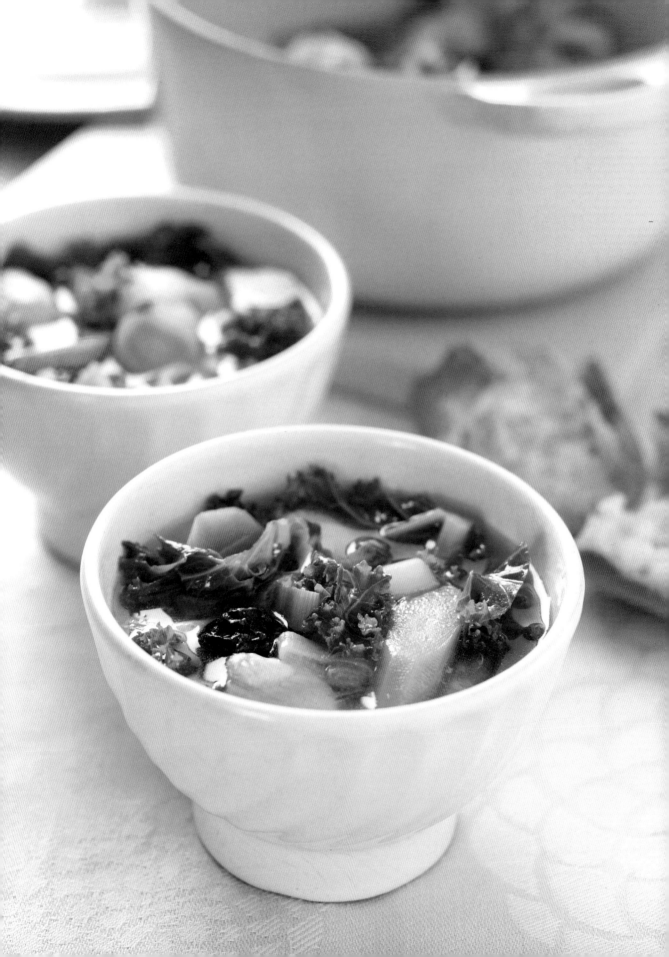

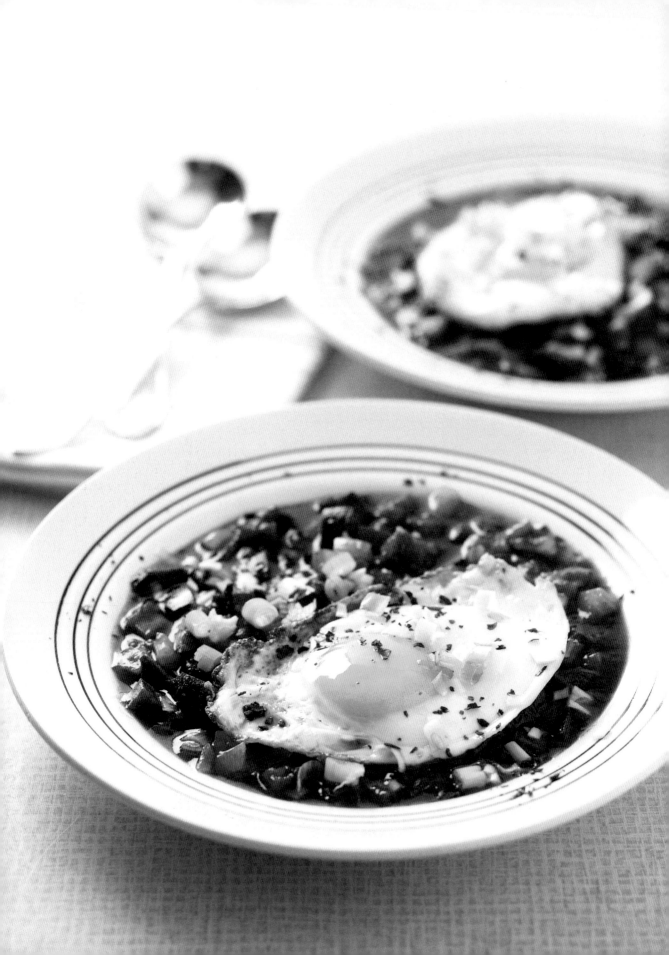

RED PEPPER AND TOMATO SOUP WITH A SPICY EGG

For a bowl of sunshine, try a rustic soup packed with the vivid goodness of tomato and red bell peppers, topped with a chile pepper-flecked fried egg. It makes a filling snack or tasty light supper.

Serves 4
Preparation 10 minutes
Cooking 25 minutes

1 onion
1 stick celery
2 red bell peppers
3 tablespoons olive oil
1 can (14½ ounces) chopped
    tomatoes
2½ cups hot chicken stock
1 scallion
4 eggs
pinch of hot pepper flakes

Each serving provides
• 251 calories • 19 g fat • 4 g saturated fat • 11 g carbohydrates • 10 g protein • 3 g fiber

ALTERNATIVE INGREDIENTS
• To boost the fiber content of this dish, drain a 14½-ounce can of cannellini beans or red kidney beans and add them in step 2.
• For a meaty soup, add ⅓ cup sliced chorizo sausage to the soup at the end of step 3 to warm through while the eggs are frying.
• For a complete meal in a bowl, add ¼ cup miniature pasta shapes in step 2 during the final 5 minutes of cooking.

1 Chop the onion and dice the celery and peppers. Put 1 tablespoon of the oil in a large saucepan over high heat. Add the onion, celery, and peppers and cook for about 30 seconds, or until sizzling. Reduce the heat to medium-high, cover, and cook for 5 minutes, shaking the pan occasionally, until the vegetables are softened.

2 Add the tomatoes and stir in the hot stock. Return to a boil. Reduce the heat, cover, and simmer the soup for 15 minutes. Trim and finely chop the scallion.

3 Heat the remaining 2 tablespoons of oil in a large frying pan over medium-high heat. Break in the eggs and fry for 1–2 minutes, or until the whites are set but the yolks are soft. Season the soup to taste and ladle into bowls. Float an egg on each portion and sprinkle with the chopped scallion and hot pepper flakes.

COOK'S TIP
● If you prefer, you can break the eggs directly into the soup and allow them to poach for 1–1½ minutes. The trick is to have the soup bubbling steadily when the eggs are added, then regulate the heat to keep the liquid simmering gently. Use a slotted spoon to transfer the eggs to each bowl before ladling in the soup.

SUPER FOOD

TOMATOES
The antioxidant lycopene in tomatoes gives them their wonderful rich color. Lycopene is more easily absorbed by the body from processed or cooked tomatoes, so it pays to enjoy them canned or in a paste, as well as fresh. As a rich source of potassium, tomatoes can help to regulate blood pressure, reducing the risk of stroke.

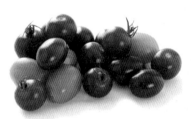

CHUNKY **FISH** AND **VEGETABLE** SOUP

Aromatic lemon and herbs blend brilliantly with leeks and lima beans to make a perfect match for pieces of succulent white fish. This robust soup is low in fat and really satisfying.

Serves 4
Preparation 10 minutes
Cooking 20 minutes

1 large leek
2 tablespoons olive oil
2 cloves garlic, crushed
4 sprigs fresh thyme
2 bay leaves
2 cans (14½ ounces each) chopped
   tomatoes
2½ cups hot fish stock
1 pound skinless firm white fish, such
   as snapper, cod, or halibut
1 small cucumber
1 cup frozen baby lima beans
grated zest of 1 lemon
½ cup store-bought croutons

Each serving provides
• 312 calories • 10 g fat • 1 g
saturated fat • 29 g carbohydrates
• 28 g protein • 7 g fiber

ALTERNATIVE INGREDIENTS
• Try a mixture of salmon and white
fish or mixed seafood. If using frozen
mixed seafood, add an extra minute of
cooking time in step 3.
• For a subtle anise flavor, add
1 large fennel bulb, cut into slim
wedges, then slice these across into
shreds. Cook the fennel with the leek
in step 1.
• Frozen peas or sweet corn can
be used instead of the lima beans.
• For a more substantial soup,
add a drained 14½-ounce can of
cannellini or black-eyed peas with
the lima beans.

1 Finely chop the leek. Heat the oil in a large saucepan over high heat, then add the leek, garlic, thyme, and bay leaves. Cover and cook for 2 minutes, reducing the heat if the vegetables begin to brown too quickly.

2 Stir in the tomatoes and the hot stock. Return to a boil, cover, reduce the heat to low, and simmer for 15 minutes. Meanwhile, cut the fish into 1½-inch chunks and dice the cucumber.

3 Add the lima beans to the pan, cover, and return to a boil. Reduce the heat so that the soup is bubbling gently, then add the fish, lemon zest, and cucumber. Cover and simmer for 3 minutes, or until the fish is cooked through. Ladle into four bowls, add a sprinkling of croutons to each one, and serve.

COOK'S TIPS
● When buying fresh fish, choose fillets or steaks that are firm and translucent. Fish that smells fishy is probably past its prime. If you are concerned about sustainability, buy fish that is responsibly caught or farmed. If buying supermarket fish, look for a logo stating that the fish has come from a sustainable source.
● Croutons are available in different sizes and flavors, so you can add your own twist to the presentation and taste. Or, make your own: Toast four thick slices of whole-grain bread and cut into chunks just before serving.

SUPER FOOD

WHITE FISH
Government guidelines recommend that we eat more fish—at least one serving of white fish per week—to maintain good health. White fish is low in fat, high in protein, and rich in iodine, vital for a healthy metabolism.

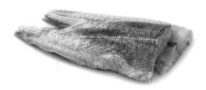

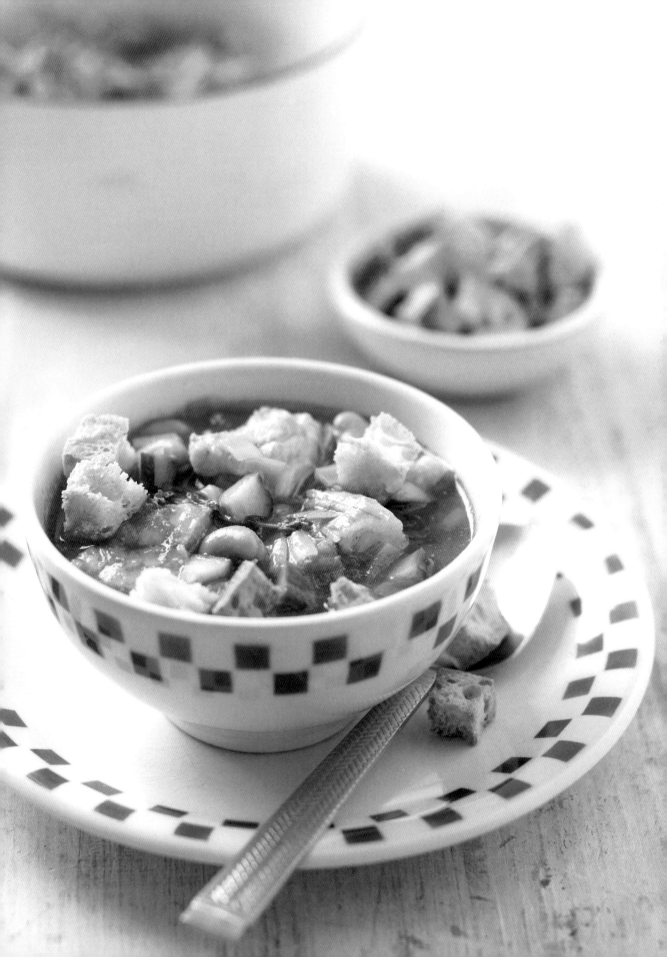

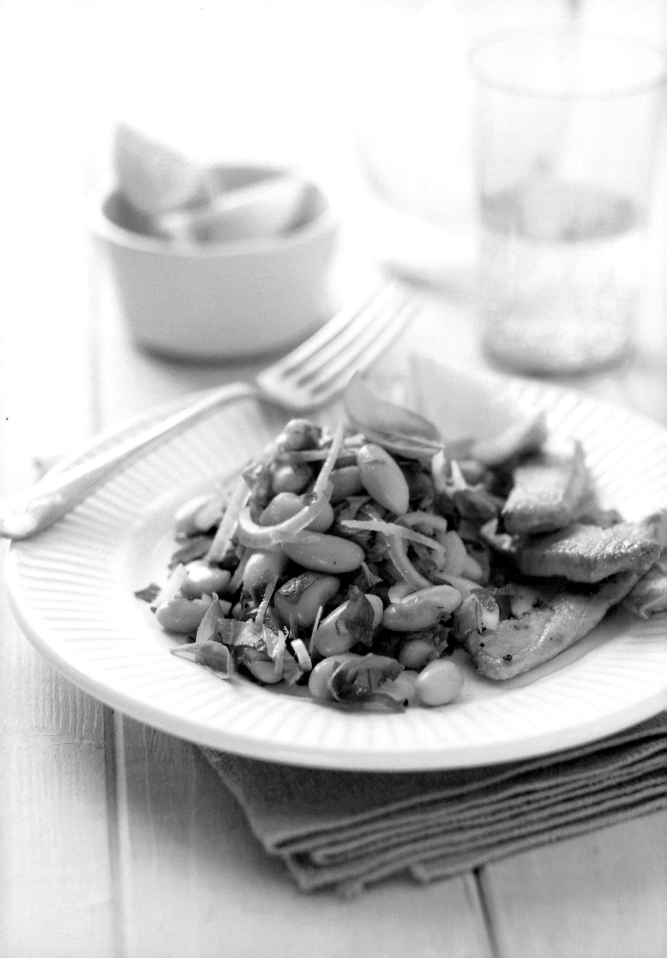

FRESH **TUNA** AND **BEAN** SALAD

What better way could there be to get those all-important omega-3 oils? Arrange strips of lightly seared tuna next to a lemony bean salad infused with garlic and basil for a tangy lunch or starter.

Serves 4
Preparation 20 minutes
Cooking 1 minute

1 small red onion
1 can (**14 ounces**) cannellini beans
1 small clove garlic, chopped
zest of 1 lemon
4 tablespoons chopped fresh parsley
8 fresh basil leaves, finely shredded,
   plus extra whole leaves, to garnish
2 tablespoons olive oil
⅓ pound tuna steak
4 lemon wedges, to garnish

Each serving provides
• 220 calories • 10 g fat • 2 g
saturated fat • 15 g carbohydrates
• 17 g protein • 5 g fiber

ALTERNATIVE INGREDIENTS
• Use ½ pound smoked mackerel,
boned and flaked, instead of the tuna.
• Grilled haloumi cheese (available at
Middle Eastern markets) is a delicious
vegetarian alternative with the bean
salad. Broil the slices on high for
30 seconds on each side.
• You can top this salad with broiled
salmon fillets. Broil them on high, skin
side down, for 1 minute until just firm.

1 Thinly slice the onion. Drain and rinse the cannellini beans. In a bowl, mix the cannellini beans with the garlic, onion, lemon zest, parsley, shredded basil, and oil. Cover and let stand for 15 minutes.

2 Meanwhile, cut the tuna steak into slices about 2 inches thick. Heat a heavy nonstick frying pan over high heat, add the tuna slices, and sear for 30 seconds. Turn the fish over and sear for another 30 seconds. Remove from the heat immediately.

3 Divide the bean salad among four plates. Arrange 3–4 tuna slices on one side, and garnish each portion with a lemon wedge and whole basil leaves.

COOK'S TIPS
● The frying pan must be very hot so that the tuna browns and cooks almost immediately. If you do not have a nonstick pan, add 1 tablespoon olive oil or canola oil before adding the tuna. Use tongs for turning the tuna, or try a spatula and fork.
● For rare tuna still pink in the middle, sear the steak whole, for 30–60 seconds on each side, then remove from the heat and slice. This method is best suited to really fresh raw tuna. Frozen tuna is better cooked until opaque.

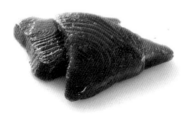

SUPER FOOD

TUNA
Unlike canned tuna, fresh tuna is rich in health-promoting omega-3 oils. In addition to their proven heart benefits, these oils can alleviate inflammatory conditions such as rheumatoid arthritis and joint stiffness. One weekly serving of oily fish, such as herring, salmon, mackerel, or fresh tuna, provides your daily requirement.

BEANS

In all its forms, from tender garden-fresh green beans to robust dried kidney beans, the humble bean soaks up flavors while contributing a generous helping of fiber for digestive health and enriching the blood with iron. Beans fill you up but are low in fat, and as most beans contain at least 20 percent protein, they are an excellent alternative to meat for vegetarians.

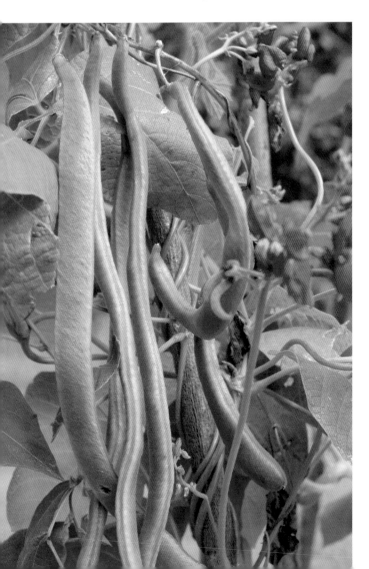

WARM CITRUS BEAN SALAD

Serves 4
Preparation 10 minutes Cooking 15 minutes

Each serving provides • 104 calories • 5 g fat
• 1 g saturated fat • 9 g carbohydrates • 6 g protein
• 7 g fiber

Boil **1¾ cups frozen baby lima beans** in a saucepan of boiling water for 3 minutes, or until just tender, then drain and set aside. Heat **1 tablespoon olive oil** in a frying pan and add **2 finely chopped shallots** and **1 crushed garlic clove**. Sauté over medium heat for 8 minutes, or until softened. Add the beans to the onions in the pan with **2 tablespoons finely chopped fresh mint, 2 tablespoons finely chopped fresh parsley** and the **juice of ½ lemon**. Cook for 2 minutes, stirring occasionally, before serving.

COOK'S TIPS

● If the lima beans are large, remove the outer pale green cases. Pour boiling water over them, leave for 2–3 minutes, then drain and refresh with cold water. Pop the beans out of their cases.
● This dish works really well with grilled chicken or smoky bacon.
● Use the juice of 1 lemon to sharpen the flavor and serve with steamed white fish fillets.

SUMMER BEAN RISOTTO

Serves 4
Preparation 5 minutes Cooking 30 minutes

Each serving provides • 596 calories • 12 g fat
• 4 g saturated fat • 110 g carbohydrates
• 19 g protein • 7 g fiber

Heat **1 tablespoon olive oil** in a large frying pan and add **1 thinly sliced large onion**. Cook over medium-low heat for 5 minutes, or until softened. Stir in **2 finely chopped cloves garlic**. Add **1¾ cups risotto rice**, turn up the heat to medium-high, and stir to coat all the rice with oil. Add **1 tablespoon fresh thyme** and the **juice of 1 lemon**. Begin to add **4 cups hot vegetable stock** to the pan ¼ cup at a time, allowing the rice to absorb each amount of stock before adding more. Drain and rinse **2½ cups canned cannellini beans** and add to the pan when half the stock is used up. Season to taste with plenty of **ground black pepper**. After about 25 minutes, or when all the liquid is absorbed, the rice grains should be soft and creamy. If the rice is not tender, continue to add more hot vegetable stock or water until cooked. Divide the risotto among four bowls and top each portion with **1 tablespoon shaved parmesan**.

COOK'S TIPS

● Replace ½ cup of the stock with dry white wine for a more sophisticated flavor.

● Add ⅔ cup chopped cooked green beans towards the end of the cooking time to boost color and nutrition.

● Serve the risotto with a crisp green salad.

MEDITERRANEAN GREEN BEANS

Serves 4
Preparation 5 minutes Cooking 15 minutes

Each serving provides • 102 calories • 7 g fat
• 1 g saturated fat • 8 g carbohydrates • 3 g protein
• 4 g fiber

Trim **1 pound green beans** and boil in a saucepan for 3 minutes, or until just cooked but still firm. Refresh the beans under cold running water, drain, and pat dry. Heat **1 tablespoon olive oil** in a frying pan and sauté **1 thinly sliced onion** over medium heat for about 8 minutes, or until softened. Stir **16 whole cherry tomatoes** and **2 teaspoons olive oil** into the onions. Cook for 2 minutes, turning the tomatoes gently once or twice. Add the cooked green beans to the pan and stir for 1 minute over the heat to warm through.

COOK'S TIPS

● This tasty and healthy side dish goes very well with beef or chicken. Add ½ pound diced cooked potatoes to the pan with the onions for a main dish.

● For extra crunch, add 2 tablespoons toasted slivered almonds to the dish before serving.

SPICY CARIBBEAN RICE

Serves 4
Preparation 15 minutes Cooking 45 minutes

Each serving provides • 540 calories • 19 g fat
• 9 g saturated fat • 81 g carbohydrates • 16 g protein
• 10 g fiber

Heat **2 tablespoons olive oil or canola oil** in a large frying pan over a medium heat and add **2 finely chopped red onions** and **2 sliced red bell peppers** to the pan. Cook for 5 minutes to soften the vegetables, then add **2 finely chopped cloves garlic** and **1 or 2 finely chopped chilies, 1 teaspoon medium pepper sauce** and

2–3 teaspoons paprika. Stir for 1 minute, or until the aromas are released, then add **1 cup long-grain brown rice**. Stir to coat all the grains of rice with oil. Pour in **1 cup hot vegetable stock** and **1¾ cups light coconut milk**. Bring to a simmer then reduce the heat, cover, and cook for 15 minutes. Drain and rinse **1 cup each canned red kidney beans** and **black-eyed peas**. Add to the rice with **2 teaspoons dried thyme** and **2 teaspoons dried oregano**. Cover again, simmer for 10 minutes then stir in **4 chopped tomatoes**. Cook uncovered for another 15 minutes, or until the rice is tender. To serve the dish moist, you may need to add more hot stock or water in order to have a small amount of liquid in the pan by the time the rice is cooked.

COOK'S TIP

● For a heartier dish, add small pieces of cooked chicken or bacon to the pan with the tomatoes.

RICH CHICKEN AND BEAN HOTPOT

Serves 4
Preparation 10 minutes Cooking 1 hour

Each serving provides • 311 calories • 8 g fat • 1 g saturated fat • 24 g carbohydrates • 37 g protein
• 7 g fiber

Heat **2 teaspoons olive oil** in a flameproof casserole dish and add **4 boneless, skinless chicken breasts**. Cook for 5 minutes, turning occasionally, until browned on both sides. Remove from the dish and keep warm. Add **1 tablespoon olive oil** to the dish with **2 sliced onions** and **1 chopped celery stalk**. Cook over a medium-low heat for 5 minutes, or until softened. Stir in **4 chopped garlic cloves, 1 cup hot chicken stock, 1 bay leaf, 1 teaspoon dried rosemary, 5 peeled chopped tomatoes** (see page 56, No-Cook Tomato Pasta Sauce, for how to peel tomatoes) and **¼ cup tomato purée**. Cover and cook over a low heat for 20 minutes. Drain and rinse **1 cup canned borlotti beans** and add them to the casserole dish with the browned chicken fillets. Simmer for another 30 minutes uncovered, stirring occasionally, until the chicken is cooked through and the sauce is thickened. Sprinkle with **2 tablespoons chopped fresh parsley**.

COOK'S TIP

● Sides of crusty bread and a green salad add extra dimensions of flavor and texture.

● Borlotti beans are a type of cranberry bean. You can use pinto beans but the flavor will be slightly different.

CARROT PANCAKES WITH PROSCIUTTO AND MANGO

Freshen up these golden pancakes and high-protein prosciutto slivers with delicious slices of firm, ripe mango. Bursting with antioxidants and vitamin C, it tastes fabulous, too.

Serves 4
Preparation 10 minutes
Cooking 10 minutes

For the pancakes
1 small carrot
²⁄₃ cup self-rising flour
1 egg
¹⁄₃ cup low-fat (1%) milk
2 tablespoons chopped fresh parsley
1 tablespoon olive oil or canola oil

For the mango salad
1 ripe mango
8 slices prosciutto
4 sprigs fresh basil, to garnish
2 tablespoons olive oil

Each serving provides
494 calories • 39 g fat • 6 g saturated fat • 27 g carbohydrates • 11 g protein • 3 g fiber

ALTERNATIVE INGREDIENTS
• Try other types of air-dried ham such as westphalian or serrano instead of prosciutto.
• Use papaya either instead of mango or combined with it. Halve the fruit, scoop out and discard the seeds, then peel and slice the papaya.
• For a lighter fruit flavor with a contrasting crunchy texture, slice 1 starfruit instead of mango, sprinkle the ham with 1 teaspoon lightly toasted pine nuts per portion, and drizzle with walnut oil instead of olive oil.

1 First make the pancakes. Finely grate the carrot. Sift the flour into a bowl, add the egg and half the milk, then stir the mixture to form a thick paste and beat until smooth. Gradually beat in the remaining milk to make a thick batter. Stir in the carrot and parsley.

2 Heat a griddle pan or heavy frying pan and brush with a little of the oil. Drop 4 separate tablespoonfuls of batter into the pan, spacing them well apart. Cook for 2 minutes, or until browned underneath and bubbling on top. Turn and cook the second side for about 1 minute. Transfer the pancakes to a plate lined with a dish towel and wrap them to keep warm. Repeat twice more to make 12 small pancakes.

3 Peel the mango and cut the flesh from the pit in small neat slices (see Cook's Tip). Divide the mango among four plates. Trim away any fat from around the edges of the prosciutto, arrange the slices on the plates, then scatter with the basil leaves. Drizzle 2 teaspoons olive oil over each portion of prosciutto and serve with the pancakes.

COOK'S TIP
● To slice mango flesh, use a large knife to make one cut straight down into the pit, then cut the fruit at an angle to remove the first slice. Work outwards, cutting off slices at an angle until the fruit is removed from one flat side. Turn the pit over and repeat for the second half. Peel each slice before serving.

SUPER FOOD

MANGOES
Thanks to its high vitamin C and carotenoid content, the mango is a great source of antioxidants, good for boosting immunity and offering protection from heart disease and some cancers.

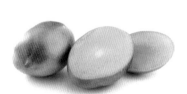

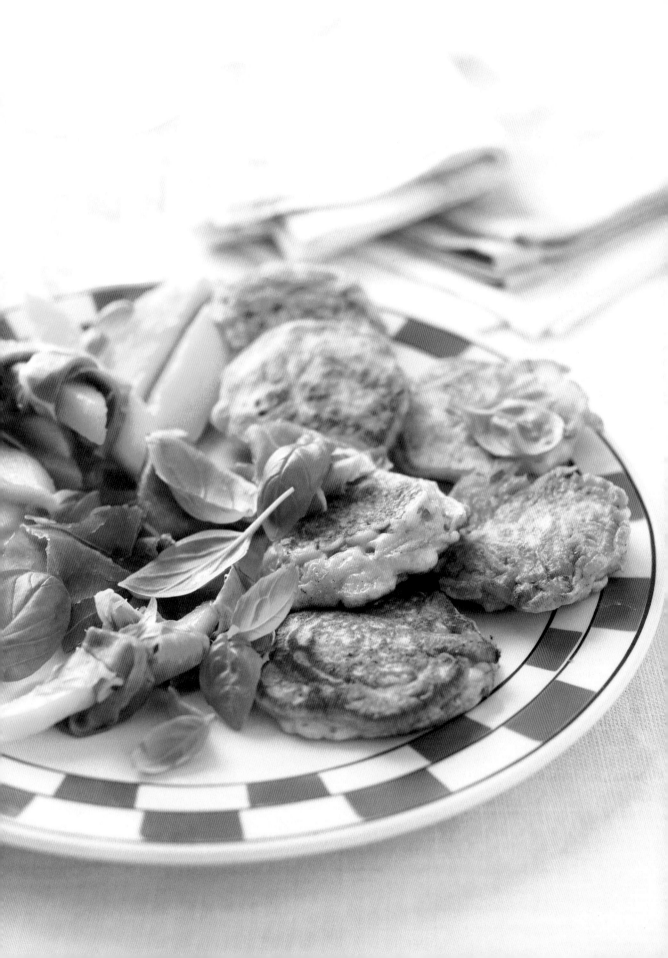

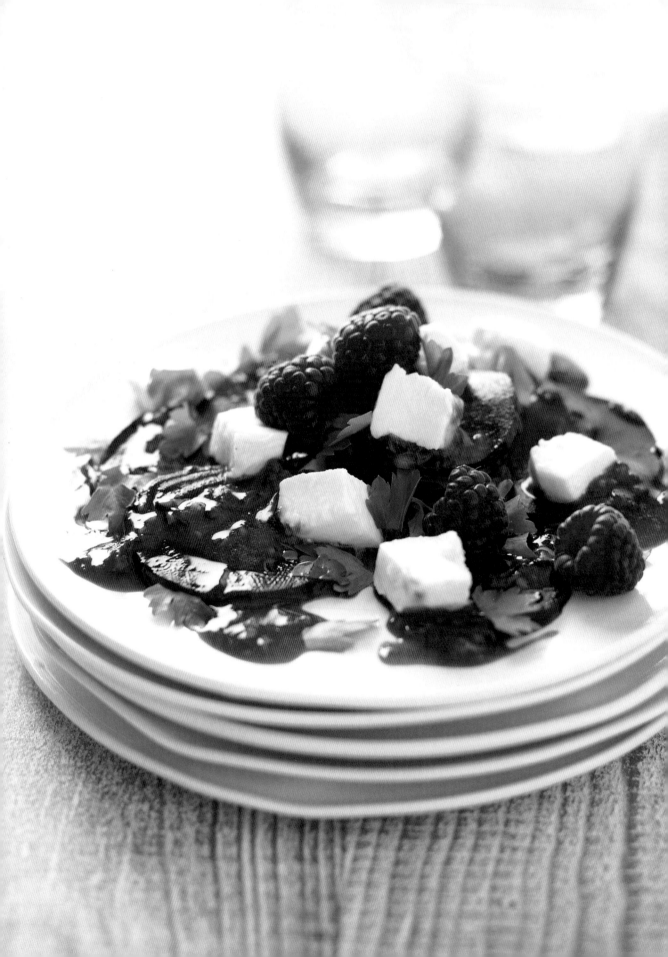

BEET AND MOZZARELLA SALAD WITH RASPBERRY DRESSING

A piquant fruit dressing spices up this salad of creamy mozzarella cheese and earthy beets. The raspberries contain natural antioxidants that may help to protect against heart disease.

Serves 4
Preparation 10 minutes

½ cup ounces raspberries
2 teaspoons honey
2 teaspoons cider vinegar
1 pound beets
6 ounces mozzarella
¼ cup chopped flat-leaf parsley
a few whole raspberries, to garnish

Each serving provides
• 167 calories • 8 g fat • 5 g saturated fat • 15 g carbohydrates
• 10 g protein • 4 g fiber

ALTERNATIVE INGREDIENTS
• Blackberries taste as good with beets as raspberries do.
• For a contrasting flavor, use a cheese with a more pronounced taste, such as roquefort or goat's cheese.
• For a tangy flavor, use feta instead of mozzarella and tender basil leaves instead of parsley.
• Add orange slices to the beets for a citrus kick. Drizzle with a little olive oil, then add the mozzarella. A few fresh oregano leaves make a tasty garnish.

1 Put the raspberries in a bowl and crush them with a fork. Drizzle in the honey, then mix in the vinegar to make a thick dressing.

2 Thinly slice the beets and arrange the slices on four plates. Dice the mozzarella into ½-inch cubes. Spoon the raspberry dressing over the beets and add the mozzarella. Sprinkle the chopped parsley leaves over the dish, then garnish with whole raspberries and serve.

COOK'S TIPS
● Make this salad as close to serving time as possible because the raspberries (and raspberry vinegar) will lose flavor if left for more than an hour.
● Frozen raspberries are ideal for this dressing. Either microwave them on high for 30 seconds, or let them defrost at room temperature for a couple of hours.
● For a more substantial salad, serve with boiled new potatoes—they are great for soaking up the lovely salad juices.
● You can cook fresh beets or, to save time, buy them pre-cooked (see Cook's Tips on page 22).

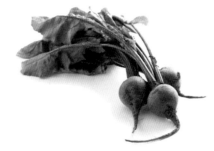

SUPER FOOD

BEETS
Known for their distinctive, deep purple color, beets contain a range of essential vitamins and minerals, including vitamin C, magnesium, potassium, and folate. Betaine, a compound important for heart health, is also abundant in beets.

TANGY **SARDINE** PÂTÉ

Lemon, garlic, and dill deliver flavor punches to a robust fish pâté that is great as a tasty starter or snack. Serve with vine-ripened tomatoes, thin cucumber sticks, and triangles of crunchy toast.

Serves 4
Preparation 5 minutes

1 can (4 ounces) sardines in olive or canola oil, drained
1 clove garlic, crushed
grated zest of 1 lemon and juice of ½ lemon
½ cup low-fat ricotta or low-fat cream cheese
1 small scallion
2 tablespoons chopped fresh dill

Each serving provides
• 83 calories • 5 g fat • 3 g saturated fat • 1 g carbohydrates • 7 g protein • 0 g fiber

ALTERNATIVE INGREDIENTS
• For a fabulous, firm-textured mustard and dill pâté, reduce the quantity of low-fat ricotta or low-fat cream cheese to ¼ cup and omit the scallions. Use 2 tablespoons whole-grain mustard instead of the garlic, and reduce the zest to ½ lemon and the juice to 1 tablespoon.
• Use canned mackerel in oil instead of sardines. Canned smoked mackerel makes a tasty alternative to sardines.
• A number of herbs complement sardines. Try chopped fresh parsley as an alternative to dill, adding 4 finely shredded fresh basil leaves to the parsley for a distinctive aroma.

1 Use a fork to mash the sardines with the garlic and lemon zest in a bowl. Stir in the lemon juice when the sardines have a smooth consistency. Add the low-fat ricotta or cream cheese and beat the mixture until all the ingredients are combined.

2 Season to taste and divide the pâté among four ramekins, or spoon it onto plates. Finely chop the scallion and sprinkle a little over each portion together with the dill.

COOK'S TIPS
● Use leftover pâté to fill rolls or sandwiches. The pâté will keep for up to 2 days in the fridge; store in a sealed container to prevent the strong smell of garlic and fish from infusing other food.
● Make double the quantity of pâté and freeze half to use on another occasion. Store in an airtight container for up to 2 months.

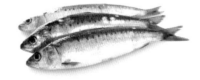

SUPER FOOD

SARDINES
One of the few foods rich in vitamin D, sardines help to boost dietary intake of this essential vitamin. Vitamin D is needed for the formation and maintenance of bones and the absorption of calcium into the body. It may also play a role in protecting against breast, prostate, and colon cancers and heart disease.

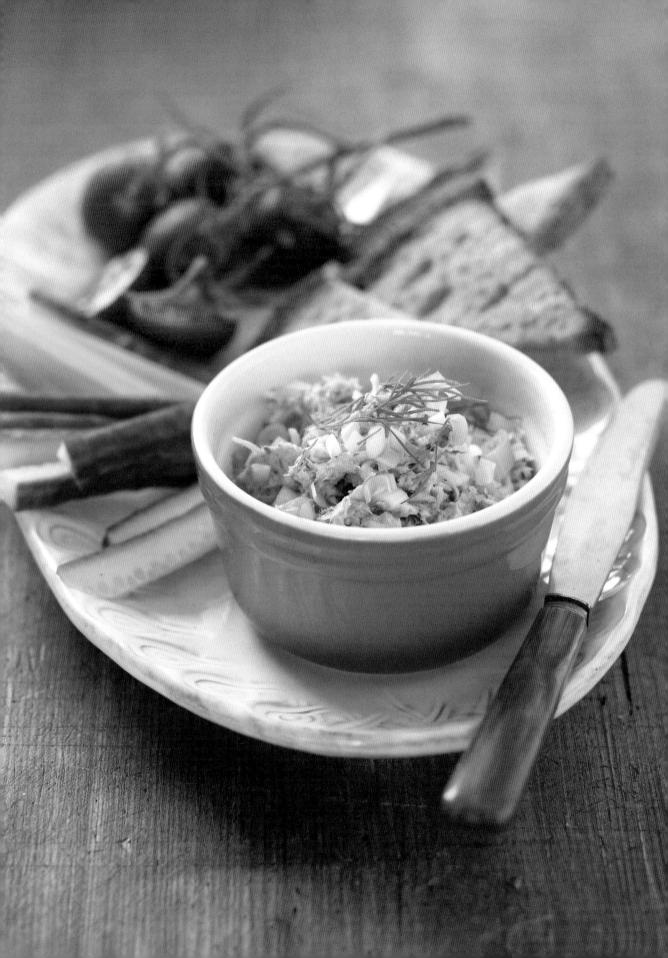

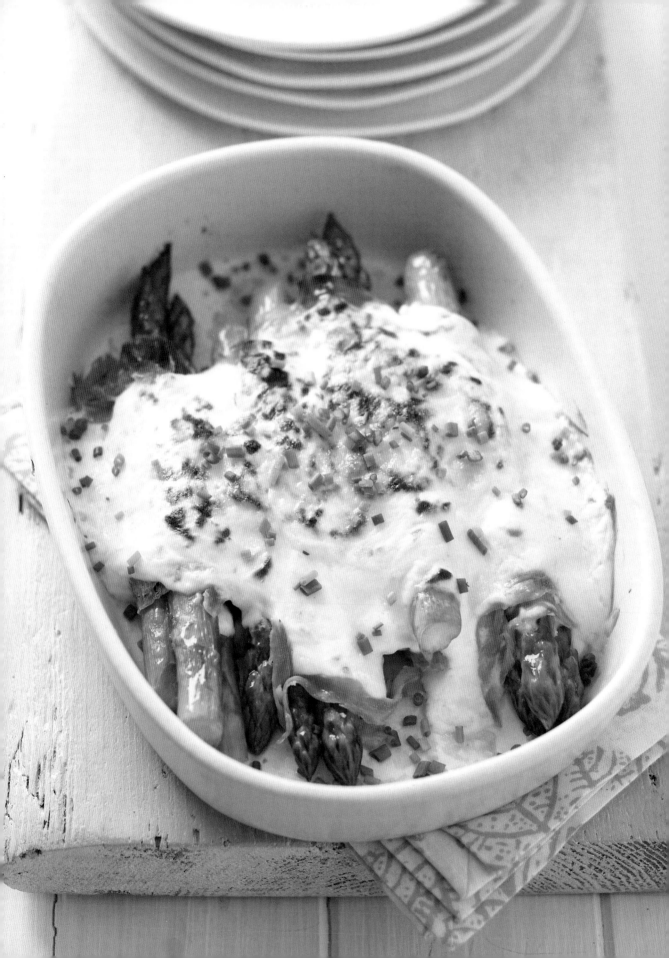

ASPARAGUS AND HAM GRILL

Quick to prepare with a no-fuss cheesy sauce, this grill is sure to become a favorite for a tasty hot lunch. Asparagus provides a host of health benefits, so make the most of it when it is in season.

Serves 4
Preparation 5 minutes
Cooking 12 minutes

12 asparagus spears
4 large slices cooked ham,
    about 6 ounces
⅔ cup low-fat ricotta or
    low-fat cream cheese
1 teaspoon cornstarch
¼ cup parmesan
3 tablespoons milk
2 tablespoons snipped fresh chives

Each serving provides
• 170 calories • 10 g fat • 6 g saturated fat • 3 g carbohydrates • 17 g protein • 1 g fiber

ALTERNATIVE INGREDIENTS
• Try baby leeks instead of asparagus. Allow 2–3 leeks per portion and poach them in a pan of boiling water for 3–5 minutes, or until tender.
• Use crumbled blue cheese instead of parmesan.

1 Trim off any tough ends from the asparagus (see Cook's Tip) and lay the spears in a large frying pan. Add just enough boiling water to cover, then return to a boil over high heat. Reduce heat, cover the pan, and simmer for about 5 minutes, or until the spears are just tender.

2 Meanwhile, lay the ham on a work surface. Preheat the broiler to medium-high and have a large ovenproof dish or four gratin dishes ready for step 3. In a bowl, mix the ricotta or low-fat cream cheese and cornstarch. Finely grate the parmesan. Reserve 1 tablespoon of the parmesan and stir the rest into the mixture. Whisk in the milk.

3 Drain the asparagus and place three spears over each slice of ham. Roll up and place in the prepared dish. Spoon the cheese mixture over the ham and sprinkle with the remaining 1 tablespoon of parmesan. Cover any protruding asparagus tips with foil.

4 Broil the asparagus and ham rolls for 5–6 minutes, or until the cheese topping is bubbling and browned. Sprinkle with the snipped chives before serving.

COOK'S TIP
● If the spears have slightly tough ends, trim them off with a knife or snap them off—the stems will break at their weakest point—where the tender spear meets the woody end. Use the woody parts to flavor a stock, straining and discarding them before use.

SUPER FOOD

ASPARAGUS
This colorful vegetable is a good source of energy-releasing B vitamins, including folate, which lowers the risk of heart disease and stroke. With calcium and magnesium to maintain strong bones, asparagus is an all-round super food.

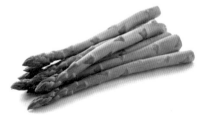

GARLIC **MUSHROOMS** WITH **SUN-DRIED TOMATOES**

Great for soaking up the garlic flavor and as a contrast to the sweetness of the tomatoes, mushrooms are also low in calories and a good source of fiber. It all adds up to a mouthwatering, satisfying dish, wonderful hot or cold.

Serves 4
Preparation 5 minutes
Cooking 5 minutes

2 cups button mushrooms, about a pound
4 tablespoons olive oil
4 cloves garlic, crushed
12 sun-dried tomato halves
2 tablespoons chopped fresh flat-leaf parsley
lemon wedges, to garnish

Each serving provides
• 205 calories • 16 g fat • 2 g saturated fat • 10 g carbohydrates • 5 g protein • 6 g fiber

ALTERNATIVE INGREDIENTS
• Use cremini mushrooms instead of button mushrooms for a slightly stronger flavor.
• Try nut oils instead of olive oil. Cook the garlic in the olive oil then add walnut or hazelnut oil in step 2.
• Add sunflower seeds to the ingredients. Roast 2–3 tablespoons sunflower seeds in a dry pan and remove them before adding the oil and garlic. Sprinkle the seeds over the mushrooms before serving.

1 Halve the mushrooms and trim any long stems. Heat 1 tablespoon of the oil in a large saucepan. Add the garlic and cook for 1 minute over high heat until it begins to sizzle.

2 Add the mushrooms and continue to cook, stirring occasionally, for 4 minutes. When the mushrooms begin to brown, remove the pan from the heat and toss them in the remaining oil.

3 Slice the sun-dried tomatoes and stir them into the mushrooms together with the parsley. Season to taste and garnish with lemon wedges before serving.

COOK'S TIPS
● To serve cold, add the sun-dried tomatoes in step 3, then transfer the mushroom mixture to a bowl, cover, and marinate for 15 minutes. Add the parsley just before serving.
● Larger mushrooms also work well in this recipe if they are quartered, but do not use open-cap mushrooms—with the soft gills exposed, they are not firm enough.

SUPER FOOD

MUSHROOMS
A useful source of fiber, mushrooms contain energy-releasing B vitamins and minerals, too. They are rich in selenium, an important antioxidant that may help to prevent heart disease and cancer, as well as being high in folate for healthy blood and circulation.

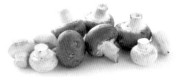

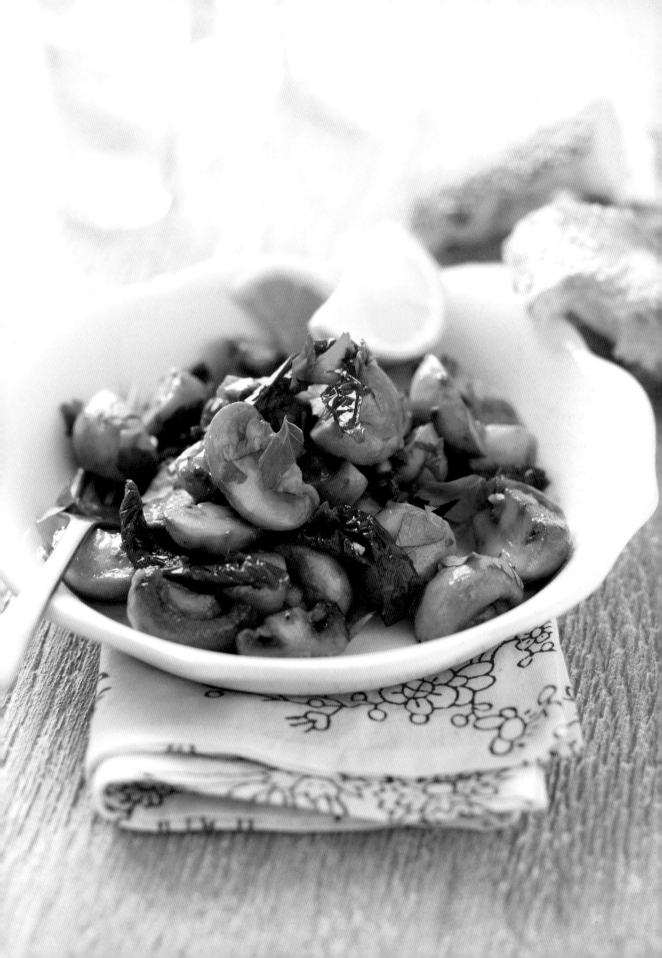

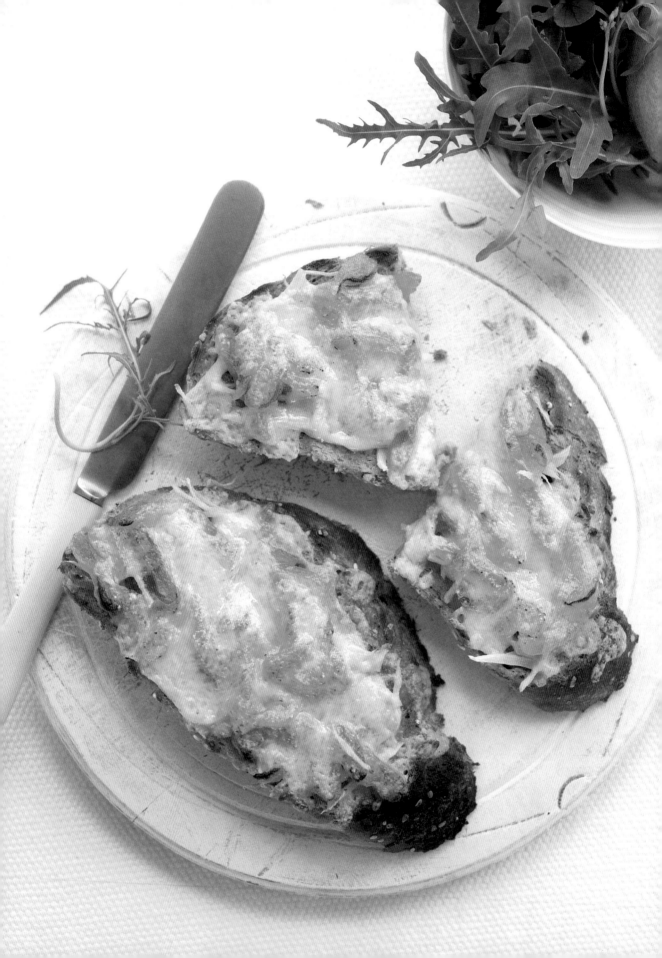

GINGER AND APRICOT CHEESE TOAST

Here is a lively and unusual version of an old favorite that combines the zing of ginger and the succulence of apricots with a high-calcium cheese for a really nutritious snack.

Serves 4
Preparation 10 minutes
Cooking 5 minutes

1 medium piece fresh ginger
⅓ cup dried apricots, sliced
4 thick slices whole-grain bread
½ cup grated cheddar
1 small bunch arugula
1 small bunch watercress
lemon wedges, to garnish

Each serving provides
• 272 calories • 12 g fat • 7 g saturated fat • 29 g carbohydrates • 13 g protein • 3 g fiber

ALTERNATIVE INGREDIENTS
• To help you achieve your seven servings of fruit and vegetables per day, dice an apple and add it to the toast in addition to the ginger and apricots.
• Leave out the ginger and use ¼ cup chopped dates instead of the apricots.
• Top with crumbled feta instead of cheddar.

1 Preheat the broiler to high. Cut the ginger into fine strips. Toast the bread slices on one side under the broiler. Turn the slices and lay them close together in the broiler pan.

2 Scatter the ginger and apricots evenly over the bread, then sprinkle with the cheese, right up to the edges. Toast for 5 minutes, or until the cheese is bubbling and golden.

3 Divide the cheese toasts among four plates and serve with the arugula and watercress leaves garnished with lemon wedges.

COOK'S TIPS
● Adding the topping to the untoasted side of the bread means that the crusts do not burn before the cheese has melted. The result is a crisp base with a moist top.
● Instead of grating the cheese, pare off thin slices using a potato peeler to get a more even covering.

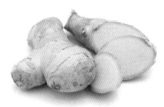

SUPER FOOD

GINGER
Ginger has traditionally been used to stimulate appetite and soothe the digestive system. It is also used for reducing nausea.

MINTED **CELERY** HUMMUS

Celery gives a lovely light crunch to this high-fiber chickpea dip, while mint imparts a clean, fresh flavor. Serve with vegetable sticks and warm pita bread for a quick, healthy, low-fat snack.

Serves 4
Preparation 10 minutes

1 can (14 ounces) chickpeas, drained
4 large leaves fresh mint
1 clove garlic
1 tablespoon tahini
4 tablespoons olive oil
1 stalk celery
grated zest and juice of 1 lemon
mint sprigs, to garnish

Each serving provides
• 251 calories • 19 g fat • 3 g saturated fat • 13 g carbohydrates • 7 g protein • 1 g fiber

ALTERNATIVE INGREDIENTS
• Fennel is delicious and delicate in hummus instead of celery. Use a quarter of a fennel bulb, finely diced, and don't use mint. For a more pronounced anise flavor, use the top of the fennel bulb—the remains of the stalk and any feathery leaves—chop, and add them to the hummus with the garlic and chickpeas.
• For a hummus with a rich tomato flavor, finely chop 4 sun-dried tomatoes (drained, if packed in olive oil) and add them with the celery in step 3. Leave out the mint leaves but stir in a finely shredded basil sprig. Let the hummus stand for 30 minutes and stir before serving.

1 Put the chickpeas, mint, garlic, and tahini in a food processor and reduce to a chunky mixture.

2 With the motor running, gradually pour in the oil until the mixture forms a thick paste. Continue to process, adding 2 tablespoons of water to thin the hummus if it is too thick.

3 Dice the celery and add it to the processor with the lemon zest and half of the lemon juice. Process for 3 seconds to avoid mashing the celery. Stir in the remaining lemon juice, season to taste, and transfer the hummus to a bowl. Serve garnished with mint sprigs.

COOK'S TIPS
● Tahini is sesame seed paste. It is thick and pale, usually with a layer of oil on the surface that has separated from the ground seeds. Stir well before use.
● If you do not have a food processor, make the hummus in a blender. Use a spatula to scrape the mixture down the sides occasionally so that it processes evenly. Stir in the celery with the remaining lemon juice.
● This hummus will keep in a sealed container in the fridge for 3 days.

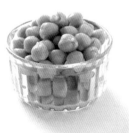

SUPER FOOD

CHICKPEAS
A low-fat, starchy, high-fiber food, chickpeas are good for digestive health. They also contain calcium, which helps to maintain healthy bones and teeth, and are a useful source of iron, making them a great alternative to red meat.

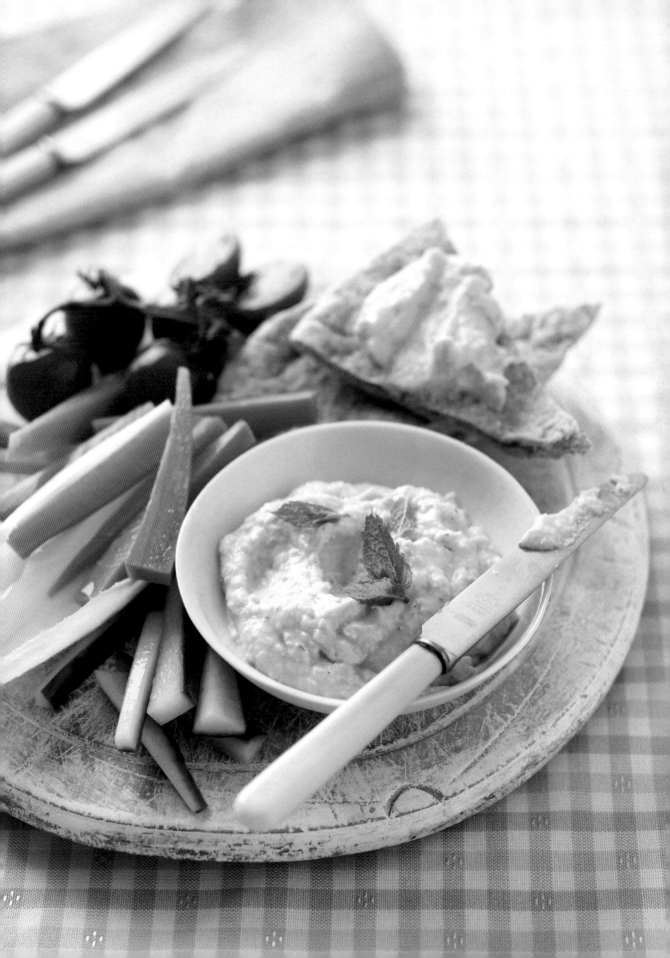

CHEESY **VEGETABLE** FRITTATA

Tender baby turnips add peppery punch, and plenty of fiber, to the zucchini and tomatoes in a layered pan omelet. A topping of toasted brie slices adds a delectable creaminess.

Serves 4
Preparation 10 minutes
Cooking 25 minutes

1 onion
½ pound baby turnips
2 zucchini
2 tablespoons olive oil
1 clove garlic, crushed
5 eggs
3 tablespoons chopped fresh parsley
2 large plum tomatoes
7 ounces brie

Each serving provides
• 388 calories • 31 g fat • 13 g saturated fat • 8 g carbohydrates • 21 g protein • 3 g fiber

ALTERNATIVE INGREDIENTS
• Use 1 cup small cauliflower florets instead of the baby turnips. When cooking, check that they are tender, but not soft, by piercing with the tip of a sharp knife before adding the zucchini.
• Celeriac makes a nice change from turnips. Use 1 cup diced celeriac and top the frittata with roquefort, gorgonzola, or a smoked cheese.
• Butternut squash goes well with turnip instead of zucchini. Add 1⅓ cups peeled, diced butternut squash with the turnips in step 1.

1 Finely chop the onion. Peel, halve, and thinly slice the turnips. Finely slice the zucchini. Heat 1 tablespoon of the oil in a large covered frying pan over high heat. Add the onion, garlic, and turnips then turn down the heat to medium-low. Cover and cook for 5 minutes, stirring occasionally, until the turnip slices are tender. Stir in the zucchini, cover and cook for another 4 minutes, or until the zucchini are tender and beginning to brown in places.

2 Preheat the broiler to high. Beat the eggs with salt and pepper to taste and add the parsley. Add the remaining oil to the pan with the vegetables and heat for a few seconds until sizzling. Pour in the eggs, cover and cook for 10 minutes. After 2 minutes of cooking, using a spatula, lift the set egg mixture off the bottom of the pan.

3 Slice the tomatoes and cut the brie into four wedges. Place the frying pan under the broiler, with the handle sticking out, and broil the frittata for 1 minute to set any uncooked egg. Arrange the tomatoes and the brie slices on top. Broil for another 4 minutes, or until the brie is lightly golden. Cool for 2–3 minutes before cutting into wedges.

COOK'S TIPS
• The trick with pan omelets—Italian frittata or Spanish tortilla—is to cover the pan to keep in the heat, which helps to set the egg mixture and prevent the underneath from overbrowning in the pan. Regulate the heat—and be patient—for good results.
• This frittata is also great cold for picnics or in lunchboxes. Cool the cooked frittata for 20–30 minutes, cover, and chill in the fridge until needed or for up to 24 hours.

SUPER FOOD

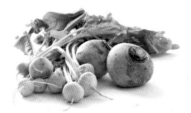

TURNIPS
A winter root crop, turnips contain more energy-giving carbohydrates than many other vegetables. They are a good source of fiber, which makes them beneficial for digestive health, and their potassium content can help to regulate blood pressure.

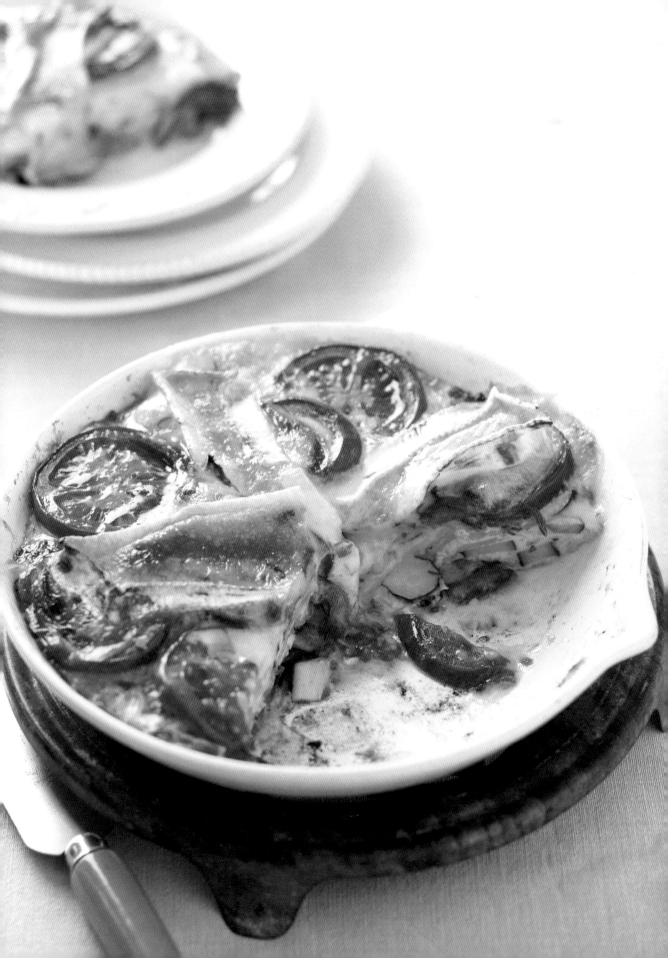

TOMATOES

Fruit or vegetable? Who cares, when tomatoes are jam-packed with health-giving nutrients? Eat just one large tomato and you get over half of your daily vitamin C needs, potassium to aid the control of high blood pressure, a rich supply of carotenes, and lycopene, which may help to reduce the risk of cancer.

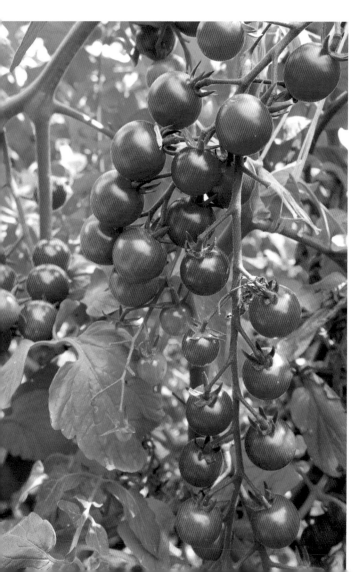

CHEESY-CRUST BAKED TOMATOES

Serves 4
Preparation 10 minutes Cooking 45 minutes

Each serving provides • 180 calories • 7 g fat • 2 g saturated fat • 26 g carbohydrates • 6 g protein • 3 g fiber

Preheat the oven to 375°F. Cook **⅓ cup brown rice** in a saucepan of boiling water with **½ teaspoon saffron threads** for 20 minutes, or until tender. Slice the tops off **4 large tomatoes** and scoop out the insides, leaving the walls intact. Reserve any juice. Heat **1 tablespoon olive oil** in a frying pan and fry **1 small finely chopped onion** for 5 minutes over medium heat, or until softened. Add **⅔ cup chopped cremini mushrooms** and cook for 1 minute. When the rice is cooked, drain and combine with the onion and mushroom mixture, **2 tablespoons chopped fresh parsley** and any **reserved tomato juice**. Fill the tomatoes with the mixture. Combine **2 tablespoons fresh breadcrumbs** with **2 tablespoons grated parmesan**, then sprinkle over the tomato tops. Place on a lightly oiled baking sheet and brush the tomato skins with a little olive oil or canola oil. Bake in the oven for 20 minutes, or until the tomatoes are tender.

COOK'S TIP

● The stuffed tomatoes are ideal as a starter or a light lunch served with salad greens.

NO-COOK TOMATO SAUCE WITH PASTA

Serves 4
Preparation 10 minutes, plus 15 minutes standing
Cooking 12 minutes

Each serving provides • 406 calories • 15 g fat • 2 g saturated fat • 56 g carbohydrates • 11 g protein • 6 g fiber

Peel **6 ripe tomatoes**. The best way to do this is to remove any stems, make a cross with a sharp knife on the bottom end and blanch (submerge the tomatoes in boiling water) for 1–2 minutes, or until the skins start to split. Drain and peel off the skins. Chop the tomatoes and transfer to a bowl. Crush **2 cloves garlic** with **1 teaspoon sea salt** in a mortar and pestle or small bowl and mix until you have a paste, then add this to the tomatoes. Stir in **2 tablespoons chopped fresh parsley, 2 tablespoons finely shredded fresh basil leaves, 3 tablespoons olive oil, 1 tablespoon red** wine vinegar, and add **ground black pepper** to taste. Let stand for 15 minutes at room temperature, covered, then stir again. Cook **10 ounces pasta** for 12 minutes, or according to the package directions. Drain pasta, return to the pan, and stir in the tomato sauce. The heat of the pasta will warm the sauce.

COOK'S TIP

● If you prefer, you can heat the sauce for a short while in a bowl in the microwave or in a saucepan.

SUMMER SEAFOOD SALAD

Serves 4
Preparation 10 minutes Marinating 30 minutes

Each serving provides • 349 calories • 28 g fat
• 5 g saturated fat • 9 g carbohydrates • 15 g protein
• 4 g fiber

Thaw **1⅓ cups frozen mixed cooked seafood** in the fridge or, if available, use 1⅓ cups of fresh cooked mussels, shrimp, and squid. Halve **¾ pound of ripe cherry tomatoes** and place in a large bowl. Rinse and drain the seafood and add to the bowl with **1 thinly sliced small red bell pepper** and **2 peeled sliced ripe avocados**. In a small bowl combine **3 tablespoons olive oil** with **2 teaspoons hot sauce** (optional), **2 teaspoons white wine vinegar, a pinch of paprika**, and **ground black pepper** to taste. Cover and set aside in a cool place for 30 minutes to allow flavors to develop at room temperature. Place a handful of baby salad greens on four plates then spoon a quarter of the seafood mixture onto each plate. Garnish with **1 tablespoon chopped fresh cilantro** per portion.

COOK'S TIPS

● Using a mixture of golden, orange, and red tomato varieties will make this salad even more appetizing.
● Replace the seafood with the same quantity of shrimp or crab meat for a more conventional salad.

CLASSIC TOMATO SOUP

Serves 4
Preparation 35 minutes Cooking 30 minutes

Each serving provides • 145 calories • 7 g fat
• 2 g saturated fat • 16 g carbohydrates • 4 g protein
• 3 g fiber

Peel and chop **2 pounds firm ripe tomatoes** (see opposite page, No-Cook Tomato Sauce with Pasta, for how to peel tomatoes). Heat **1 tablespoon olive oil** over medium heat and add **1 finely chopped onion**. Sauté the

onions for 3 minutes, or until just softened. Add **1 large chopped clove garlic** and **1 teaspoon paprika** and continue to stir-fry for 1 minute. Stir in **2 tablespoons tomato paste**, then cook for another 2 minutes. Add the chopped tomatoes, without their juice if too watery, **2 teaspoons superfine sugar, 1 bay leaf, 2½ cups hot vegetable stock** and **½ cup low-fat (1%) milk**. Bring the soup to a simmer and cook, uncovered, for 20 minutes. Remove the bay leaf, allow the soup to cool a little, then purée in a blender (or in the pan using a stick blender) until smooth. Reheat, season to taste, and ladle into four bowls. Sprinkle each serving with **1 teaspoon snipped fresh chives**.

COOK'S TIPS

● Classic tomato soup is often made with cream instead of milk, but the low-fat milk still gives a creamy texture to the finished soup and is lower in fat.
● Drizzle 1–2 teaspoons of heavy cream into each bowl for a touch of indulgence.

TRICOLOR TOMATO TOWERS

Serves 4
Preparation 15 minutes

Each serving provides • 447 calories • 35 g fat
• 17 g saturated fat • 8 g carbohydrates • 25 g protein
• 3 g fiber

Lightly crush **2 tablespoons pine nuts** in a bowl and combine with **3 tablespoons store-bought basil pesto** and **4 finely chopped scallions**. Rinse and pat dry **2 fresh mozzarella balls** and carefully cut each one into 8 thin slices. Slice the bottom off each of **4 large tomatoes** to make a flat base, then cut each tomato into five horizontal layers. Re-assemble each tomato on a serving plate, spreading a little pesto mixture and adding a slice of mozzarella between each tomato layer. Slowly drizzle **½ teaspoon olive oil** over each tomato and garnish with **2–3 small fresh basil leaves**.

COOK'S TIPS

● Make sure that the tomatoes are ripe yet firm, or they will be hard to slice evenly and will not retain their shape when stacked.
● If you are concerned about the layers slipping, insert a cocktail toothpick down through the center of the tomato, but be sure tell your diners before serving.

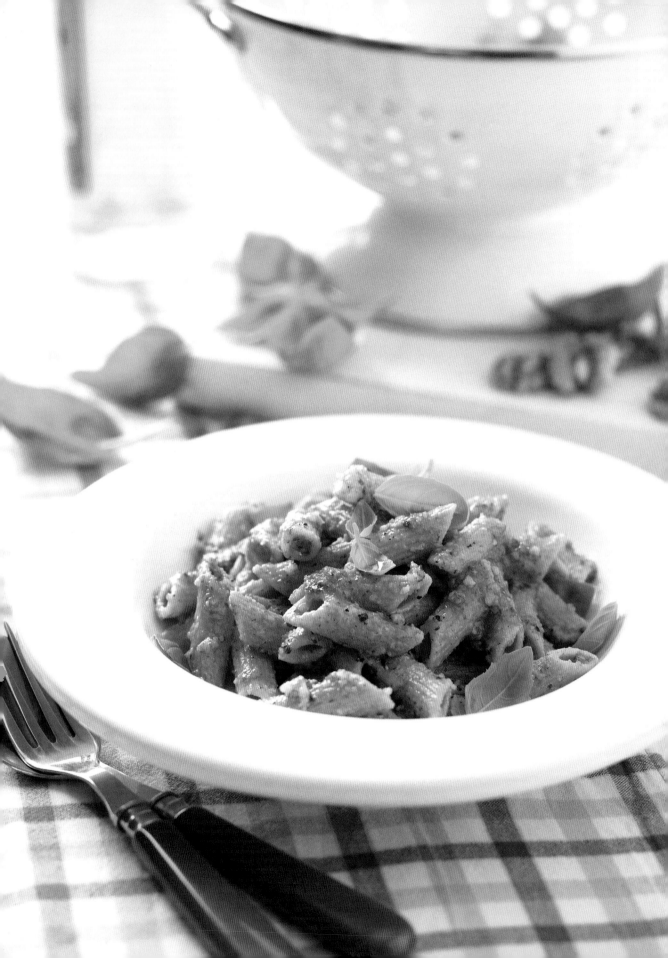

WALNUT AND BASIL PESTO PASTA

Packed with Italian flavor and the intense aroma of basil, pesto sauce makes a brilliant partner for whole-wheat pasta. For a tasty twist, this pesto uses walnuts instead of the more traditional pine nuts.

Serves 4
Preparation 5 minutes
Cooking 15 minutes

2 tablespoons parmesan
1 small clove garlic
¼ cup walnuts
½ cup fresh basil leaves
4 tablespoons olive oil
10 ounces whole-wheat pasta,
    such as fusilli, penne, or spaghetti

Each serving provides
• 510 calories • 27 g fat • 4 g saturated fat • 58 g carbohydrates • 13 g protein • 3 g fiber

ALTERNATIVE INGREDIENTS
• For a traditional pesto, replace the walnuts with ¼ cup pine nuts.
• Rather than serving the pesto with pasta, use it in rolls, sandwiches, or wraps. Spread the pesto thinly instead of butter or mayonnaise as a base for lettuces, tomatoes, sliced hard-boiled eggs, or cooked, diced chicken.
• For a more substantial meal with added protein, broil four fish steaks, such as cod, salmon, or tuna, and top each portion of pesto pasta with fish just before serving.

1 Cut the parmesan into ½-inch pieces. Mix the garlic, parmesan, walnuts, and basil (reserving a few leaves to garnish) in a food processor or blender until reduced to a chunky paste.

2 With the motor running, gradually pour in the oil to create a coarse, thick paste.

3 Fill a large saucepan with boiling water. Add the pasta, return to a boil and cook for 12–15 minutes, or follow the package directions for specific cooking times.

4 Drain the pasta in a colander and return it to the pan. Add the pesto and toss to coat evenly. Transfer the pesto pasta to four warmed plates, garnish with the reserved basil leaves, and serve.

COOK'S TIPS
● To test if the pasta is cooked, carefully remove a piece with a slotted spoon, cool under cold running water, and taste. It should be firm but not crunchy in the middle—and definitely not mushy.
● Pesto freezes well and is a great way of preserving home-grown basil. Freeze the pesto in containers that contain enough sauce for one meal. Thaw it in the fridge overnight or at room temperature for 2–3 hours before use.

SUPER FOOD

OLIVE OIL
Eighty percent of the fats in olive oil are heart-healthy monounsaturated and polyunsaturated fats, containing vitamin E, which helps protect against heart disease. Virgin olive oil, and particularly extra virgin, is high in antioxidants. Like all oils, olive oil is high in calories, so use sparingly if you're watching your weight.

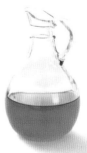

BANANA AND DATE BREAKFAST BAGEL

Bananas and whole-grain bagels release energy slowly, so this satisfying snack is guaranteed to keep you alert and stave off hunger until lunchtime. The mixed seeds are full of protein.

Serves 4
Preparation 10 minutes
Cooking 5 minutes

4 whole-grain bagels
½ cup low-fat ricotta or low-fat
   cream cheese
2 large bananas
12 large pitted dates
8 tablespoons mixed seeds
   (see Cook's Tips)
4 teaspoons honey

Each serving provides
• 453 calories • 17 g fat • 4 g
saturated fat • 60 g carbohydrates
• 17 g protein • 9 g fiber

ALTERNATIVE INGREDIENTS
• Allow 2 pitted sliced fresh apricots
per bagel instead of banana.
• Try using different bread bases.
English muffins have a softer, breadier
texture compared to bagels, while
French brioche rolls are richer and
slightly sweet. Thin slices of dark rye
or pumpernickel bread also work well.
Increase the quantity of honey to
6 teaspoons when using firmer breads.
• For added fiber, include 1 tablespoon
each of wheat germ and whole rolled
oats in the seed mix before sprinkling
over the bagels.

1 Preheat the broiler to the hottest setting. Cut the bagels in half horizontally and toast them, cut sides down, for 2 minutes until warm but not overly browned.

2 Spread the untoasted sides of the bagels with ricotta or cream cheese, then place them, cheese side up, in a large ovenproof dish or cover the broiler pan with foil before adding the bagels. Be careful as the pan will be hot.

3 Slice the bananas at a slight angle and arrange the slices over the bagels. Chop the dates into thirds and place the pieces on and around the banana. Sprinkle each bagel half with seeds then drizzle with honey. Broil the bagels for 3 minutes, or until the topping is hot. Watch carefully so the seeds do not burn.

COOK'S TIPS
● There are many brands of mixed seeds in health food stores and supermarkets and most contain sunflower, sesame, and pumpkin seeds as the main ingredients. Store any leftover seeds in an airtight container.
● Buy raw seeds and toast them lightly in a dry, heavyweight frying pan over medium heat, stirring frequently until lightly browned. Cool completely before storing in an airtight container.

SUPER FOOD

BANANAS
Ripe bananas are great energy boosters, and with their low to moderate glycemic index (GI), provide a sustained energy supply. Full of essential potassium, bananas can help to regulate blood pressure, reducing the risk of a stroke.

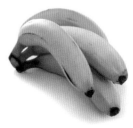

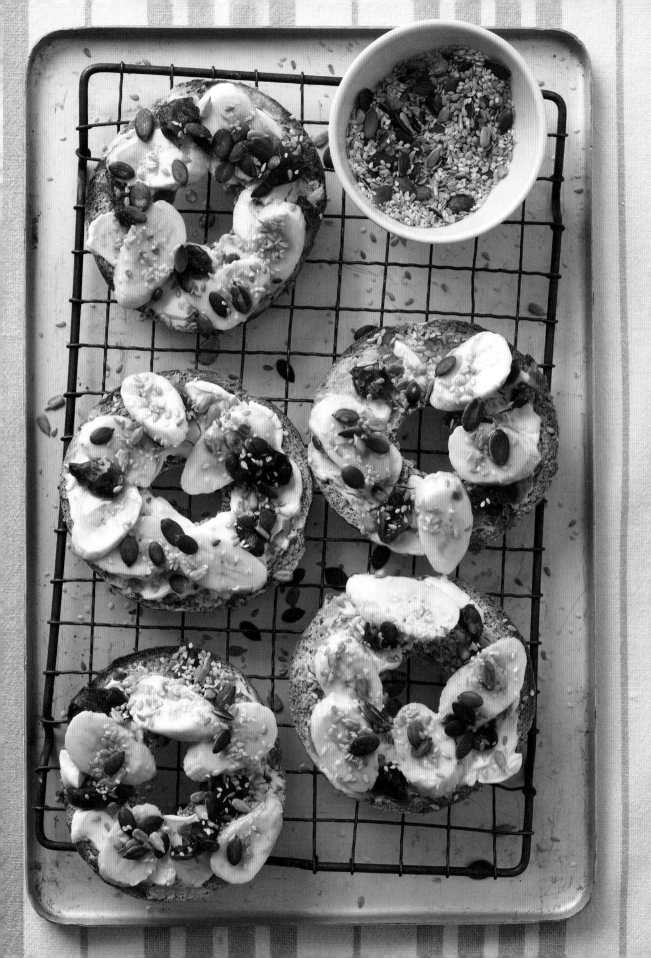

RASPBERRY, BANANA, AND **OAT** SMOOTHIE

Beautiful to look at and delightful to taste, this feel-good high-fiber drink provides both quick-release and slow-burning energy that lasts for hours. Raspberries are high in antioxidants, too.

Serves 4
Preparation 5 minutes

2 large bananas
¼ cup rolled oats
1 cup raspberries
1 tablespoon honey
8 raspberries, to garnish

Each serving provides
• 150 calories • 2 g fat • 0 g saturated fat • 32 g carbohydrates • 3 g protein • 3 g fiber

ALTERNATIVE INGREDIENTS
• Use 1 cup blackberries, red currants, or strawberries instead of the raspberries for an equally refreshing and good-for-you smoothie.
• For a chilled smoothie, substitute frozen mixed berries for fresh raspberries.

1 Peel the bananas and cut them into 1½-inch chunks. Put the bananas, oats, and raspberries in a blender. Add the honey and 1 cup cold water. Purée until smooth, then add another 1 cup water and blend for another 4–5 seconds.

2 Pour the smoothie into four tall glasses. Garnish with 2 raspberries per glass and serve immediately.

COOK'S TIPS
● For a refreshing raspberry drink that is tangy rather than sweet, use just-ripe bananas, which contain less sugar than very ripe ones.
● Rolled oats are large flakes sometimes sold as traditional or original oats. Do not buy fine, medium, or coarse oatmeal as it will not blend well in the drink.

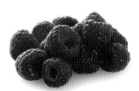

SUPER FOOD

RASPBERRIES
Raspberries are full of nutrient goodness—they are a valuable source of fiber, contain potassium, which helps to regulate blood pressure, and pack an antioxidant punch thanks to their high levels of vitamin C and flavonoids.

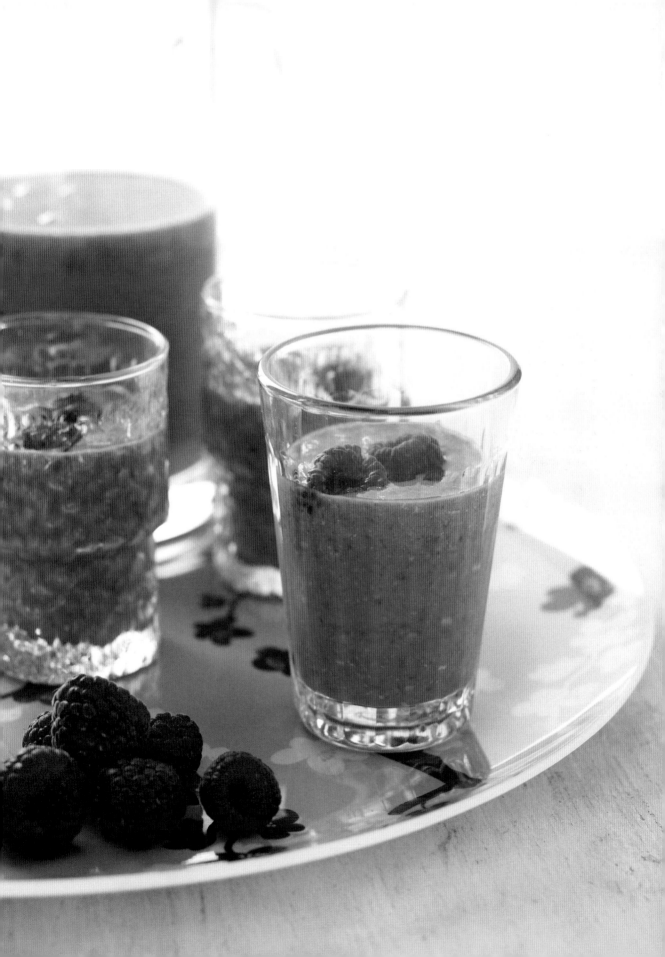

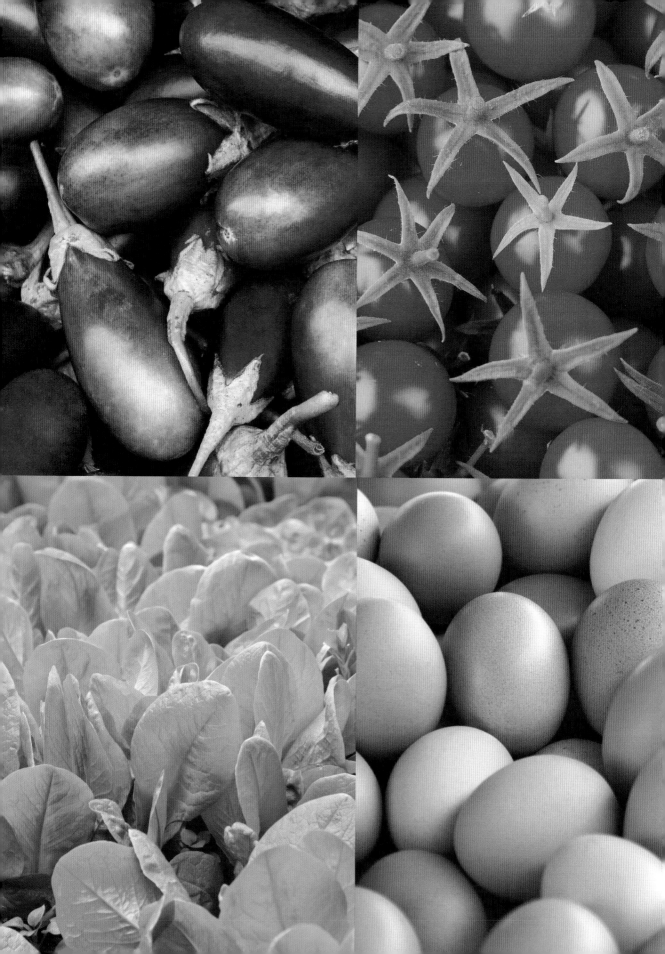

VEGETABLES
and
SALADS

BUTTERNUT SQUASH WITH BELL PEPPERS AND ALMONDS

Succulent is the word for a sunny medley of vitamin-rich butternut squash and yellow bell peppers in a nut and honey glaze. It's ideal as a side dish or a vegetarian main course with country-style bread.

Serves 4
Preparation 10 minutes
Cooking 20 minutes

½ butternut squash,
   about 1¼ pounds
2 cloves garlic
2 tablespoons olive oil
8 sprigs fresh thyme
2 large yellow bell peppers
¼ cup whole almonds
1 tablespoon honey
finely pared zest and juice of
   1 lemon

Each serving provides
• 195 calories • 9 g fat • 1 g saturated fat • 25 g carbohydrates
• 6 g protein • 6 g fiber

ALTERNATIVE INGREDIENTS
• When in season, use 2–3 small yellow pattypan squash, halved, per portion instead of the butternut squash slices. Add 10 minutes to the cooking time.
• Eggplant slices work well in place of butternut squash. Allow 3 large slices per portion or 2 large eggplant in total. When available, use white-skinned eggplant for a change.
• Try pistachios instead of almonds and add ¼ cup sliced pitted black olives.

1 Preheat the oven to 400°F. Peel the butternut squash and scoop out the seeds. Cut the squash into 12 slices, each about ½-inch thick. Transfer the slices to a shallow roasting pan. Slice the garlic. Drizzle the squash slices with 1 tablespoon of the oil and add the garlic and thyme. Roast in the oven for 20 minutes, or until softened and beginning to brown.

2 Meanwhile, slice the bell peppers into ½-inch strips. When the squash has just 5 minutes of cooking time left, heat the remaining tablespoon of oil in a frying pan over a medium-high heat. Add the bell pepper strips and fry for 5 minutes, stirring frequently, until they are tender and beginning to brown. Transfer the bell pepper strips and squash slices to a warmed serving dish.

3 Add the almonds, honey, and lemon zest and juice to the frying pan. Stir-fry over a high heat for a few seconds until the mixture is bubbling and the lemon juice and honey have thickened to form a glaze. Spoon over the vegetables and serve.

COOK'S TIPS
● Butternut squash will continue to soften after it has been removed from the oven. To test if it is done, carefully prick with a fork—it should be tender but firm.
● To measure out honey, dip the spoon into the jar; then scrape off the excess honey from the sides of the spoon and level the top with a knife.

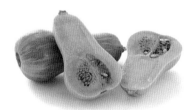

SUPER FOOD

BUTTERNUT SQUASH
A source of both types of fiber—soluble and insoluble—butternut squash helps to promote digestive health and lower blood cholesterol. The nutrient-packed orange flesh is bursting with antioxidants alpha- and beta-carotene, as well as vitamin E.

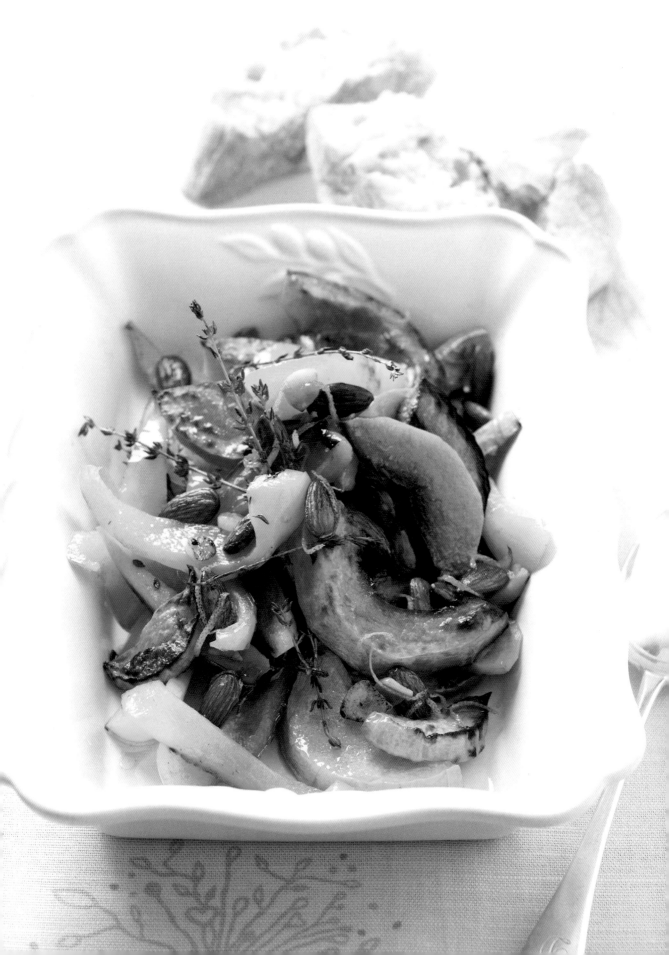

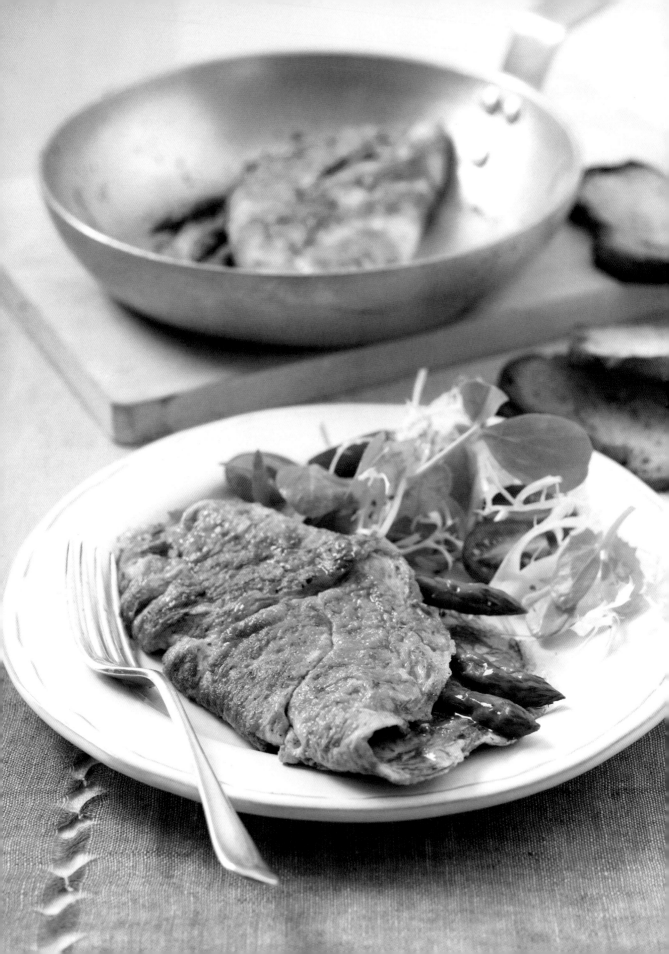

HERBED **ASPARAGUS** OMELETS

The delicate flavor of asparagus combines perfectly with light fluffy eggs in a nutritious dish that can be rustled up in minutes. Serve with a salad and sliced tomato drizzled with olive oil.

Serves 2
Preparation 5 minutes
Cooking 8 minutes

8 asparagus spears
4 eggs
4 tablespoons chopped fresh dill
2 teaspoons butter

Each serving provides
• 257 calories • 20 g protein • 18 g fat
• 3 g saturated fat • 5 g carbohydrates
• 20 g protein • 3 g fiber

ALTERNATIVE INGREDIENTS
• If you are concerned about your cholesterol levels, use 1 teaspoon of olive oil per omelet instead of butter. Heat it in the pan until hot rather than adding it to a hot pan.
• Use chopped mixed fresh herbs instead of dill—fennel, parsley, chives, thyme, and tarragon all go well with eggs.
• For a fish and herb omelet, add 2 tablespoons chopped smoked salmon per portion, scattering it over the egg in step 3 before adding the asparagus.

1 Trim or snap any tough ends from the asparagus (see Cook's Tip on page 47) and lay the spears in a frying pan. Add just enough boiling water to cover, return to a boil, then reduce the heat. Cover and simmer for 3 minutes, or until the asparagus are just tender. Drain.

2 Meanwhile, beat 2 eggs in a bowl with 1 tablespoon of water and 2 tablespoons of dill. Heat a frying pan or omelet pan until very hot. Add 1 teaspoon of the butter and swirl it around the pan. Over high heat, pour the beaten eggs into the pan and cook for 1–2 minutes, lifting the edge of the omelet as it cooks to allow the egg to run onto the hot pan.

3 When the egg is almost set, add 4 asparagus spears. Fold the omelet over the asparagus, turn out onto a plate, and keep warm. Repeat with the remaining ingredients to cook the second omelet.

COOK'S TIPS
● To be sure that your omelets are hot when you eat them, prepare warm plates for serving and have accompaniments ready on the table.
● Use a heavy pan to make the omelets, making sure that it is evenly coated with butter or oil to prevent the eggs from sticking.

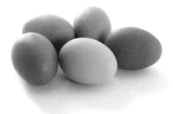

SUPER FOOD

EGGS
The ultimate natural fast food, eggs are easy to cook, nutritious, and versatile. Rich in vitamins A and D for eye and bone health, eggs also contain the pigments zeaxanthin and lutein, which may help to prevent degenerative eye disease.

TOFU-STUFFED **PEPPERS**

Sweet grilled bell peppers are filled with bite-sized tomatoes and marinated tofu pieces for a vivid, juicy Mediterranean-style dish. Serve with baked new potatoes.

Serves 4
Preparation 5 minutes
Marinating 1 hour
Cooking 15 minutes

3 tablespoons olive oil
pinch of grated nutmeg
½ teaspoon paprika
½ teaspoon dried marjoram
2 large cloves garlic, crushed
1 package (14 ounces) firm tofu
4 large green bell peppers
24 cherry tomatoes
1 teaspoon fennel seeds
¼ pound herbed mixed salad, such as arugula, watercress, and basil

Each serving provides
• 218 calories • 17 g fat • 2 g saturated fat • 8 g carbohydrates
• 10 g protein • 5 g fiber

ALTERNATIVE INGREDIENTS
• Add a pinch of red pepper flakes to the tomatoes for a hint of heat.
• Use cumin seeds instead of fennel and sprinkle the tofu with tandoori seasoning or good-quality curry powder rather than nutmeg.
• You can use haloumi or Indian paneer cheese instead of tofu, although this will increase the amount of saturated fat per portion.
• For a more delicate flavor, try yellow bell peppers with yellow cherry tomatoes, and basil leaves in place of garlic.

1 Mix the oil, nutmeg, paprika, marjoram, and 1 crushed garlic clove in a shallow dish just large enough to hold the block of tofu. Add the tofu and turn it to coat all sides, then cover and set aside to marinate for 1 hour.

2 Preheat the broiler to high. Cut each bell pepper in half and remove the seeds. Broil, cut sides down, for 3–4 minutes, until blistered but not blackened. Turn the pieces, cut sides up, and broil for another 2 minutes, or until juicy and just tender.

3 Cut each tomato in half and mix with the fennel seeds and remaining crushed garlic clove in a bowl. Remove the tofu from the marinade and slice it into eight slices, then cut these across in half.

4 Divide the tomatoes among the bell pepper halves and broil for 2 minutes. Place two pieces of tofu in each bell pepper half, setting them at an angle among the tomatoes. Drizzle the remaining marinade over the tofu and grill for another 4–5 minutes, or until the tofu is just beginning to brown. Divide the salad among four plates, place the bell pepper halves on top and serve.

COOK'S TIPS
● Before cutting the bell peppers in half, put them on your cutting board or work surface to check the best place to slice so that they sit flat.
● As well as the fresh tofu used in this recipe, which has a relatively short shelf-life and must be stored in the fridge, look for sealed packages of tofu, which make a good pantry ingredient. Smoked tofu also works well in this recipe.

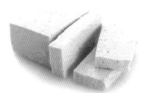

SUPER FOOD

TOFU
Also known as soybean curd, tofu is a low-fat, high-protein food. Soy protein helps to lower blood cholesterol levels, making tofu good for heart health. A source of calcium, tofu can also play a role in maintaining strong bones.

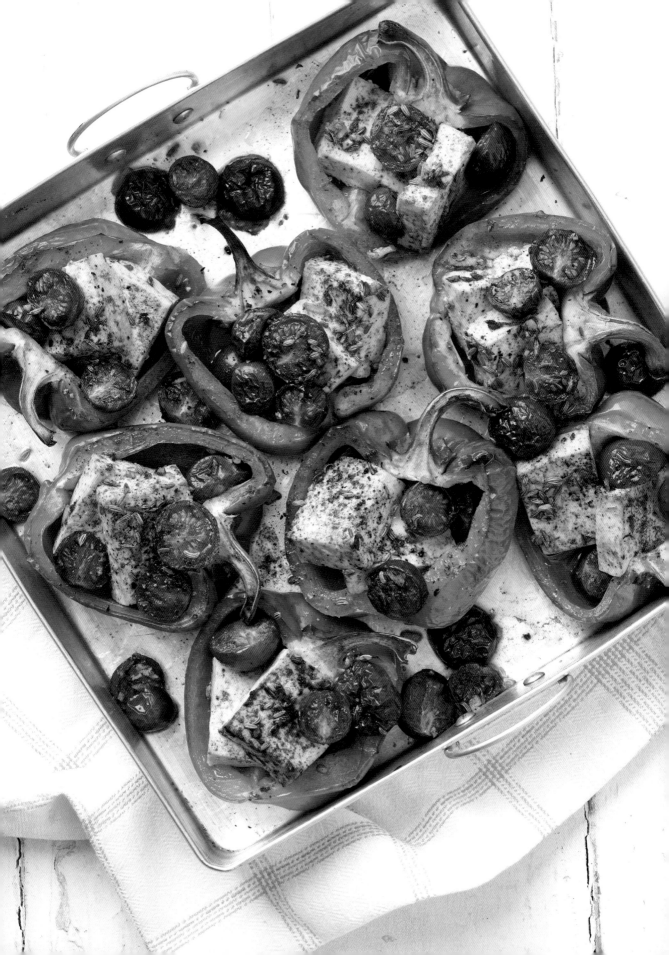

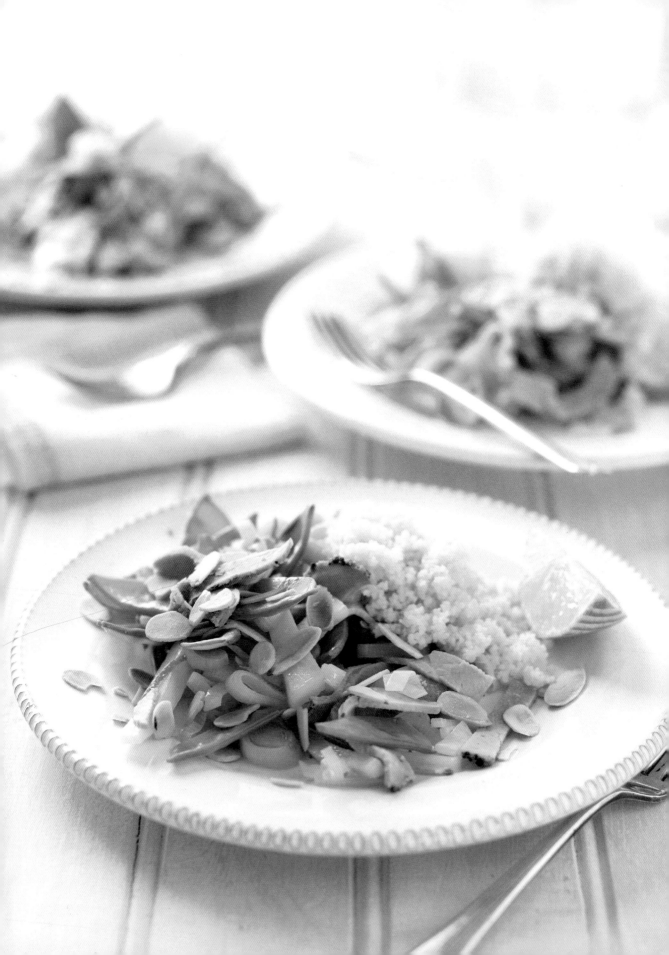

SPRING **GREENS** STIR-FRY WITH **HAM** AND TOASTED **ALMONDS**

Simply stir-fry leeks, cucumber, and snow peas with lime zest, heart-friendly toasted almonds, and lean ham and you have a super-quick light dish, great with couscous.

Serves 4
Preparation 10 minutes
Cooking 12 minutes

1½ cups snow peas
¼ cup slivered almonds
2 leeks
½ cucumber
½ pound lean cooked ham
2 tablespoons olive oil
grated zest of 1 lime
4 lime wedges, to garnish

Each serving provides
• 300 calories • 21 g fat • 4 g saturated fat • 7 g carbohydrates
• 21 g protein • 5 g fiber

ALTERNATIVE INGREDIENTS
• Sugarsnap peas make a good substitute for snow peas. They are more substantial and often have a fuller flavor.
• Try pastrami or smoked pork loin, chicken, or turkey as an alternative to the ham.
• For a vegetarian meal, leave out the ham and add ½ cup frozen soybeans or shelled lima beans in step 3. Use cashew nuts instead of almonds, increasing the quantity to ⅓ cup.

1 Put the snow peas in a large frying pan and add just enough boiling water to cover. Return to a boil, cover, and cook over high heat for 1 minute until the snow peas are bright green and slightly puffed. Drain and set aside.

2 Roast the almonds in a dry frying pan over a medium-high heat for 2 minutes. Shake the pan frequently so the nuts cook evenly and do not burn. Transfer to a plate.

3 Slice the leeks. Peel the cucumber and cut it into ½-inch wide sticks. Cut the ham into 1-inch strips. Add the oil to the frying pan and stir-fry the leeks over a medium-high heat for 3 minutes. Add the lime zest and cucumber and cook for another 5 minutes, or until the leeks are reduced and the cucumber is cooked.

4 Stir in the snow peas, ham, and almonds and stir-fry for 1 minute to heat through. Serve garnished with lime wedges.

COOK'S TIPS
● Carefully zest the lime using a zester and you can use the leftover lime, minus the zest, as a garnish rather than buying two limes.
● Do not cook the snow peas for too long or they will get soft and turn a dull green color. They should be bright green with a crunchy texture.
● Air-dried, uncooked ham, such as westphalian, prosciutto, parma, or serrano, is not recommended for a stir-fry.

SUPER FOOD

ALMONDS
With high levels of cholesterol-lowering monounsaturated fats, almonds are especially good for keeping the heart healthy. They are also rich in essential vitamin E, an important antioxidant that may help to fight the free radical damage that can eventually lead to cancer or heart disease.

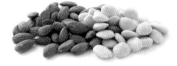

BROCCOLI MASHED POTATOES WITH POACHED EGG

Melt-in-your-mouth mashed potatoes team with vitamin C–rich broccoli and tangy black olives for a great alternative to plain mashed potatoes. Top with a poached egg for extra protein and flavor.

Serves 4
Preparation 15 minutes
Cooking 25 minutes

2 pounds potatoes
2 cloves garlic
1 cup rough-chopped broccoli spears
¼ cup pitted black olives, sliced
4 eggs
2 tablespoons olive oil
4 tablespoons low-fat (1%) milk
grated zest of 1 lemon
4 tablespoons chopped fresh parsley

Each serving provides
• 341 calories • 16 g fat • 3 g saturated fat • 36 g carbohydrates • 15 g protein • 5 g fiber

ALTERNATIVE INGREDIENTS
• Use sweet potatoes instead of regular potatoes, or a mixture of half sweet and half regular.
• Add 1 cup each rutabaga and carrots to the potatoes as a change from the broccoli. Cut the rutabaga into 1-inch chunks and cook for 5 minutes before adding the carrots and potatoes.

1 Peel the potatoes and cut them into 1-inch cubes. Peel the garlic. Put the potatoes and garlic in a large saucepan and pour in just enough boiling water to cover. Return to a boil over high heat, reduce the heat to low, cover, and simmer for 15 minutes or until tender.

2 Meanwhile, pour 1-inch of boiling water into a large shallow pan set over medium heat. Return to a boil and carefully break the eggs, one at a time, into the water, keeping them separate until the white is set. Simmer for 8–10 minutes or until done.

3 Drain the potatoes in a colander. Pour the oil into the potato saucepan, add the broccoli, and sauté over a medium-high heat for 2 minutes before adding the milk. Bring to a boil, cover, and cook for another 2 minutes. Transfer the broccoli mixture to a bowl.

4 Return the potatoes to the saucepan (off the heat) and mash them. Stir in the broccoli and milk once the potatoes are thoroughly mashed. Gently mix in the lemon zest, olives, and parsley. Carefully remove the eggs from the pan with a slotted spoon and place one on top of each portion of mashed potatoes before serving.

COOK'S TIPS
● Use potatoes suitable for boiling, such as russets or Yukon golds.
● To poach an egg, keep the water at a bare simmer throughout cooking. Cook until the white is set—this will take 5–10 minutes over low heat. You can use an egg poacher for a uniform shape.

SUPER FOOD

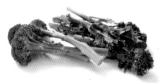

BROCCOLI
An original super food hero, broccoli is one of the top-scoring antioxidant vegetables. It contains sulforaphane, a phytochemical known to activate enzymes that may destroy cancer-causing chemicals. And it takes only one 3-ounce serving of lightly cooked broccoli to provide up to 100 percent of your daily vitamin C requirements.

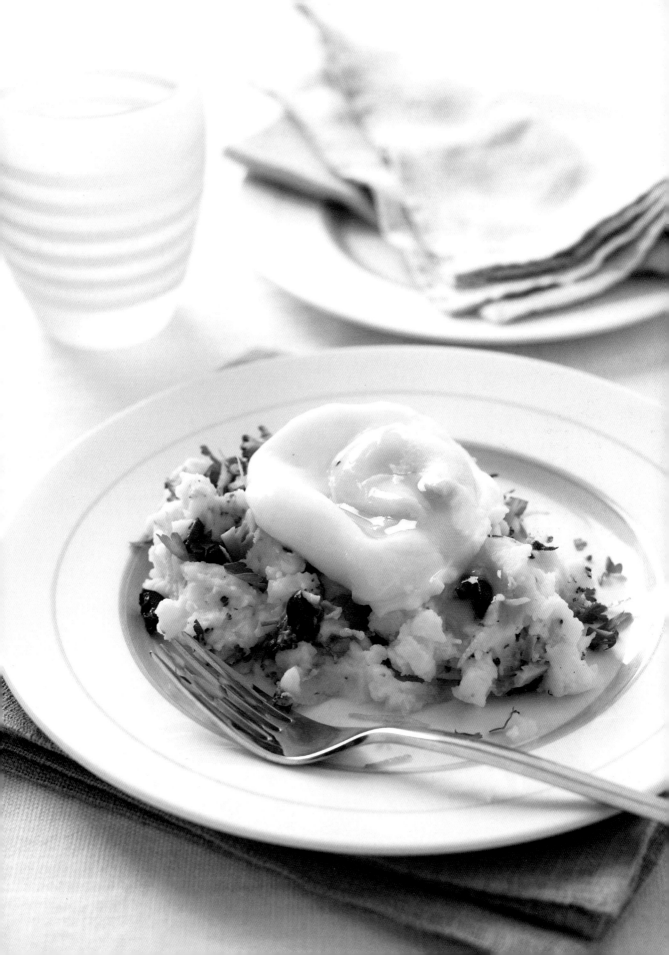

BROCCOLI

A versatile vegetable in the kitchen, broccoli is also rich in a number of nutrients. These include phytochemicals, or plant chemicals, which may help to prevent some cancers and heart disease as well as protect against the signs of ageing. Broccoli contains plenty of vitamin C, too, boosting the immune system.

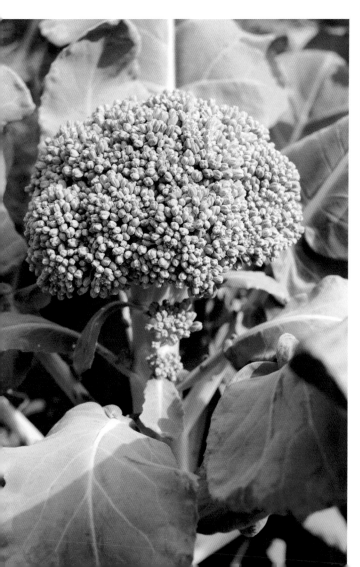

BROCCOLI PÂTÉ

Serves 4
Preparation 15 minutes Cooking 28 minutes

Each serving provides • 157 calories • 11 g fat • 3 g saturated fat • 3 g carbohydrates • 1 g protein • 3 g fiber

Preheat the oven to 350°F. Cook **1½ cups broccoli florets** in a pan of boiling water for 3 minutes, or until barely cooked. Drain, refresh under cold running water, and pat dry with paper towels. Transfer the broccoli to a large bowl and lightly mash. Stir in **3 beaten eggs, ¼ cup low-fat (1%) milk, 3 tablespoons grated parmesan** and **2 finely chopped scallions**. Season to taste. Lightly brush four ramekins with **olive oil or canola oil** and fill each with a quarter of the broccoli mixture. Place the ramekins on a baking sheet and bake in the oven for 25 minutes or until set and golden. Let cool, then serve.

COOK'S TIP
● Garnish with cherry tomatoes or basil leaves and serve with a sliced baguette or whole-grain crackers.

SUMMER BROCCOLI AND LEMON SOUP

Serves 4
Preparation 10 minutes Cooking 32 minutes

Each serving provides • 150 calories • 6 g fat • 1 g saturated fat • 18 g carbohydrates • 8 g protein • 5 g fiber

Heat **1 tablespoon olive oil** in a large frying pan. Add **1 finely chopped onion** and sauté gently over low heat for 5 minutes, or until softened. Add **2 crushed cloves garlic** and stir for 1 minute before adding **2 cups broccoli florets**, cut in half if large, and **1 cup finely diced potato**. Pour in **4 cups vegetable stock**, bring to a boil, then lower the heat immediately, cover, and simmer for 25 minutes. Cool a little, then purée in a blender. Return the soup to the pan, add the **juice of ½ lemon** and reheat gently. Stir **1 tablespoon plain yogurt** into each bowl of soup and sprinkle each with **½ tablespoon finely snipped fresh chives** before serving piping hot.

COOK'S TIP
● Do not boil the soup, except to bring the stock up to temperature, otherwise it will lose its vibrant green color, making it less appetizing.

WHOLE-WHEAT PASTA WITH PINE NUTS

Serves 4
Preparation 10 minutes Cooking 15 minutes

Each serving provides • 552 calories • 27 g fat
• 5 g saturated fat • 62 g carbohydrates • 20 g protein
• 10 g fiber

Cook **10 ounces whole-wheat spaghetti** in a saucepan of boiling water according to package directions, or until tender. Add **1¾ cups broccoli florets**, cut in half if large, to the pan for the last 5 minutes of cooking. Meanwhile, heat **3 tablespoons olive oil** in a small frying pan and add **4 crushed cloves garlic** and **1 finely chopped red chile**. Stir over a medium heat for 2 minutes. Drain the pasta and broccoli and transfer them to a serving dish. Pour the garlic and chile oil over the hot pasta and toss thoroughly to coat. Mix **4 tablespoons toasted pine nuts, 2 tablespoons grated parmesan** and **2 tablespoons breadcrumbs**. Sprinkle the crumb topping over the pasta before serving.

COOK'S TIP
● To make breadcrumbs, process 1 slice of whole-grain bread in a food processor and until it turns to crumbs. Transfer to a baking sheet and toast the crumbs under the broiler, turning often, until golden.

SWEET POTATO, BROCCOLI AND LENTIL SALAD

Serves 4
Preparation 15 minutes Cooking 25 minutes

Each serving provides • 472 calories • 28 g fat
• 4 g saturated fat • 43 g carbohydrates • 14 g protein
• 9 g fiber

Preheat the oven to 400°F. Peel **about 1 pound sweet potatoes** and cut into 1-inch cubes. Toss the cubes in **3 tablespoons olive oil** and arrange on a baking sheet. Bake for 25 minutes, or until cooked through and golden. Meanwhile, cook **⅔ cup brown** or **green (puy) lentils** in a pan of boiling water for 25 minutes, or until tender, then drain. Cook **1¼ cups broccoli florets** in a pan of boiling water for 5 minutes. Transfer to a colander and refresh under cold running water, then pat dry. Halve **⅔ cup cherry tomatoes** and chop **1 small bunch fresh cilantro leaves**. Make a dressing by mixing together **2 tablespoons olive oil, 2 tablespoons sesame oil, 2 tablespoons light soy sauce, ½ teaspoon hot sauce** and **½ teaspoon finely grated fresh ginger**. Toss the broccoli, potatoes, and lentils with the tomatoes, cilantro, and dressing. Serve warm or cold.

COOK'S TIP
● This salad is ideal as a starter or part of a buffet. It would also make a nice accompaniment to grilled chicken breasts.

BROCCOLI, CARROT, AND MUSHROOM STIR-FRY

Serves 4
Preparation 10 minutes Cooking 6 minutes

Each serving provides • 201 calories • 13 g fat
• 2 g saturated fat • 15 g carbohydrates • 6 g protein
• 4 g fiber

Heat **1 tablespoon olive oil or canola oil** in a wok or non-stick frying pan. Add **1 cup broccoli florets** and **⅔ cup carrots**, cut into thin julienne strips (see Cook's Tip). Stir-fry over high heat for 2 minutes and add **8 scallions**, sliced lengthwise, and cook for another 2 minutes. Stir in another **1 tablespoon olive oil or canola oil**, plus **½ cup sliced button mushrooms** and **2 crushed cloves garlic**. Stir-fry for 1 minute then pour in **2 tablespoons light soy sauce, 2 teaspoons honey** and **1 tablespoon rice vinegar**. Heat through for 1 minute and serve sprinkled with **4 tablespoons cashew nuts**.

COOK'S TIP
● To make julienne strips, first peel the carrots. Trim four sides of each carrot to create a rectangle. Cut the rectangle lengthwise into ⅛-inch slices then stack the slices and cut lengthwise to make ⅛-inch strips.

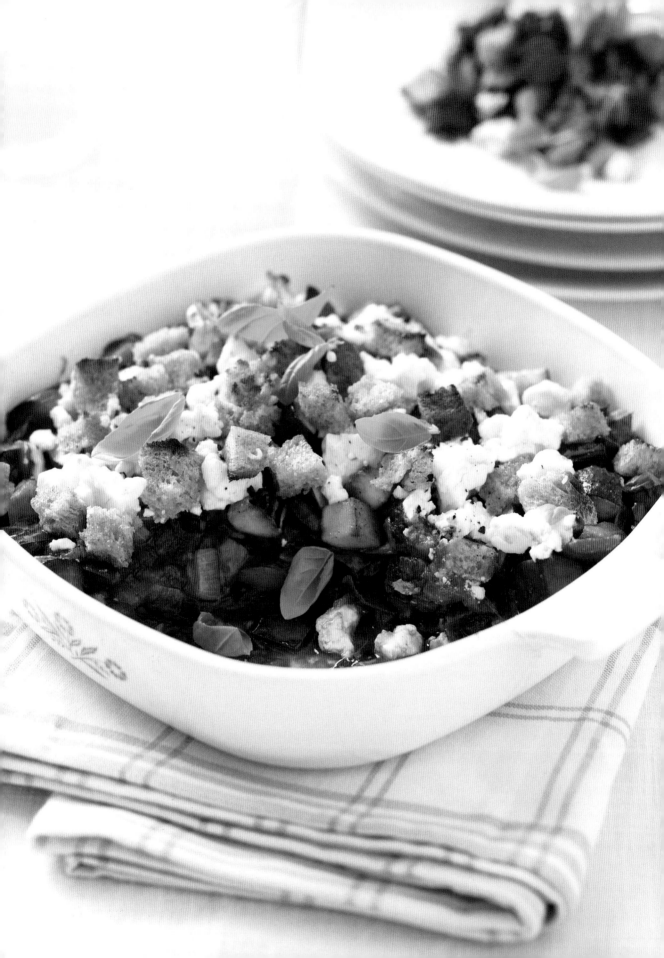

RATATOUILLE WITH FETA GRATIN

A light version of a classic dish that contains all the goodness of eggplant, zucchini, and tomatoes. The topping of bread and Greek feta turns a side dish into a vegetarian main meal.

Serves 4
Preparation 20 minutes
Cooking 20 minutes

1 medium eggplant, about ⅔ pound
1 onion
2 tablespoons olive oil
1 clove garlic, crushed
2 zucchini
4 large tomatoes
2 tablespoons tomato paste
4 tablespoons chopped fresh parsley
4 fresh basil sprigs

Topping
2 slices whole-grain bread
⅔ cup crumbled feta
1 tablespoon olive oil

Each serving provides
• 294 calories • 20 g fat • 7 g
saturated fat • 19 g carbohydrates
• 10 g protein • 5 g fiber

ALTERNATIVE INGREDIENTS
• For a more traditional ratatouille, add
1 diced green bell pepper with the
onion in step 1.
• Use a 14½-ounce can of chopped
tomatoes instead of fresh tomatoes.

1 Trim and discard the stem end of the eggplant and cut the flesh into ½-inch cubes. Chop the onion. Heat the oil in a large saucepan over high heat, add the onion and garlic, and cook for 1 minute. Add the eggplant, reduce the heat to medium, and cook for 5 minutes, stirring occasionally, until softened.

2 Meanwhile, cut the zucchini into ½-inch cubes. Add them to the pan and continue to cook for another 2 minutes, stirring occasionally until the vegetables start to brown.

3 Preheat the broiler to high. Dice the tomatoes then add them with the tomato paste to the pan. Stir in ⅓ cup of cold water. Heat the mixture until simmering, cover, and cook over a medium to medium-low heat for 8–10 minutes. Stir in the parsley and transfer to a shallow ovenproof dish.

4 For the topping, cut the bread into ½-inch cubes. Add the feta to a bowl with the bread, then pour in the oil and toss to coat. Sprinkle the topping over the ratatouille and broil for 1–2 minutes, or until the cheese softens and the bread browns. Strip the leaves from the basil sprigs and sprinkle them over the ratatouille before serving.

COOK'S TIP
● Don't worry about salting the eggplant before use. In the past, eggplant cultivars were bitter and had to be salted (known as degorging) to draw out the sour juices, but varieties available in supermarkets today have been bred to avoid this and can therefore be added straight into the ratatouille.

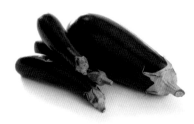

SUPER FOOD

EGGPLANT
Rich in antioxidants, eggplant may help to protect against cancer and heart disease. It also contains vitamin K, needed to regulate blood clotting, some folate for heart health, and a useful amount of fiber.

MIXED GRILL WITH TOMATOES

Ripe tomatoes have unbeatable flavor and are crammed with antioxidants that help to protect cells. Combine them with green beans, mushrooms, a fried egg, and bread for a big, tasty, meat-free breakfast.

Serves 4
Preparation 10 minutes
Cooking 20 minutes

½ pound green beans
4 tablespoons olive oil
1 garlic clove, crushed
½ teaspoon mixed dried herbs
12 slices baguette
6 tomatoes
8 medium portbello mushrooms
4 eggs
2 tablespoons snipped fresh chives
2 tablespoons chopped fresh parsley

Each serving provides
• 423 calories • 24 g fat • 4 g saturated fat • 37 g carbohydrates
• 16 g protein • 5 g fiber

ALTERNATIVE INGREDIENTS
• You can serve baked beans instead of green beans.
• Try poached or scrambled eggs as a change from fried eggs.
• For a main meal, omit the fried bread, and serve with mashed potato.
• Top each mushroom with a ½-inch-thick slice of haloumi cheese or tofu, and leave out the egg.

1 Preheat the broiler to high and line the broiler pan with foil. Trim the beans and put them in a saucepan. Pour in boiling water to cover, then return to a boil, reduce the heat, cover, and cook for 5 minutes, or until tender. Drain and keep warm.

2 Mix the oil, garlic, and herbs, and brush a little on one side of the baguette slices. Fry, oiled sides down, in a dry frying pan over medium heat for 4 minutes, or until browned. Set aside.

3 Halve the tomatoes and place them on the broiler pan, cut sides down. Place the mushrooms on the broiler pan, stem sides up. Brush everything with the flavored oil and broil for 3 minutes. Turn over, brush with more oil and broil for another 3 minutes. Add the bread, untoasted sides up, and brush sparingly with the oil. Broil for 1–2 minutes.

4 Meanwhile, heat the remaining garlic-and-herb oil in the frying pan over high heat. Break in the eggs and cook for 1–2 minutes. Transfer the eggs to four plates. Add the mushrooms, tomatoes, and green beans. Sprinkle with chives and parsley before serving with the bread.

COOK'S TIP
● Slice tomatoes in half horizontally rather than down through the stems so they sit flat on the broiler pan and cook evenly.

SUPER FOOD

TOMATOES
The antioxidants in tomatoes may help to combat the effects of free radicals in the body. These molecules can damage cells, which researchers think may lead to cancer and some other diseases. Antioxidants are able to 'mop up' the free radicals and so protect cells.

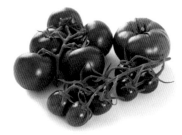

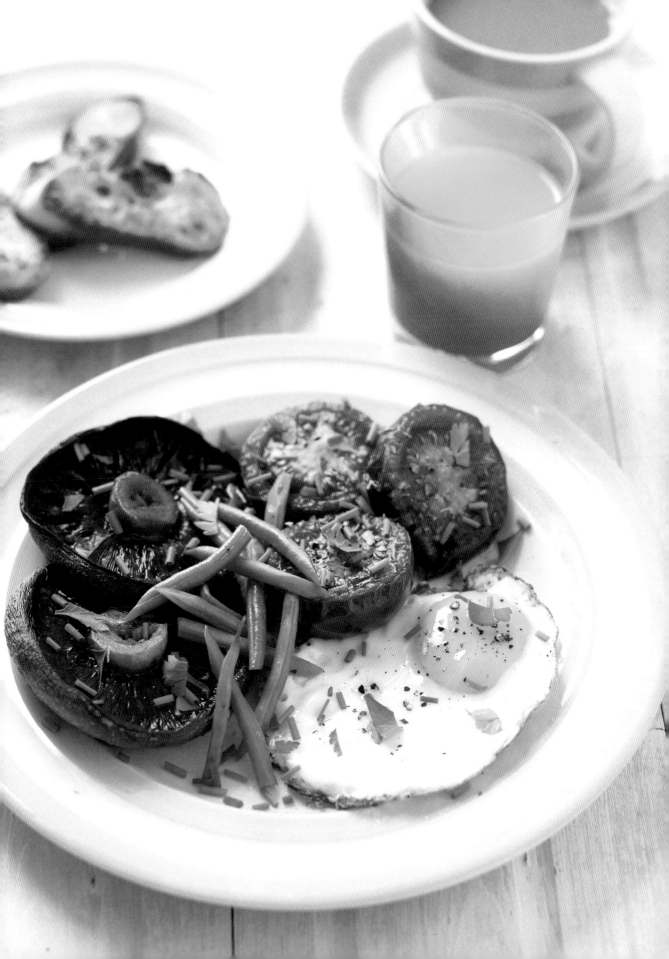

AVOCADO AND EGGPLANT STACKS

A topping of haloumi cheese adds a taste of Cyprus to little towers of tender sun-ripened vegetables for an enticing mix of textures and flavors. Just add a tomato salad.

Serves 4
Preparation 10 minutes
Cooking 12 minutes

1 large eggplant, about 1 pound
2 tablespoons olive oil
1 clove garlic, crushed
grated zest of 1 lemon and
    juice of ½ lemon
2 firm ripe avocados
½ pound haloumi cheese
2 tablespoons slivered almonds

Each serving provides
• 465 calories • 42 g fat • 15 g saturated fat• 6 g carbohydrates
• 16 g protein • 6 g fiber

ALTERNATIVE INGREDIENTS
• Try Indian paneer or mozzarella cheese instead of the haloumi. Paneer retains a similarly firm texture during cooking, but the mozzarella will melt.
• If you don't have fresh lemon, use 2 tablespoons of bottled lemon juice. The recipe will taste just as good but with a slightly less zingy flavor.
• You can use pine nuts instead of slivered almonds.
• Sliced tomatoes can be broiled on top of the eggplant—substitute them for the almonds or the avocado slices. Use 1–2 tomato slices for each slice of eggplant.

1 Preheat the broiler to high and line the broiler pan with foil. Trim and cut the eggplant into 12 slices. Place the eggplant on the foil. Mix the oil and garlic and brush sparingly over the eggplant. Broil for 4 minutes, or until just beginning to brown. Turn over, brush with more oil and broil for another 4 minutes, or until tender.

2 Put the lemon zest and juice in a shallow non-metallic dish. Cut the avocados into quarters. Peel and cut each quarter into three slices, coating them in the lemon juice to prevent discoloration. Cut the haloumi into 12 slices.

3 Sprinkle the almonds over the eggplant and arrange three avocado slices, with the lemon zest, on each. Top each stack with a slice of haloumi and brush with any remaining oil. Broil for 4 minutes, or until the cheese browns.

COOK'S TIPS
● For a balanced stack, layer a large slice of eggplant, then a medium slice of avocado, and finally a small slice of cheese. If top-heavy, the stacks will topple over.
● If the heat is not evenly distributed under the broiler, rearrange the eggplant slices when turning them so they brown all over.

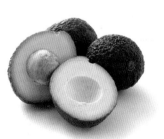

SUPER FOOD

AVOCADOS
Unusually for a fruit, avocados are high in fat—20 g in half an avocado—though most of the fat is the healthy, monounsaturated kind that helps to lower blood cholesterol and keep hearts healthy. Avocados are also rich in fiber. Half an avocado provides one-quarter of your total daily fiber needs.

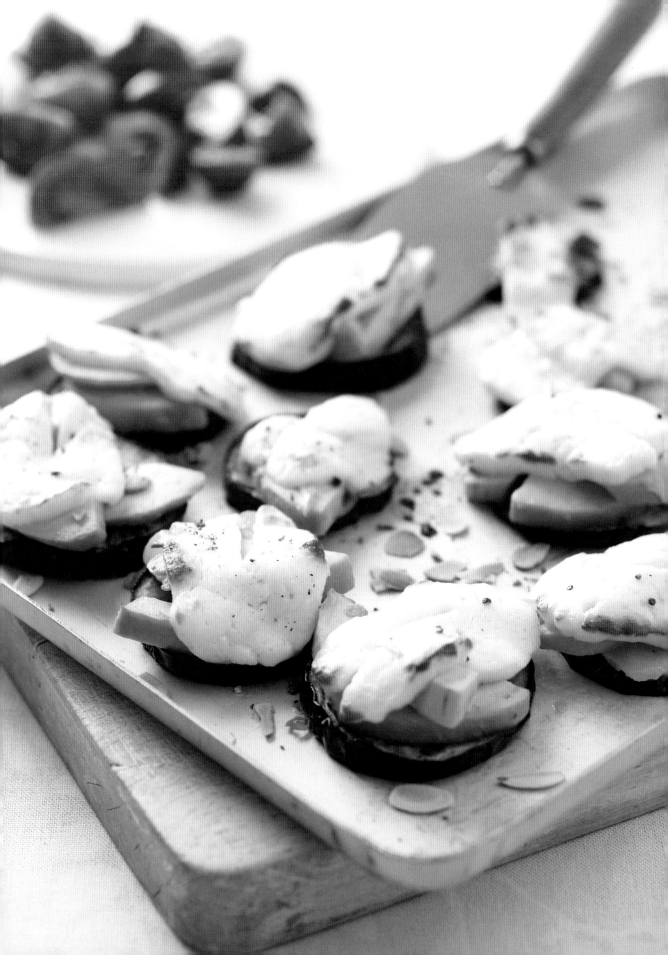

GLAZED PEARS WITH FETA

Salty feta offsets the sweetness of honey-glazed pears for a refreshingly different and healthy salad. Toasted pumpkin seeds add extra bite—as well as zinc and selenium—to boost the immune system.

Serves 4
Preparation 10 minutes
Cooking 10 minutes

½ head of crunchy lettuce,
  such as romaine or iceberg
1 bunch arugula
juice of 2 limes and grated zest
  of 1 lime
1 tablespoon honey
4 large firm, just-ripe pears
4 tablespoons pumpkin seeds
1 cup crumbled feta

Each serving provides
• 327 calories • 17 g fat • 8 g saturated fat • 32 g carbohydrates • 13 g protein • 5 g fiber

ALTERNATIVE INGREDIENTS
• A blue cheese, such as stilton, is a delicious alternative to feta here. Or try a gorgonzola dolce or cambozola for a creamy texture.
• Firm apples with a sweet-sharp flavor can be used instead of the pears for a crunchier salad. Use lemon zest with apples rather than lime.
• Pine nuts make a good substitute for pumpkin seeds.
• Peppery arugula is delicious with the lime and feta, but watercress also works well, as would the slightly bitter red leaves of radicchio.

1 Coarsely shred the lettuce and divide it among four large plates, together with the arugula. Stir together the lime juice, honey, and 4 tablespoons of water in a frying pan.

2 Peel, core, and slice the pears, removing the stems. Add to the frying pan and bring to a boil over high heat. Cook, turning the pear slices, for 3–5 minutes, or until the liquid has evaporated and the slices are slightly golden. Remove the pan from the heat, add 2 tablespoons of water, and stir to glaze the pears.

3 Toast the pumpkin seeds by sprinkling them into a separate dry frying pan and cook over a medium heat for 3–4 minutes. Stir occasionally to prevent the seeds from burning.

4 Arrange the pears on top of the leafy salad. Divide the crumbled feta among the plates of salad leaves. Sprinkle the lime zest and toasted pumpkin seeds over the top, then serve.

COOK'S TIPS
● Peel the pears whole, quarter them lengthwise, and then you will be able to cut the core out easily. Cut each quarter lengthwise into neat slices. Have the juices ready in the pan, adding the pears as they are prepared so they don't discolor.
● Use a spatula and fork to turn the pears in the frying pan. The cooking time will depend on the type of pan. For instance, the juices may evaporate and begin to caramelize more quickly in a thin metal pan. Take care when adding water to a hot pan as it may spit.
● A zester is a useful kitchen tool for removing the zest from citrus fruit, such as lime, but if you don't have one, use a vegetable peeler.

SUPER FOOD

PEARS
Like most fruits, pears are excellent for effective weight control. They are low in calories, yet have a good fullness factor, great for staving off hunger. Pears also have a low glycemic index (GI) rating, so they help to keep blood glucose steady.

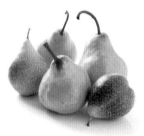

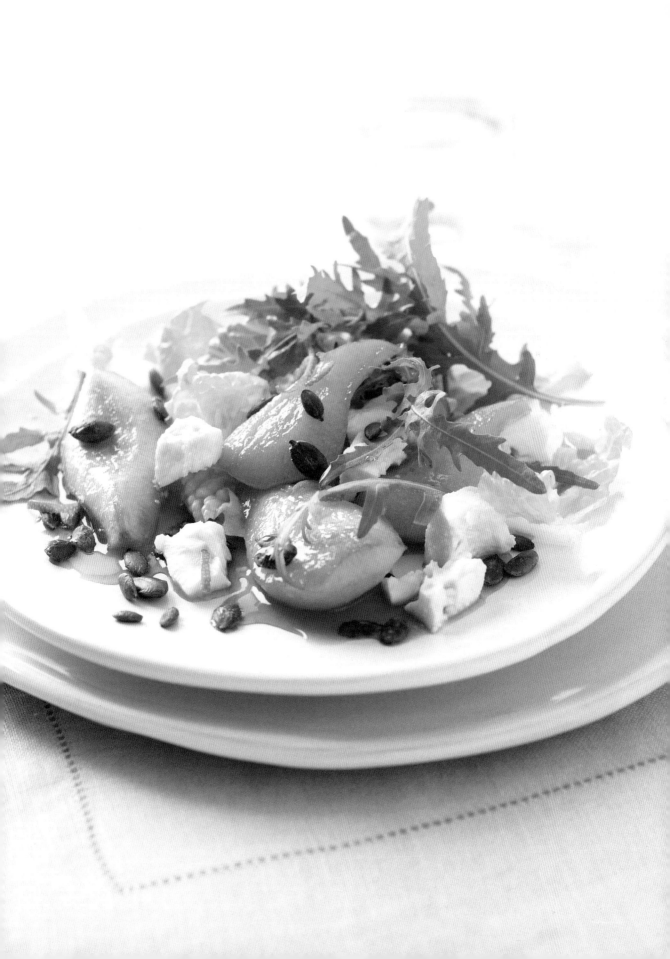

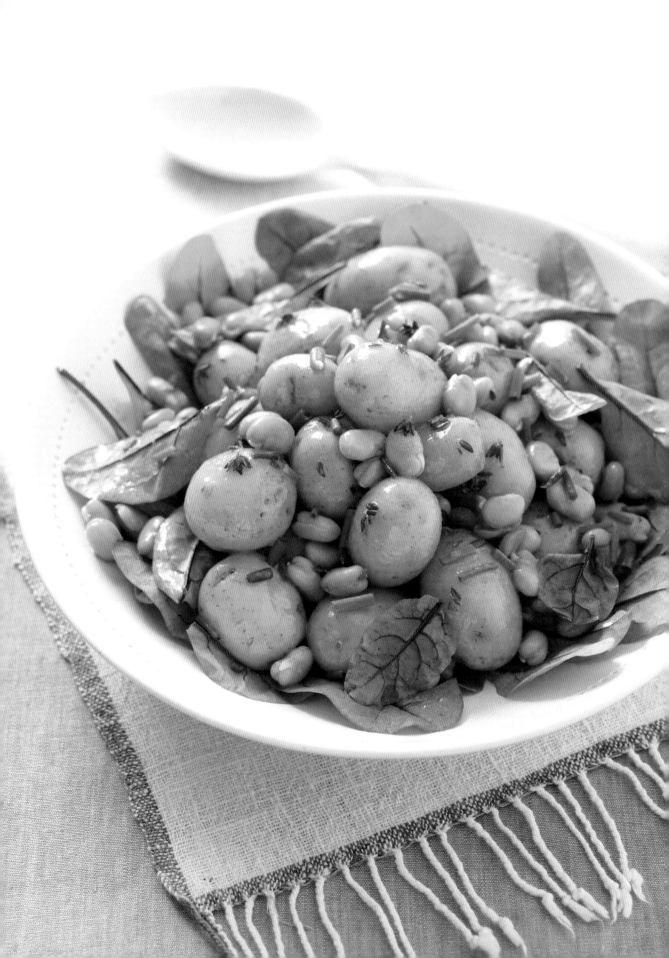

WARM **POTATO** AND **LIMA BEAN** SALAD

For an elegant, flavor-drenched, warm salad, take nutty new potatoes and high-fiber lima beans, drizzle them with a herby vinaigrette, then serve on salad greens.

Serves 4
Preparation 15 minutes
Cooking 15 minutes

1 pound baby new potatoes
4 cups fresh lima beans or
  1²/₃ cups frozen baby lima beans
1 teaspoon sugar
1 teaspoon English mustard
1 teaspoon cider vinegar
3 tablespoons olive oil
3 large sprigs thyme
4 ounces beet leaves or mixed
  salad leaves
4 tablespoons snipped fresh chives

Each serving provides
• 247 calories • 13 g fat • 2 g saturated fat • 28 g carbohydrates • 7 g protein • 6 g fiber

ALTERNATIVE INGREDIENTS
• Freshly cooked baby beets work well in this salad with the lima beans. Trim off the leaves but keep the roots and stems in place. Wash and boil ²/₃ pound beets for 20 minutes until tender. Drain and soak in cold water until cool enough to handle, then rub off the skins under water. Cook the lima beans separately. Add the hot beets to the dressing and then add the lima beans.

1 Put the potatoes in a large saucepan and add boiling water to cover. Return to a boil, reduce heat, cover and cook for 10 minutes. Meanwhile, shell the lima beans, if using fresh ones. Soak the shelled beans in a bowl of hot water for 3–4 minutes before peeling off the pale green outer skins. Add the beans to the potatoes, return to a boil, cover, and cook for 4 minutes until tender.

2 Make a vinaigrette by whisking the sugar, mustard, and vinegar in a large bowl until the sugar has dissolved. Whisk in the oil and rub the thyme leaves off the stalks and into the bowl. Season to taste.

3 Make a bed of salad greens on four plates. Drain the potatoes and beans and stir them into the vinaigrette. Sprinkle with chives and mix again. Top the greens with the potato and bean salad.

COOK'S TIPS
● Sugar does not dissolve in oil, so to avoid a grainy vinaigrette, combine the sugar with the mustard and vinegar before adding the olive oil.
● Some salad greens have a slightly bitter taste that is pleasant in young leaves but can be a little too strong in older ones. Choose small, young leaves, or if only older ones are available, reduce their quantity by half and mix them with 'sweeter' leaves, such as lamb's lettuce (mâche), oakleaf lettuce, or finely shredded Chinese cabbage.

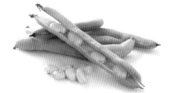

SUPER FOOD

LIMA BEANS
Part of the legume family, lima beans are a good source of both soluble and insoluble fiber to keep the digestive system in good order. They also contain energy-releasing B vitamins, including folate, which helps to maintain healthy blood and circulation.

ENDIVE AND APPLE SALAD

Apples and dates add sweetness to the subtle flavors of celeriac and crisp endive to create a fresh, light salad lunch or an accompaniment to broiled poultry or pork.

Serves 4
Preparation 15 minutes

1 tablespoon cider vinegar
2 tablespoons olive oil,
  plus 1 tablespoon for serving
1 cup peeled, coarsely grated celeriac
2–3 apples, about ½ pound
¼ cup chopped pistachios
⅔ cup chopped medjool dates
3–4 heads endive

Each serving provides
- 334 calories • 20 g fat • 3 g saturated fat • 37 g carbohydrates
- 5 g protein • 7 g fiber

ALTERNATIVE INGREDIENTS
- Try ¼ cup walnuts or pecans instead of the pistachios.
- Fresh dates are fine if you can't find medjool dates.
- Dried apricots or dried cranberries make good alternatives to the dates.
- For a more substantial meal, top the salad with ⅓ cup crumbled feta. For a meat option, sauté ¼ pound sliced chorizo or other cured sausage for a minute before adding to the salad.
- This salad is great served in wraps. Spread whole-wheat tortillas with low-fat ricotta or low-fat cream cheese flavored with garlic and herbs. Top with the salad, omitting the endive, and roll up.

1 Whisk the vinegar and 2 tablespoons of oil together in a large bowl to make a dressing. Add the celeriac to the dressing, and mix thoroughly.

2 Cut apples into quarters, remove the cores, then cut each quarter into two wedges. Slice the wedges widthwise and mix with the celeriac. Stir the nuts and dates into the celeriac mixture.

3 Separate the individual endive leaves and arrange them on a serving plate. Drizzle with the remaining oil. Pile the salad onto the plate and use the endive leaves to scoop up the salad.

COOK'S TIPS
● The coarsest disc on a food processor is ideal for grating celeriac, also known as celery root. Alternatively, use the coarse blade on a box grater and press firmly to remove good-sized shreds.
● Prepare the salad up to 2 hours in advance of serving. Cover the serving plate with plastic wrap and store in the fridge until needed.

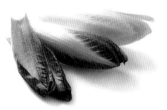

SUPER FOOD

BELGIAN ENDIVE
A mildly bitter salad leaf, Belgian endive is high in fiber, vitamin C, and a variety of minerals. The red variety provides good amounts of beneficial antioxidants.

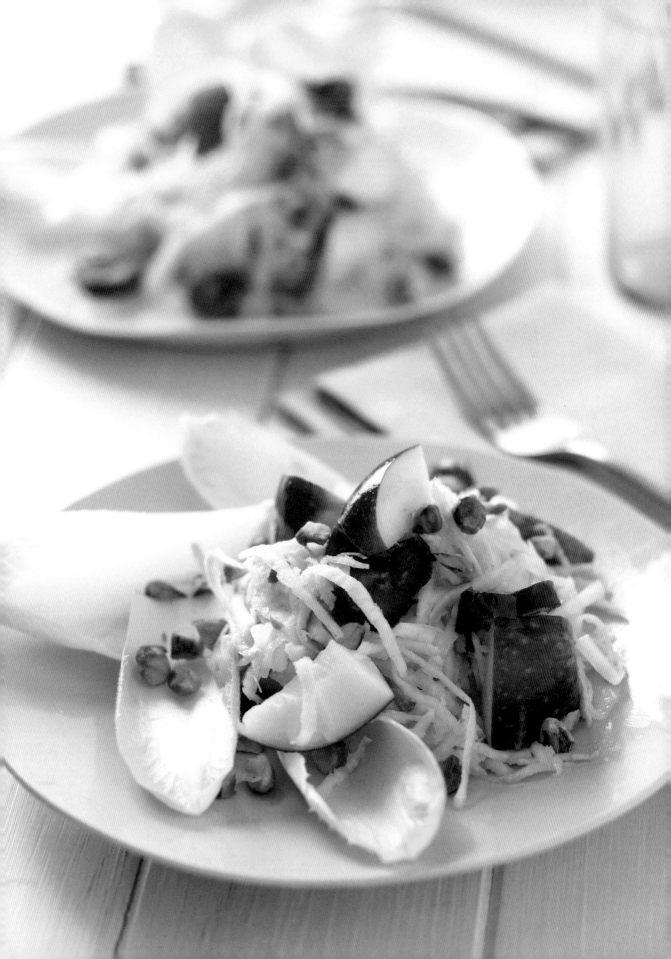

APPLES

Easily available, apples offer many nutritional benefits and may even help to sharpen mental alertness. They also contain plenty of soluble fiber that can contribute to lower blood cholesterol. And, with an average of only 65 calories, an apple is the perfect healthy snack.

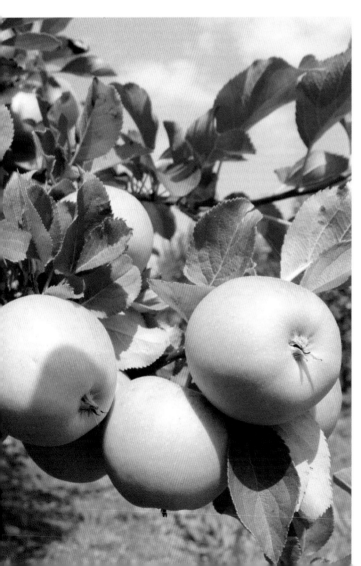

BAKED OATY APPLES

Serves 4
Preparation 10 minutes, plus 15 minutes standing
Cooking 40 minutes

Each serving provides · 249 calories · 7 g fat · 4 g saturated fat · 48 g carbohydrates · 2 g protein · 5 g fiber

Preheat the oven to 350°F. Put ⅓ **cup golden raisins** in a heatproof bowl and cover with hot water and let them plump up for 15 minutes. Meanwhile, warm **2 tablespoons honey** in a small saucepan with **2 tablespoons rolled oats** and ½ **teaspoon ground mixed spice**. Drain the raisins and stir them into the oats. Core **4 baking apples** and score them horizontally with a sharp knife to penetrate the skin. Place the apples in an ovenproof dish and fill each cavity with the raisins and oats. Place a **dollop of butter** on the top of each apple. Pour **1 cup of water** around the apples in the dish. Bake for 40 minutes, or until the apples are soft. Baste the apples with the juices halfway through cooking to keep them moist.

COOK'S TIPS

● Try to use unblemished apples, as bruises will spoil the appearance of your dessert and may affect the dish's nutritional content. Choose from a variety of baking apples, such as Granny Smith or Honeycrisp.
● Vary the sweet filling by using chopped dried apricots instead of raisins, and replace the oats with chopped or slivered almonds.

WALNUT AND APPLE STUFFING

Serves 4
Preparation 10 minutes Cooking 40 minutes

Each serving provides · 148 calories · 5 g fat · 1 g saturated fat · 24 g carbohydrates · 4 g protein · 4 g fiber

Preheat the oven to 350°F. Heat **1 tablespoon olive oil** in a frying pan and cook **1 large finely chopped onion** over a medium-low heat for 5 minutes, or until softened. Meanwhile, process **enough slices of stale whole-grain bread** in a food processor to make ½ cup of breadcrumbs. Finely chop **2 red apples**, leaving on the nutritious skins, and add them to the pan. Stir for 2 minutes, remove from the heat, and add the whole-grain breadcrumbs, **3 tablespoons chopped fresh parsley, 1 tablespoon chopped fresh sage, 2 tablespoons chopped walnuts** and **2 tablespoons dried cranberries**. Mix and let cool for 1 minute before stirring in **1 beaten egg yolk**. Season to taste then spoon the mixture into a shallow ovenproof dish. Dissolve **1 vegetable stock cube** in ⅓ **cup boiling water** and pour it over the stuffing. Bake in the oven for 25 minutes, or until golden.

COOK'S TIP

● If you don't have a food processor, use a blender to make the breadcrumbs, or rub the stale bread against the coarse side of a grater until it crumbles.

APPLE AND GINGER SMOOTHIE

Serves 4
Preparation 10 minutes

Each serving provides · 312 calories · 3 g fat
· 2 g saturated fat · 64 g carbohydrates · 9 g protein
· 2 g fiber

Roughly chop **4 apples**. Place them in a blender, or in a bowl if you have a stick blender. Add **1 cup apple juice** and **2 tablespoons finely grated fresh ginger**. Blend until smooth, then add **2 cups frozen vanilla low-fat yogurt** and **1¼ cups apple juice**. Blend again until smooth and pour the smoothie into four tall glasses.

COOK'S TIPS

● This smoothie works well with any type of apple, but the flavor is best with tangy green apples, such as Granny Smith.

● Try 1 teaspoon ground ginger or 2 tablespoons finely chopped crystalized ginger instead of the fresh ginger.

CARROT, APPLE, AND BEET SALAD

Serves 4
Preparation 15 minutes Marinating 30 minutes

Each serving provides · 131 calories · 11 g fat
· 2 g saturated fat · 6 g carbohydrates · 1 g protein
· 2 g fiber

Grate **2 carrots** and **1 small cooked beet** into a large serving bowl. Make a dressing by mixing **3 tablespoons olive oil, ½ tablespoon white wine vinegar, ½ tablespoon balsamic vinegar, ½ teaspoon dijon mustard, a pinch of sugar** and a little salt and pepper. Add **3 tablespoons raisins, 2 tablespoons cashew nuts** and **4 tablespoons bottled French dressing** to the serving bowl. Finely chop **2 red apples**, leaving on the skins. Toss the apples with the salad, making sure that they are coated with the dressing to

prevent them from discoloring. Marinate the salad for 30 minutes before serving.

COOK'S TIP

● To cook a raw beet, place it in a fine-meshed sieve over a pan of boiling water and steam for 15 minutes, or until cooked but still firm. Drain and run it under cold water, then peel off the skin. Let cool before grating. Don't overcook the beet because it will not grate easily if soft, and the crunchy texture of the salad will be lost.

FIG, APPLE, AND CINNAMON COMPOTE

Serves 4
Preparation 5 minutes Cooking 22 minutes

Each serving provides · 143 calories · 6 g fat
· 0 g saturated fat · 22 g carbohydrates · 2 g protein
· 4 g fiber

Slice **2 eating apples** (such as McIntosh or Red Delicious) and **1 baking apple** (such as Granny Smith). Put them in a saucepan with ½ **cup orange juice, 4 chopped dried figs** and **1 level teaspoon ground cinnamon**. Bring to a boil, then reduce the heat and simmer, uncovered, for 20 minutes, or until the apples are tender when gently pressed with the back of a spoon. Sprinkle with **2 tablespoons toasted pine nuts** before dividing among four bowls to serve.

COOK'S TIPS

● Cinnamon is a sweet spice and using it in this fruity dish means that there is no need for added sweeteners, such as sugar. You can also add half a cinnamon stick to the compote instead of ground cinnamon, but remember to remove it before serving.

● Vanilla or butterscotch ice cream, or a spoonful of crème fraîche, would taste great with this compote.

LIGHTLY SPICED **VEGETABLE** MEDLEY

This creative combination of flavors will brighten a simple fish, meat, or poultry dish. The warm and aromatic cardamom seeds add a delicate hint of spice to the tender vegetables.

Serves 4
Preparation 20 minutes
Cooking 25 minutes

1 onion
2 celery stalks
1 large carrot
1 eggplant
1 pound potatoes
1 cup cauliflower florets
10 green cardamom pods
2 tablespoons olive oil or canola oil
4 cloves garlic, crushed
2 tablespoons ground coriander
8 ounces spinach
2 tablespoons chopped fresh cilantro
finely grated zest of 1 lemon
1⅓ cups plain yogurt

Each serving provides
• 286 calories • 13 g fat • 3 g saturated fat • 36 g carbohydrates
• 13 g protein • 7 g fiber

ALTERNATIVE INGREDIENTS
• Try sweet potatoes instead of regular potatoes.
• Leave out the eggplant and add 2 chopped parsnips together with the cauliflower.
• For a different take on spiced vegetables, add 1 finely chopped fresh green chile to the onion mixture in step 2, add a 14½-ounce can of chopped tomatoes in step 3, and reduce the water to ¼ cup.

1 Thinly slice the onion and celery. Halve and slice the carrot. Chop the eggplant into small chunks. Dice the potatoes. Break any large cauliflower florets in half or into quarters. Scrape out the seeds from the cardamom pods.

2 Heat the oil in a large pan over a medium-high heat. Add the onion, celery, carrot, garlic, and cardamom seeds. Stir, cover, and cook for 3 minutes. Stir in the eggplant and add the ground coriander without stirring. Cover and cook for another 3 minutes.

3 Add the potatoes. Stir in 1 cup of boiling water, cover, and return to a boil. Reduce the heat so that the mixture simmers steadily, then cook for 10 minutes. Stir in the cauliflower and cook for another 8 minutes, or until all the vegetables are tender.

4 Shred the spinach and stir it thoroughly into the vegetable mixture. Cook, stirring, for 1 minute, or until the spinach has wilted. Stir in the fresh cilantro and lemon zest. Divide the vegetables among four plates or bowls and serve with the yogurt.

COOK'S TIP
● To remove the small seeds from cardamom pods, slit the papery pods with the point of a knife and scrape out the small black or beige seeds with the blade.

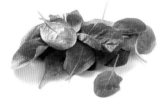

SUPER FOOD

SPINACH
A superstar among green vegetables, spinach is bursting with the colorful carotenoids lutein, zeaxanthin, and beta-carotene. These natural chemicals are great for eye health and cancer protection. Rich in folate, spinach is also good for the heart.

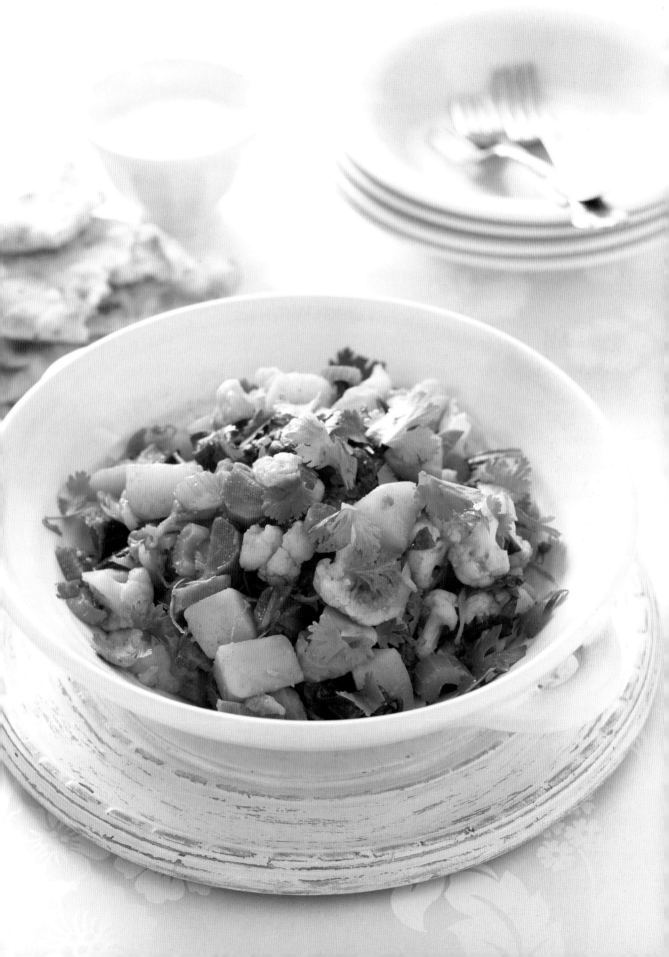

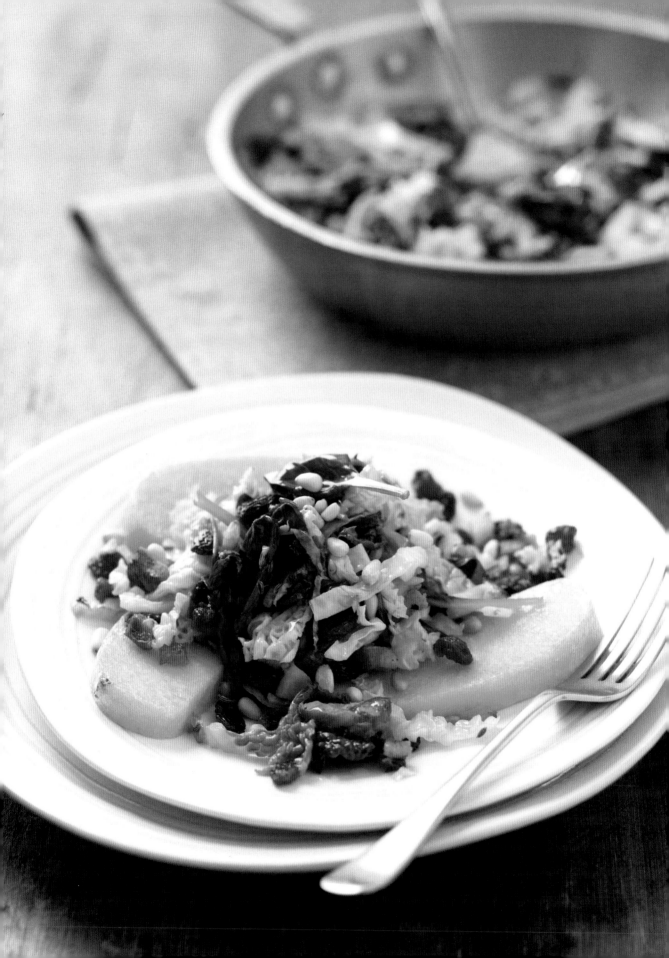

WILTED **GREENS**, CRISP **BACON,** AND **PINE NUTS** ON **POLENTA CAKES**

Savor tender, iron-rich spinach and cabbage with crisp bacon on a bed of baked polenta cakes. Garlic, fennel seeds, golden raisins, and pine nuts provide color and texture.

Serves 4
Preparation 10 minutes
Cooking 15 minutes

¼ **pound smoked bacon or pancetta**
1½ **cups finely shredded cabbage**
3 **tablespoons olive oil**
2 **cloves garlic, crushed**
1 **teaspoon fennel seeds**
¼ **cup golden raisins**
⅓ **cup pine nuts**
8 **ounces baby spinach**
16 **ounces ready-made polenta**
  (see Cook's Tip)

Each serving provides
• 403 calories • 26 g fat • 4 g saturated fat • 32 g carbohydrates • 1 g protein • 4 g fiber

ALTERNATIVE INGREDIENTS
• Cavolo nero, a dark-leafed Italian cabbage, is ideal in this recipe, but any green cabbage, such as savoy, works well.

1 Preheat the broiler to high and cover the broiler pan with foil. Dice the bacon. Heat 2 tablespoons of the oil in a large frying pan over high heat. Add the smoked bacon or pancetta to the pan with the garlic and fennel seeds. Reduce heat to medium and cook for 3 minutes, or until the bacon begins to crisp.

2 Add the raisins, pine nuts, and cabbage to the frying pan. Mix well, cover, and cook for 3 minutes, or until the cabbage has softened slightly. Stir in the spinach. Cover and cook for another 2 minutes, or until the spinach has wilted and the cabbage is tender.

3 Meanwhile, cut the polenta into ½-inch slices and arrange them on the broiler pan. Brush with ½ tablespoon of the remaining oil and broil for 5 minutes, or until golden. Turn over, brush with the rest of the oil and broil for another 5 minutes. Allowing 2–3 slices of polenta cake per portion, spoon the cabbage and spinach mixture on top.

COOK'S TIP
● To make your own polenta, add 6 cups of water to a saucepan and bring to a boil. Gradually stir in 1½ cups coarsely ground corn meal. Return to a boil, reduce the heat, and simmer for 35–40 minutes, stirring continuously, until the polenta is thick and smooth. Brush a baking sheet with olive oil and evenly spread the polenta onto it with a spatula and let it cool. Use a sharp, wet knife to cut the polenta as needed.

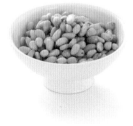

SUPER FOOD

PINE NUTS
Like most nuts, pine nuts are a good source of both polyunsaturated and monounsaturated fats, which help to lower harmful cholesterol in the blood. Pine nuts also contain vitamin E and folate, which help to protect the heart.

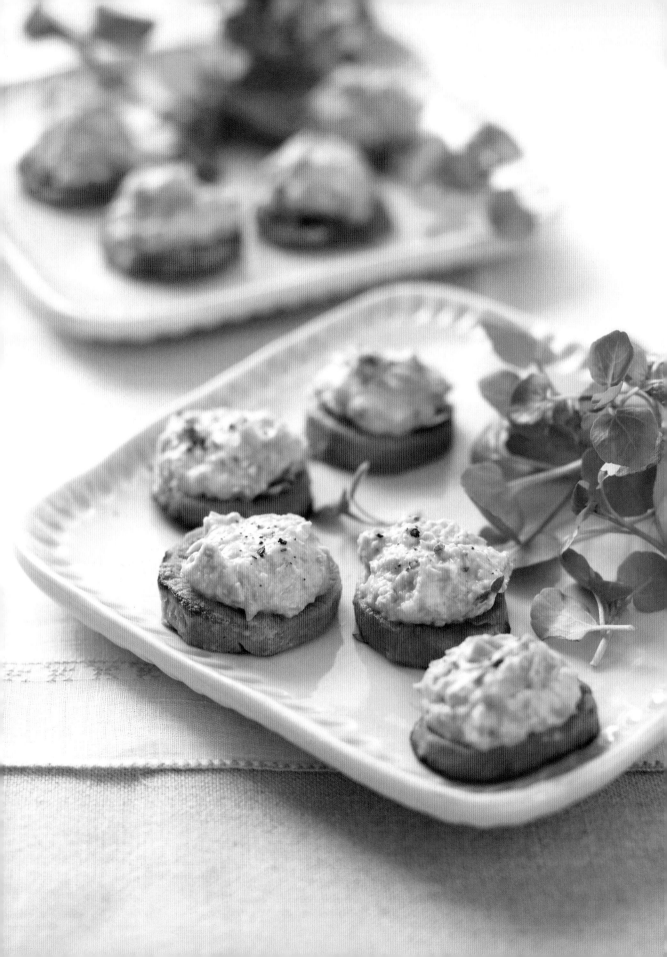

SWEET POTATO MEDALLIONS WITH MINTED PEA PURÉE

Colorful baby peas puréed with mint make a creamy topping for roasted sweet potato slices. Brimming with carotenoids and other antioxidants, this lovely dish is a powerhouse of goodness.

Serves 4
Preparation 10 minutes
Cooking 32 minutes

2 tablespoons olive oil or canola oil
1 large sweet potato
1 cup frozen baby peas
⅓ cup low-fat ricotta or low-fat cream cheese
8 large shredded fresh mint leaves
2 tablespoons snipped fresh chives
4 sprigs of fresh marjoram

Each serving provides
- 211 calories • 12 g fat • 3 g saturated fat • 17 g carbohydrates
- 8 g protein • 2 g fiber

ALTERNATIVE INGREDIENTS
- Use ordinary potatoes instead of sweet potatoes.
- Try slices of celeriac instead of sweet potato. Omit the mint from the pea purée.
- For a tasty lunch dish, top the potatoes with sliced mozzarella or thin slices of goat's cheese for the final 3 minutes of cooking. Add the pea purée and heat for 1–2 minutes.

1 Preheat oven to 400°F. Brush a baking sheet with a little of the oil or line it with parchment paper. Peel the potato, cut it into slices ½-inch thick, and place them on the baking sheet. Carefully brush the potato slices with oil, season to taste, and bake for 30 minutes, or until beginning to brown.

2 Meanwhile, put the baby peas in a saucepan. Add boiling water, return to a boil, cover, and cook for 2 minutes. Drain and purée in a blender or food processor. Mix the peas with the ricotta or cream cheese, mint, and chives. Season to taste.

3 Remove the roasted potato medallions from the oven. Strip the leaves from the marjoram, sprinkle on the potatoes, and top with the pea purée. Warm through in the oven for 2 minutes, then add freshly ground black pepper to each medallion before serving.

COOK'S TIPS
- Baby peas are better than regular peas for this recipe because they have tender skins. Standard frozen peas or mature fresh peas won't produce a fine purée.
- If you don't have a blender or food processor, you can mash the baby peas with a potato masher.

SUPER FOOD

SWEET POTATOES
Antioxidant carotenes give nutrient-packed sweet potatoes their orange color. The potatoes also contain vitamin E, which helps to protect against heart disease, and are a good source of fiber, especially if you eat the skins.

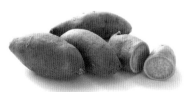

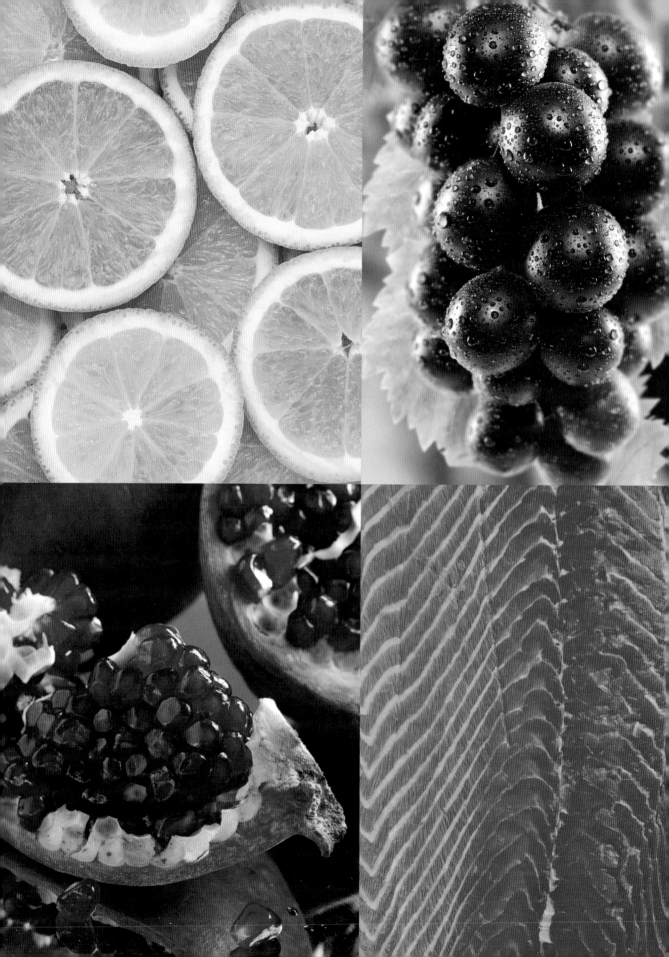

FISH
and
SEAFOOD

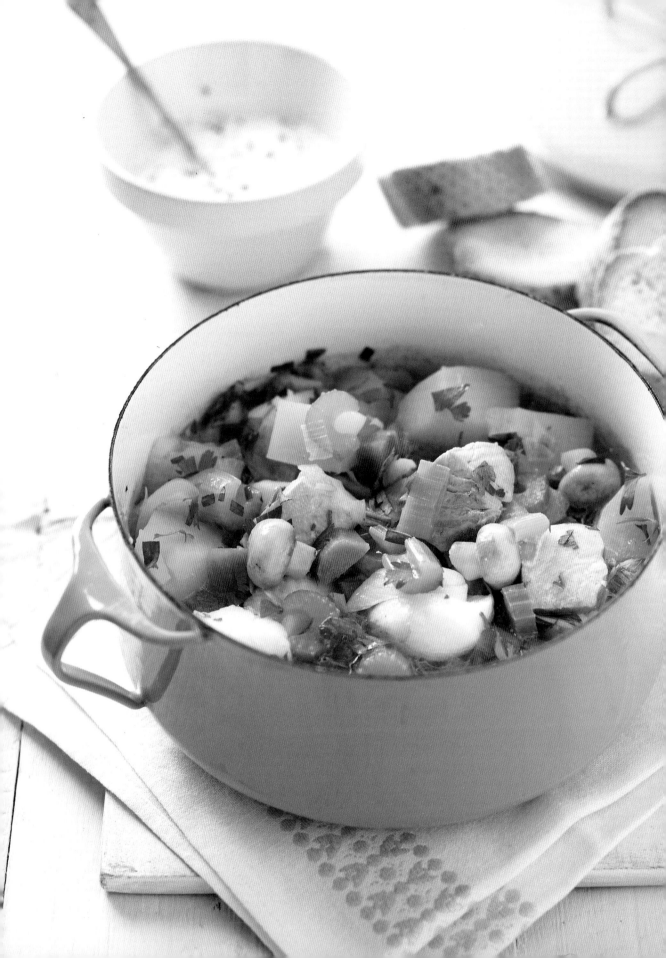

ONE-POT **FISH** CASSEROLE WITH SPICY **YOGURT**

This chunky vegetable-laden fish casserole has toasty croutons served with a piquant yogurt topping to give a tangy crunch to every scrumptious mouthful.

Serves 4
Preparation 15 minutes
Cooking 20 minutes

1 leek
2 celery stalks
1 carrot
1½ pounds potatoes
2 tablespoons olive oil
½ cup button mushrooms
2½ cups hot fish stock
½ pound skinless white fish fillet
½ pound skinless salmon fillet
1 tablespoon chopped fresh tarragon
2 tablespoons chopped fresh parsley

Spicy yogurt
¼ cup mayonnaise
¼ cup plain yogurt
1 clove garlic, crushed
½ teaspoon paprika
pinch of chili powder
1 baguette

Each serving provides
• 565 calories • 24 g fat • 4 g saturated fat • 26 g carbohydrates
• 34 g protein • 6 g fiber

ALTERNATIVE INGREDIENTS
• Make this casserole with mixed fresh or frozen seafood instead of, or in addition to, the fish.
• Try fresh sardine or mackerel fillets instead of the salmon.

1 Preheat the broiler to high. Slice and rinse the leek. Slice the celery, dice the carrot, and cut the potatoes into 1½-inch chunks. Heat the oil in a large saucepan over high heat. Add the leek, celery, and carrot, reduce heat to medium, cover, and cook for 3 minutes.

2 Add the potatoes and mushrooms to the pan and stir in the hot stock. Return to a boil, cover, and simmer for 10 minutes, or until the potatoes are tender. Cut the white fish and salmon into 1-inch pieces and stir them into the casserole. Return to a simmer, cover, and cook for another 5 minutes, or until the fish is cooked.

3 Meanwhile, mix the mayonnaise, yogurt, garlic, paprika, and chili powder. Slice the baguette and broil both sides for 2–3 minutes, or until golden. Stir the tarragon and parsley into the casserole just before transferring it to four large bowls. Serve with the spicy yogurt and toasted baguette slices.

COOK'S TIP
● Select boiling potatoes rather than baking potatoes, as the pieces will hold their shape rather than breaking down.

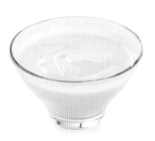

SUPER FOOD

YOGURT
With an ideal combination of protein and carbohydrate, low-fat yogurt can help fight fatigue and keep hunger at bay—good news for weight control. Yogurt is also an excellent source of calcium—important to help prevent osteoporosis. A one-cup serving provides about a third of your daily calcium needs.

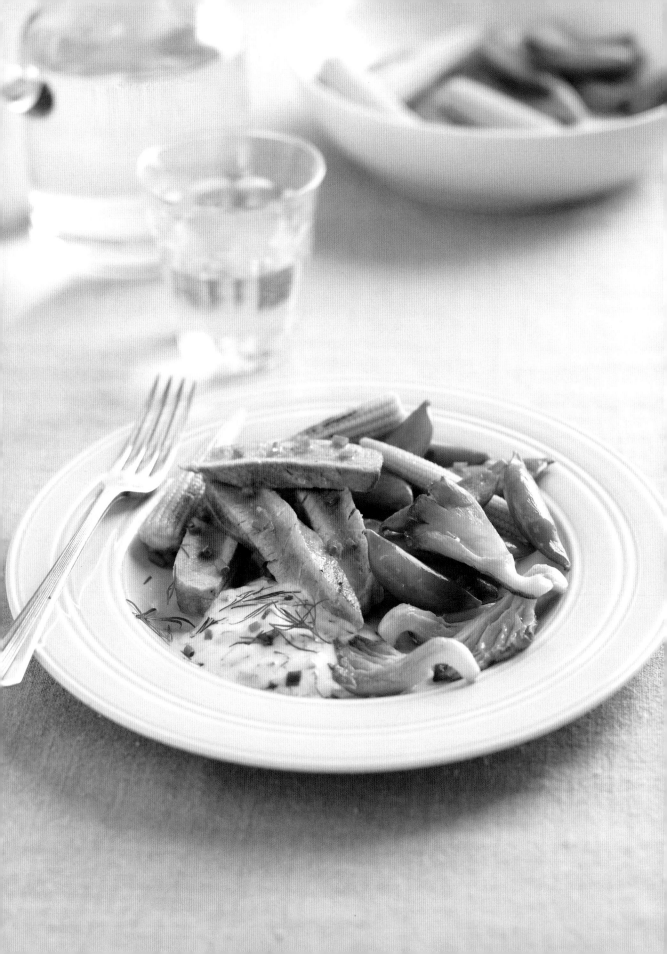

SEARED **TUNA STEAKS** IN A WARM **HERB** DRESSING

A punchy dill and horseradish sauce adds bite to this delicate combination of fresh vegetables and lightly seared tuna. It's a great way to raise your energy levels and safeguard your heart.

Serves 4
Preparation 10 minutes
Cooking 8 minutes

⅔ cup sliced oyster mushrooms
1 cup baby corn
1 cup sugarsnap peas
2 tablespoons olive oil or canola oil
4 fresh tuna steaks, about
   1¼ pounds total
2 tablespoons horseradish sauce
⅓ cup low-fat plain yogurt
4 tablespoons snipped fresh chives
2 tablespoons chopped fresh dill

Each serving provides
• 362 calories • 19 g fat • 5 g saturated fat • 5 g carbohydrates • 42 g protein • 3 g fiber

ALTERNATIVE INGREDIENTS
• Try enoki or other mushrooms instead of oyster, cooking them over high heat for 1 minute until softened.
• Fresh sardine or mackerel fillets work well as an alternative to tuna when flash-fried. Use 4 sardine or mackerel fillets and cook them skin side up for 1 minute, turn them over, and cook for another 2 minutes, or until the skin is crisp.

1 Put the baby corn in a saucepan and cover with boiling water. Return to a boil over high heat, cover, and cook for 1 minute. Add the sugarsnap peas, cover, return to a boil, then drain immediately.

2 Heat a large frying pan and swirl 1 tablespoon of the oil around the pan. Add the tuna steaks and cook over high heat for 2 minutes on each side, or until just firm and browned. The fish should feel slightly springy, not hard, and still be pink in the middle. Transfer the tuna to a dish, cover, and keep warm.

3 Add the remaining tablespoon of oil to the frying pan and sauté the corn and sugarsnap peas for 1 minute. Divide the vegetables among four warmed plates. Add the mushrooms to the pan and cook over high heat for 30 seconds. Transfer to the plates.

4 Add the horseradish, yogurt, chives, and dill to the pan. Stir to combine then immediately remove from the heat. Slice the tuna steaks and put them on the plates. Add a spoonful of sauce and serve.

COOK'S TIP
● Tuna is an oily fish that quickly goes past its prime. When buying tuna, choose steaks that have been neatly trimmed, with firm, dense red flesh. Avoid steaks with a strong smell or ones that are dull brown.

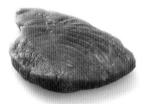

SUPER FOOD

TUNA
Fresh tuna is packed with essential omega-3 oils. Proven to help to protect against heart disease, these oils are also good for joint and brain health. Tuna contains iodine, needed for a healthy metabolism, plus vitamins D and B_{12} to help to fight fatigue.

TROUT WITH ALMONDS AND PEPPERS

Savor these succulent broiled trout fillets, combined with vitamin-packed sweet bell peppers and toasted almonds, and enjoy the anti-aging benefits of this dish. Serve with a green salad.

Serves 4
Preparation 5 minutes
Cooking 6 minutes

1½ tablespoons olive oil or canola oil
4 trout fillets, about 1½ pounds total
2 large bell peppers (1 red, 1 yellow)
¼ cup sliced almonds
4 lemon wedges, to garnish

Each serving provides
• 369 calories • 22 g fat • 3 g saturated fat • 6 g carbohydrates • 38 g protein • 4 g fiber

ALTERNATIVE INGREDIENTS
• Add a chopped mild or medium-hot fresh green chile to the sweet bell peppers and garnish the dish with lime instead of lemon.
• Green bell peppers work just as well as yellow bell peppers. Sprinkle with plenty of chopped fresh parsley before serving.
• Fresh sardine or mackerel fillets are a good alternative to the trout.

1 Preheat the broiler to high. Line a broiler pan with a layer of foil and brush with a little of the oil. Lay the trout fillets in the middle of the pan, skin side down. Cut the peppers into ½-inch slices and arrange them around the edges of the fish.

2 Brush the trout and peppers with a little more oil and then broil for 2–3 minutes, or until the fish is firm and opaque. Turn the fillets over and brush the skin with the remaining oil. Broil for another 2 minutes, or until the skin is bubbling and beginning to crisp.

3 Sprinkle the almonds over the fish and broil for 30–60 seconds until browned. Transfer to plates and serve the fish skin side up, so the skin can be eaten or discarded, and garnish with lemon wedges.

COOK'S TIP
● Watch the almonds closely as they cook—they brown quickly and will taste bitter if they burn. Remove the fish from under the broiler as soon as the almonds are golden.

SUPER FOOD

TROUT
The freshwater trout is a good source of high-quality protein and vitamins A and D. As with other oil-rich fish, it is an excellent source of omega-3s, which help to lower the risk of heart disease and stroke. These oils can also help to alleviate symptoms of rheumatoid arthritis and help to maintain mental alertness.

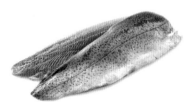

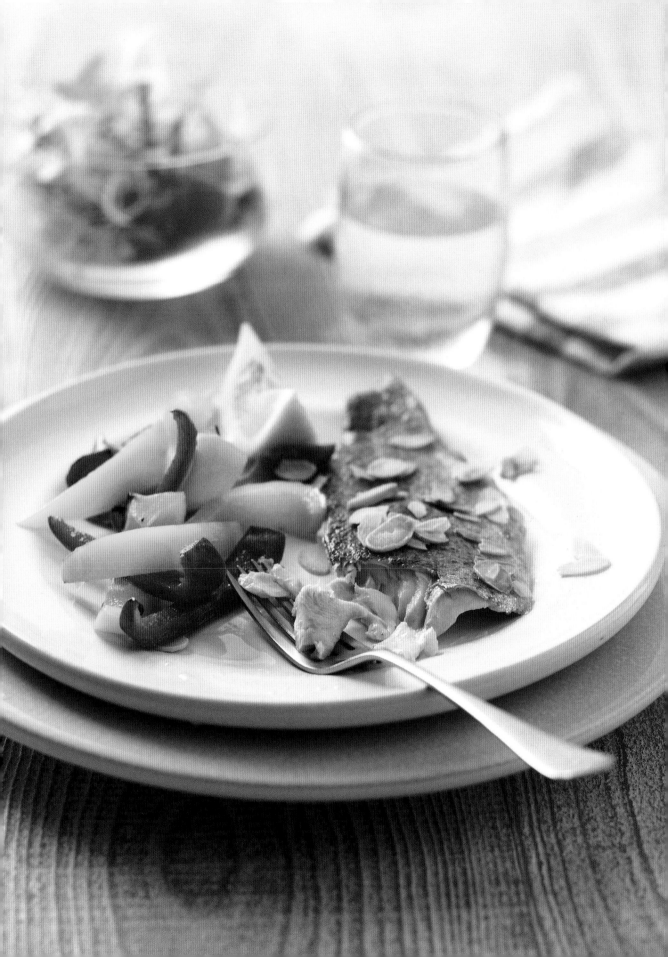

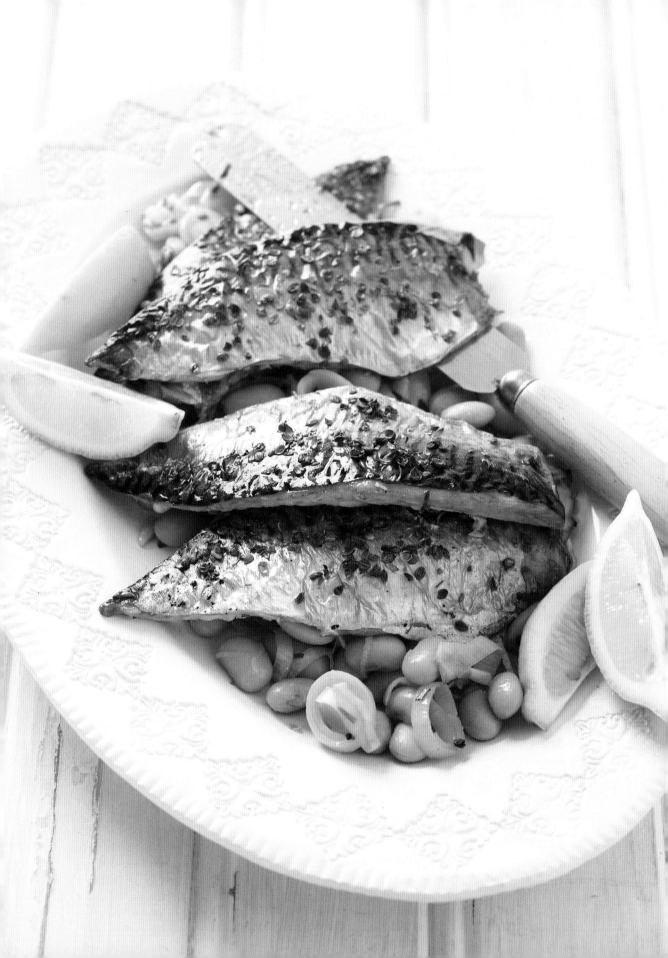

CRISP CORIANDER **FISH**
WITH ZESTY **BEANS**

Lemon and rosemary transform a dish of creamy butter beans into the perfect foil for robustly flavored broiled fish. Ready in under half an hour, this brain-power booster is the smart choice for a quick, tasty meal.

Serves 4
Preparation 10 minutes
Cooking 10 minutes

1 leek
1 tablespoon olive oil
2 sprigs rosemary, finely chopped
1 can (14 ounces) butter beans, drained
finely grated zest of 1 lemon
4 large or 8 small sardine or mackerel fillets, 1 pound total (see Cook's Tips)
1 tablespoon olive oil or canola oil
1 tablespoon crushed coriander seeds (see Cook's Tips)
8 lemon wedges, to garnish

Each serving provides
• 394 calories • 25 g fat • 5 g saturated fat• 15 g carbohydrates • 29 g protein • 5 g fiber

ALTERNATIVE INGREDIENTS
• Butter beans are mature lima beans as opposed to the more familiar immature fresh green lima beans. Other white beans, such as cannellini beans, would make an excellent substitute for butter beans.
• To serve the bean and leek mixture as a base for broiled sausages, steaks, or burgers, use canned mixed beans instead of butter beans.

1 Preheat the broiler to high and line the broiler pan with foil. Slice the leek. Heat the olive oil in a large frying pan over high heat. Add the rosemary and leek to the pan, reduce the heat, and cook for 5 minutes, or until the leek is tender. Stir in the butter beans and lemon zest. Set aside and keep warm.

2 Place the fish fillets, skin side down, on the broiler pan then brush each one with a little olive oil or canola oil. Sprinkle with half the crushed coriander seeds and broil for 2 minutes, or until just firm.

3 Turn the fish over and brush the skin with the rest of the oil. Broil for 1 minute and sprinkle with the remaining coriander seeds. Cook for another 2 minutes to crisp the skin.

4 Transfer the butter bean and leek mixture to a serving plate. Top with the fish fillets and pour the juices from the foil over the fish. Garnish with lemon wedges and serve.

COOK'S TIPS
● Use a mortar and pestle to crush the coriander seeds. To prevent the seeds from escaping, put the mortar in a plastic bag, gather the edges around the pestle, and pound the seeds. If you don't have a mortar and pestle, put the coriander seeds in a bowl and crush them with the end of a rolling pin.
● Buy gutted and cleaned fish and open them flat for broiling.

SUPER FOOD

OILY FISH
The omega-3s found in oil-rich fish such as sardines, mackerel, and anchovies have many health benefits beyond keeping the heart healthy. Evidence is emerging about their role in maintaining mental alertness and helping to prevent the onset of dementia.

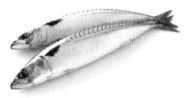

PAN-FRIED **SALMON** ON A BED OF BABY **SPINACH**

The heat from the cooked salmon is all that it takes to wilt fresh spinach leaves and enhance their flavor. Serve with tagliatelle pasta for a warm, vitamin-rich, multi-textured salad.

Serves 4
Preparation 10 minutes
Cooking 5 minutes

10 ounces tagliatelle pasta
1 pound skinless salmon fillet
¼ cup green pimento-stuffed olives
2 scallions
1 cup cherry tomatoes
4 ounces baby spinach
20 fresh basil leaves
2 tablespoons olive oil
grated zest and juice of 1 lemon

Each serving provides
• 532 calories • 20 g fat • 3 g saturated fat • 54 g carbohydrates • 34 g protein • 5 g fiber

ALTERNATIVE INGREDIENTS
• Use mixed greens instead of spinach. Try arugula, lamb's lettuce (mâche), mizuna, or watercress.
• Use scallops and pancetta instead of the salmon. Dry-fry ¼ pound diced smoked bacon or pancetta before adding the oil and cook ⅔ pound bay scallops for just until opaque.
• Cook 1 pound of squid rings instead of salmon. You can buy squid from the fish counter and ask to have it sliced into rings. Cook as for the salmon in step 2.

1 Cook the tagliatelle in a large saucepan of salted boiling water until tender but still firm to the bite.

2 Meanwhile, cut the salmon fillet into 1½-inch square chunks. Slice the stuffed olives in half, finely chop the scallions, and cut the cherry tomatoes in half. Divide the spinach among four plates and top each portion with 5 basil leaves.

3 Heat the oil in a large frying pan over high heat. Add the salmon chunks and cook for 4 minutes, turning occasionally, until they are opaque but soft. Add the olives, lemon zest and juice, and scallions to the pan. Let bubble for a few seconds, then spoon the salmon and its juices over each portion of spinach and basil.

4 Add the tomatoes to the pan and stir for 30 seconds to warm through and stir to incorporate any browned bits from the bottom of the pan. Spoon the tomatoes over the salmon and serve.

COOK'S TIP
● If baby spinach leaves are not available, choose small regular spinach leaves for maximum flavor. Avoid mature spinach leaves as these are too tough to eat raw in a salad.

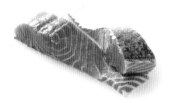

SUPER FOOD

SALMON
A rich source of protein, salmon is also high in vitamin A (great for healthy eyes and skin) and vitamin D (needed to make bones strong and guard against osteoporosis). Salmon is a beneficial source of selenium, too, which helps to boost the immune system and regulate the thyroid gland.

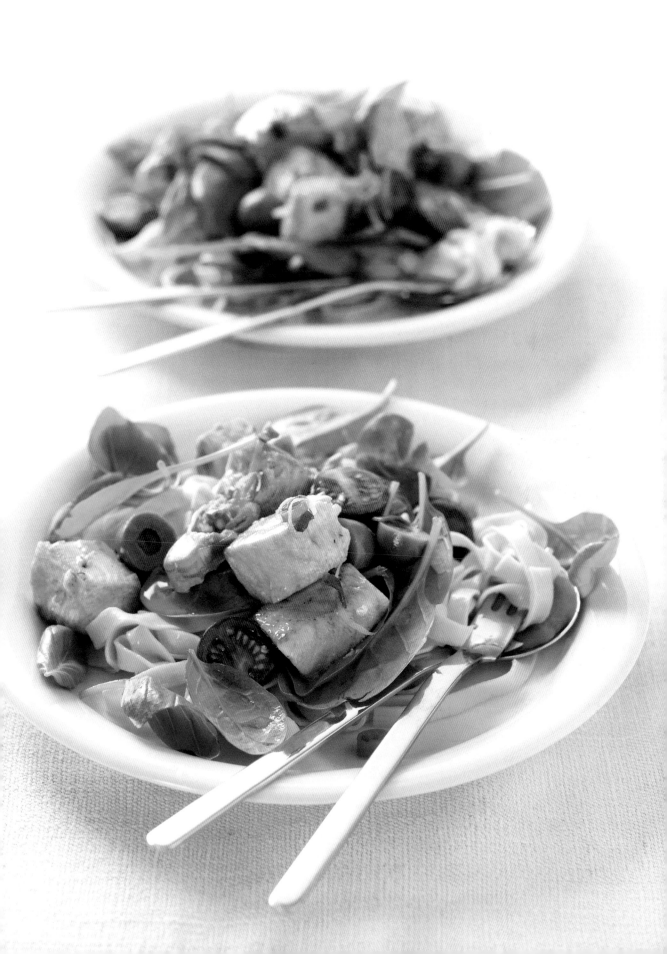

SALMON

Brimming with omega-3s, oils that are beneficial for your heart, brain, and joints, salmon is one of the healthiest fish you can buy. High in protein and an excellent source of heart-protective vitamin E, salmon is also one of the few dietary sources of vitamin D, a crucial nutrient for keeping your bones strong.

SALMON NIÇOISE

Serves 4
Preparation 10 minutes Cooking 6 minutes

Each serving provides • 326 calories • 21 g fat
• 4 g saturated fat • 6 g carbohydrates • 28 g protein
• 2 g fiber

Cook **3 eggs** in a pan of boiling water for 6 minutes, or until hard boiled. Meanwhile, steam **1 pound skinless salmon** and **⅓ cup green beans** for 5 minutes, or until the salmon is just cooked but still moist and the green beans are tender. Let cool. Drain the eggs, remove the shells and cut into quarters. Cut **8 pitted black olives** in half and halve **4 drained anchovy fillets**. Wash the outer leaves from a **head of romaine** and place them in a large salad bowl. Cut the romaine heart into 8 segments and add to the bowl. Add **3 roughly chopped tomatoes, 6 finely chopped scallions** and the green beans. Make a vinaigrette dressing by mixing **4 tablespoons virgin olive oil, 1 tablespoon red wine vinegar, ½ teaspoon dijon mustard, ½ teaspoon superfine sugar** and **1 crushed clove garlic**. Season to taste and pour over the salad. Divide the salmon into 12 large pieces and place them on the salad. Add the olives and anchovy fillets. Arrange the eggs on top of the salad before serving.

COOK'S TIP

● If you don't have a steamer, microwave the salmon and beans in a microwave-proof dish with a tight-fitting lid. Add 2 tablespoons of water to the dish, cover, and cook on high for 3–4 minutes, or until the fish is opaque and the beans are cooked but still crunchy.

SALMON AND BROCCOLI RISOTTO

Serves 4
Preparation 10 minutes Cooking 35 minutes

Each serving provides • 566 calories • 25 g fat
• 5 g saturated fat • 64 g carbohydrates • 26 g protein
• 3 g fiber

Heat **3 tablespoons olive oil** in a large frying pan. Add **1 finely chopped onion** and fry over a medium-low heat for 5 minutes, or until softened. Add **3 crushed cloves garlic** and **1¼ cups risotto rice**. Stir for 1 minute and add **5 cups fish stock**, one cup at a time, stirring regularly and allowing each cup of stock to be absorbed by the rice before adding the next one. This will take about 25 minutes. Meanwhile, cut **⅔ pound skinless salmon fillet** into bite-sized pieces. Stir the salmon into the rice after 12 minutes of cooking time.

Continue cooking the risotto for 6 minutes, then stir in **1 cup broccoli florets**, cut in half if large. Cook for 5 minutes, or until the salmon and broccoli are cooked through and the rice is creamy but still firm to the bite in the center. Stir in **2 tablespoons grated parmesan** and transfer to four plates. Garnish with **1 tablespoon chopped fresh parsley** before serving.

COOK'S TIP
● For a change, replace the broccoli with cooked peas or asparagus tips.

CRUNCHY BAKED SALMON

Serves 4
Preparation 10 minutes Cooking 15 minutes

Each serving provides • 415 calories • 30 g fat
• 4 g saturated fat • 8 g carbohydrates • 28 g protein
• 1 g fiber

Preheat the oven to 350°F. Put **3 crushed cloves garlic, 2 tablespoons pine nuts** and the leaves from **4–5 sprigs fresh basil** in a bowl and crush them together to release the aroma of the basil. Stir in **3 tablespoons olive oil** and **¼ cup fresh breadcrumbs**. Season to taste. Place **4 salmon fillets, about ½ pound each**, skin side down, on a baking sheet. Cover each one with a quarter of the topping, spreading it evenly over the fish. Bake for 15 minutes, or until the fish is cooked through and the topping is slightly browned and crisp.

COOK'S TIP
● Serve with a mixed leaf and avocado salad, or cherry tomatoes on the vine, baked in the oven at the same time as the fish.

GINGER SALMON KEBABS

Serves 4
Preparation 10 minutes Marinating 30 minutes
Cooking 5 minutes

Each serving provides • 272 calories • 19 g fat
• 3 g saturated fat • 5 g carbohydrates • 21 g protein
• 2 g fiber

Preheat the broiler to high. Cut **1 pound skinless salmon fillets** into bite-sized cubes and put them in a shallow non-metallic dish. Cut **2 yellow bell peppers** into squares and add them to the dish. In a bowl, combine **2 tablespoons olive oil, 3 teaspoons finely grated fresh ginger, 2 crushed cloves garlic, 1 finely chopped green chile (optional)** and the **juice of ½**

lemon. Gradually spoon the marinade over the salmon and pepper, then turn to coat. Cover and marinate for 30 minutes. Thread the marinated salmon and pepper pieces alternately onto four skewers. Broil the kebabs for about 3 minutes, and then turn, brush with the remaining marinade and broil for another 2 minutes. Garnish with **2 tablespoons chopped fresh cilantro** and serve.

COOK'S TIP
● Make this dish as hot or mild as you prefer. Choose the chile according to its heat—mild, medium or very hot—or omit the chile altogether for a less spicy meal.

TROPICAL MANGO AND SALMON SALAD

Serves 4
Preparation 10 minutes Marinating 30 minutes
Cooking 5 minutes

Each serving provides • 271 calories • 12 g fat
• 2 g saturated fat • 20 g carbohydrates • 23 g protein
• 2 g fiber

Preheat the broiler to high. Place **1 pound skinless salmon fillets**, cut into 8 pieces, in a non-metallic dish. Make a marinade by combining **4 tablespoons light coconut milk, 2 teaspoons fish sauce, 1 finely chopped red chile** and **1 teaspoon ground coriander seeds**. Pour the marinade over the salmon and gently turn to coat. Cover and marinate for 30 minutes. Meanwhile, slice **½ cucumber** and **1 fresh ripe mango**. Arrange **mixed salad greens** on four plates and add the cucumber slices. In a bowl, make a dressing by mixing **4 tablespoons light coconut milk, 1 tablespoon fish sauce, juice of ½ lime, 1 crushed clove garlic, 1 teaspoon Thai chili sauce** and **½ teaspoon superfine sugar**. Remove the salmon from the marinade and broil for 5 minutes, or until cooked through in the center. Arrange salmon on the salads, drizzle with dressing, and garnish each plate with **2 fresh basil leaves**.

COOK'S TIP
● Marinate the salmon for up to an hour if you have time, but avoid leaving it any longer as the fish will begin to 'cook' in the marinade.

SALMON WITH POMEGRANATE GLAZE

Jewel-like pomegranate seeds add color and zing to salmon fillets soaked in a mouthwatering fruity marinade. A quick dish to prepare and one that is guaranteed to impress.

Serves 4
Preparation 10 minutes
Marinating 15 minutes
Cooking 12 minutes

⅓ cup pomegranate juice drink
2 tablespoons soy sauce
1 clove garlic, sliced
4 salmon fillets, about ⅓ pound each
2 tablespoons olive oil or canola oil
　seeds from ½ pomegranate
　(see Cook's Tips)

Each serving provides
• 354 calories • 24 g fat • 4 g saturated fat • 4 g carbohydrates
• 31 g protein • 0 g fiber

ALTERNATIVE INGREDIENTS
• Use tuna steaks instead of salmon, allowing about ¼ pound per portion.
• If you have a juicer, you can use it to make fresh pomegranate juice for the marinade. Juice the seeds from 1–2 fresh pomegranates to get about ⅓ cup of juice.

1 To make the marinade, pour the pomegranate juice drink and soy sauce into a large, shallow non-metallic dish. Stir the garlic into the juice. Add the salmon to the marinade and turn to coat. Cover and set aside to marinate for 15 minutes.

2 Preheat the broiler to high. Line the broiler pan with foil and brush with a little of the oil. Drain the salmon, place on the foil, skin side down, and brush with oil. Pour the marinade into a small saucepan over high heat and boil for 2–3 minutes, or until thick and syrupy.

3 Spoon a little of the reduced marinade over the salmon portions and broil for 3 minutes. Turn, baste with more marinade, and broil for another 4–6 minutes, basting again, until glazed and cooked through. Transfer the salmon to four plates, pour any glaze from the broiler pan over the fish, and sprinkle with pomegranate seeds before serving.

COOK'S TIPS
● To prepare a pomegranate, use a sharp knife to score the skin into quarters, top to bottom, without piercing deeply into the fruit. Hold the pomegranate over a large bowl and pull it apart. The membranes and seeds will separate into uneven sections. Remove the seeds from the sections with your fingers, taking care to remove all the membrane and any pith, which taste bitter.
● Serve the salmon with mixed salad greens divided among the portions.

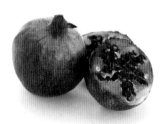

SUPER FOOD

POMEGRANATES
There is some evidence that links pomegranate juice with slowing down the effects of aging. The natural phytochemicals found in pomegranates may have anti-inflammatory properties that can help to relieve some of the symptoms of rheumatoid arthritis.

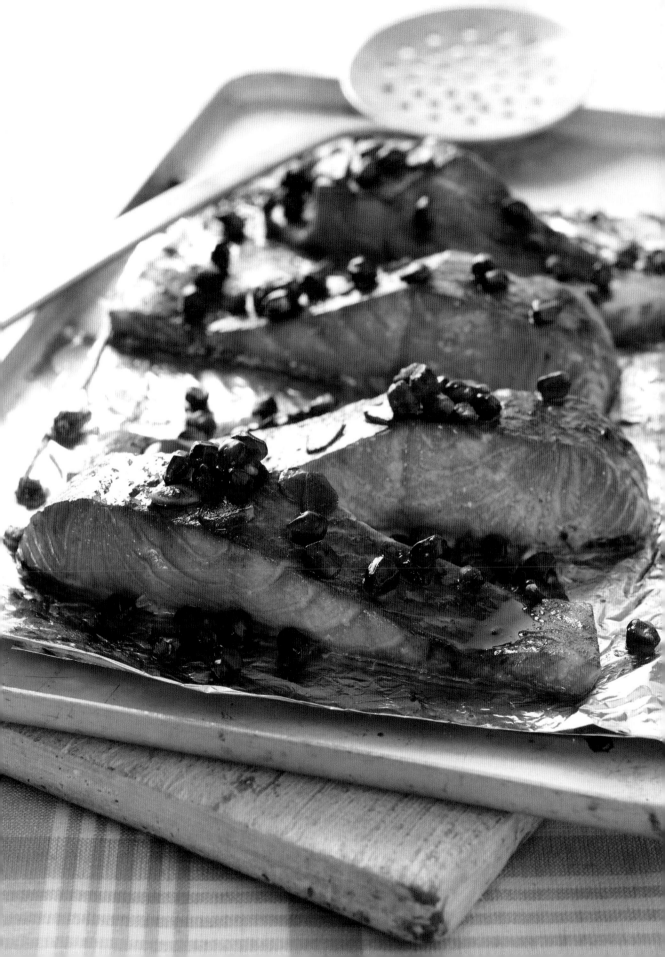

OAT-CRUSTED **FISH** WITH **AVOCADO** SALSA

Whole-grain rolled oats make a fiber-rich, crisp, golden coating for melt-in-the-mouth pan-fried fish. They're served with a tomato and avocado salsa for just the right amount of palate-cleansing bite.

Serves 4
Preparation 10 minutes
Cooking 12 minutes

1 large ripe tomato
1 small green bell pepper
1 scallion
1 clove garlic, crushed
dash of hot chili sauce
   such as Tabasco
1 ripe avocado
4 tablespoons low-fat (1%) milk
½ cup rolled oats
4 skinless white fish fillets,
   such as cod, snapper, or tilapia
2 tablespoons olive oil
lemon wedges, to garnish

Each serving provides
• 408 calories • 24 g fat • 5 g saturated fat • 12 g carbohydrates • 35 g protein • 3 g fiber

ALTERNATIVE INGREDIENTS
• Try thick pieces of flounder or sole fillets. Trout and sardines are also delicious served in this way.
• Use a pinch of dried chile flakes or a finely chopped fresh chile instead of hot chili sauce.
• For a Mediterranean flavor to the salsa, add 4–6 shredded basil leaves in step 1, plus the finely grated zest of 1 lime.

1 Dice the tomato and pepper and finely chop the scallion. Mix them with the garlic in a small bowl. Stir in the hot chili sauce. Dice the avocado and gently mix it with the other salsa ingredients.

2 Place the milk in a large shallow dish and spread half the oats on a large plate. Place the fish fillets in the milk and turn to coat them thoroughly. Transfer one fish fillet from the milk to the oats. Sprinkle 1 tablespoon of oats on top of the fillet and press them on gently to form a crust on both sides.

3 Heat a large frying pan over medium-high heat. Add 1 tablespoon oil then transfer the oat-coated fillet to the pan. Coat a second fillet and add it to the pan. Cook the fish for 3 minutes, or until the underside is crisp. Turn the fillets and cook the second side for another 3 minutes, or until crisp and golden.

4 Transfer the cooked fillets to a plate and keep them warm. Cook the remaining two fillets in the same way. Put the fish on four plates, add the salsa and garnish with lemon wedges.

COOK'S TIPS
● Use a large spatula and fork to turn the fillets. Be gentle but firm, sliding the spatula under each fillet in one movement to avoid breaking the fish.
● Rolled oats are the best variety for the oat coating because they are slightly flaky and broken, which helps them to adhere to the fish.

SUPER FOOD

OATS
With a low glycemic index (GI) value, oats provide sustained energy, helping to regulate blood glucose levels. Rolled oats and oatmeal are whole-grain foods that are packed with fiber for heart and digestive health. Oats are also plentiful in B vitamins, which are vital for maintaining a healthy metabolism.

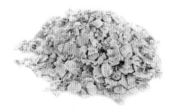

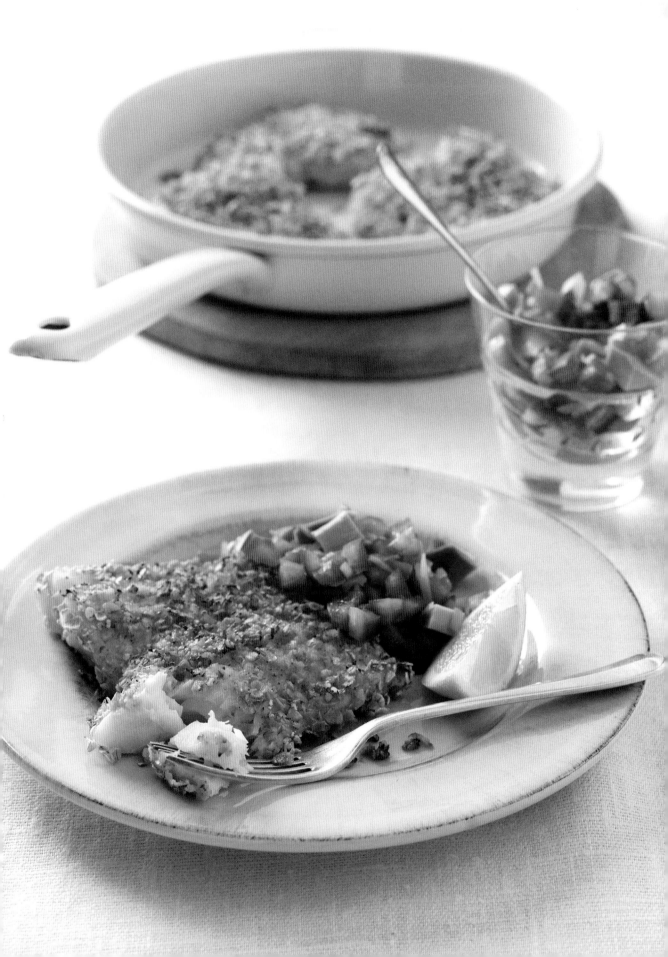

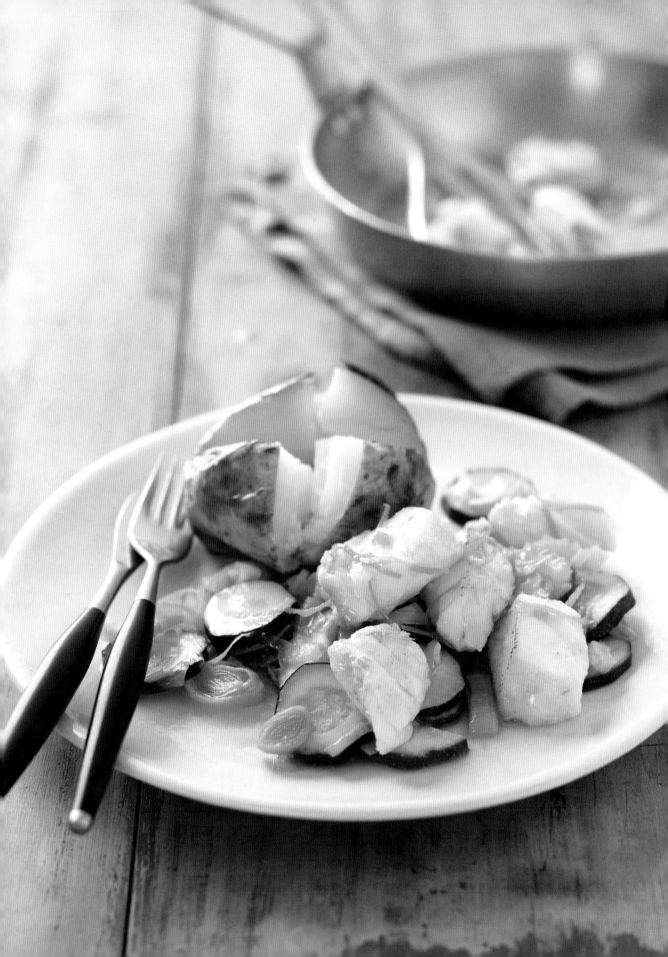

CITRUS **FISH** WITH SAUTÉED **LEEKS** AND **ZUCCHINI**

Spoon a piquant orange sauce over moist white fish resting on a bed of vegetables gently infused with garlic – and enjoy. Wholesome fish has never been more delectable.

Serves 4
Preparation 15 minutes
Cooking 15 minutes

2 leeks
2 celery stalks
4 zucchini
1 pound thick skinless white fish
    fillets, such as cod, snapper, or
    halibut
3 tablespoons olive oil
2 cloves garlic, sliced
finely pared zest and juice of
    1 orange

Each serving provides
• 242 calories • 13 g fat • 2 g
saturated fat • 7 g carbohydrates
• 24 g protein • 4 g fiber

ALTERNATIVE INGREDIENTS
• Use 1 cup mixed stir-fry vegetables
(fresh or frozen) instead of the
zucchini.
• Try salmon fillets with lemon zest
and juice instead of white fish with
orange zest and juice.
• Serve firm tofu instead of fish.
Cook 12 ounces plain or smoked tofu
in the same way as the fish in step 3.
Turn over once to brown both sides,
then slice the tofu and serve it with
the vegetables.

1 Thinly slice the leeks and rinse them in a colander. Slice the celery and zucchini. Cut the fish into 1½-inch chunks. Heat a large frying pan over a high heat and pour in 2 tablespoons oil. Add the leeks, celery, and garlic. Reduce heat to medium and cook, stirring, for 4 minutes, or until the leeks are softened.

2 Stir in the zucchini and cook for another 3 minutes, or until the zucchini begin to soften. Do not overcook as they will continue to soften when removed from the heat. Divide the vegetables among four warmed plates, set aside, and keep warm.

3 Heat the remaining tablespoon of oil in the frying pan over high heat. Add the fish and orange zest. Reduce the heat to medium and cook for 3 minutes. Add the orange juice and simmer for another 3 minutes, or until the chunks of fish are firm and opaque.

4 Use a slotted spoon to transfer the fish to the plates. Boil the pan juices over high heat for about 30 seconds, season to taste, and spoon them over the fish before serving.

COOK'S TIPS
● If you don't have a zester, peel the orange zest using a potato peeler, then cut the zest into fine strips using a small, sharp knife.
● To serve the dish with a baked potato, bake a russet or Yukon potato in the oven for 1 hour at 375°F.

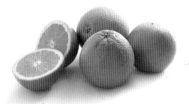

SUPER FOOD

ORANGES
Rich in vitamin C, oranges also contain more than 170 different beneficial plant compounds. The nutrients and natural chemicals in oranges are thought to help to boost the immune system, regulate blood pressure, and promote healthy skin.

HERB AND WALNUT CRUSTED FISH FILLETS

Chopped walnuts, herbs, and breadcrumbs make a satisfying topping for lightly baked fish. Serve with simple buttered vegetables—these elegant fillets should be the star of the show.

Serves 4
Preparation 10 minutes
Cooking 20 minutes

2 tablespoons olive oil, plus
    1 teaspoon for greasing
4 thick portions skinless white fish
    fillets, about ¼ pound each
¼ cup chopped walnuts
⅓ cup fresh whole-grain breadcrumbs
4 tablespoons chopped fresh parsley
2 tablespoons snipped fresh chives
4 lemon wedges, to garnish

Each serving provides
• 330 calories • 21 g fat • 3 g
saturated fat • 8 g carbohydrates
• 27 g protein • 2 g fiber

ALTERNATIVE INGREDIENTS
• Use swordfish or tuna steaks instead of white fish. Top each portion with 1–2 thick slices of tomato before adding the breadcrumb topping. Sprinkle a chopped garlic clove over the tomatoes for more flavor.
• Try cashew nuts instead of walnuts and 1 tablespoon chopped fresh tarragon instead of parsley.
• Add the grated zest of 1 lemon and a finely chopped fresh green chile to the breadcrumb mix for a citrus topping with a hint of heat.

1 Preheat the oven to 375°F. Grease a large ovenproof dish with oil and add the fish fillets.

2 Add the walnuts to a bowl with the breadcrumbs, parsley, and chives. Stir in 2 tablespoons oil, then scatter the breadcrumb topping over each portion of fish, gently pressing it down.

3 Bake in the oven for 20 minutes, or until the topping is browned and the fish is cooked through. Serve garnished with lemon wedges.

COOK'S TIPS
● If the fish fillets are thin, or have thin tail ends, fold them in half and tuck the tail ends underneath to make a thick, neat portion.
● To make ⅓ cup of fresh breadcrumbs, process 2 medium slices of whole-grain bread in a food processor or blender. Alternatively, use a chunk of stale bread and rub it against the coarse holes of a grater into a large bowl. Fresh breadcrumbs freeze well, so make a large batch if you want extra. The crumbs can be used frozen.

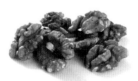

SUPER FOOD

WALNUTS
Nuts are high in fat, but most of this is the monounsaturated kind that helps to guard against heart disease and lowers blood cholesterol. Walnuts also contain health-promoting omega-3s, as well as copper and magnesium, to help to maintain strong bones and nerve and muscle function.

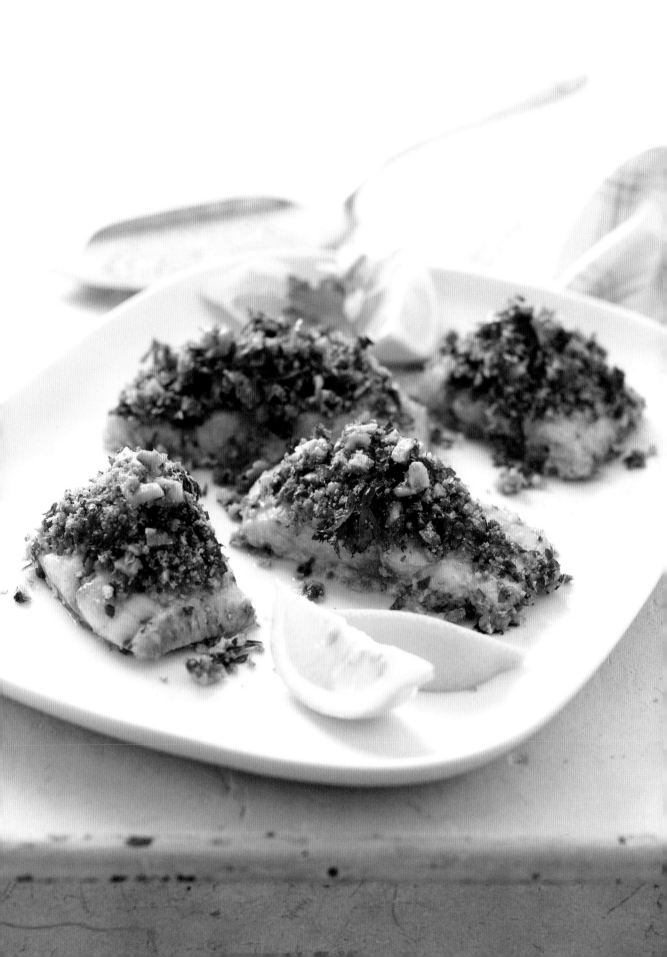

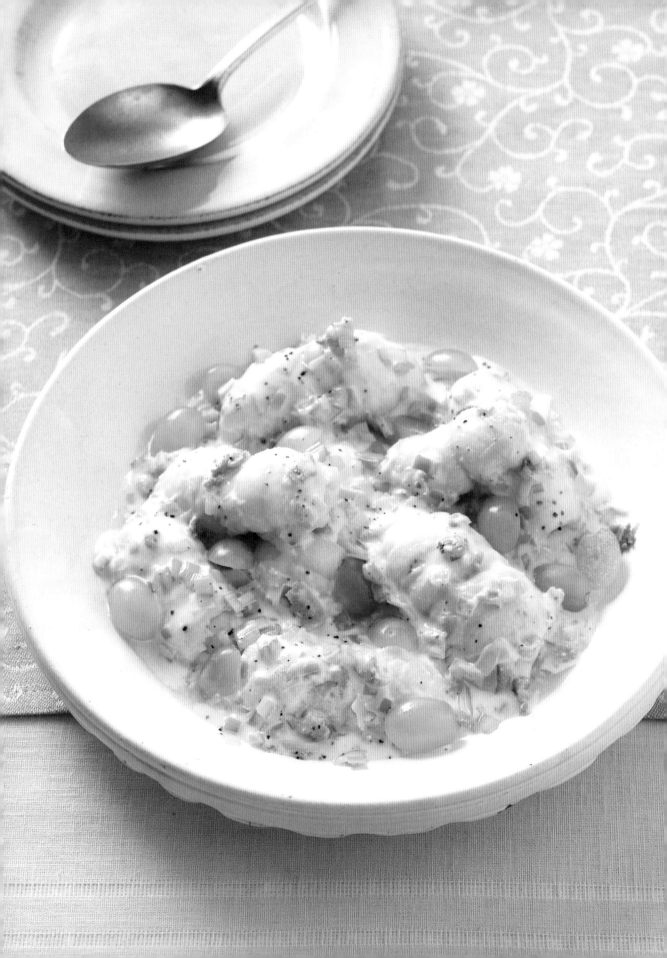

FISH WRAPS WITH GRAPES AND SAVORY WHITE SAUCE

Try this more substantial variation of the French classic, sole véronique. The generous sprinkling of green grapes melds perfectly with mild fish and a light, creamy sauce.

Serves 4
Preparation 10 minutes
Cooking 18 minutes

¼ cup diced lean bacon
1 celery stalk
1 small leek
1 tablespoon olive oil
1¾ cups dry white wine
8 skinless fish fillets such as sole or
    flounder, 1½ pounds total
    (see Cook's Tips)
2 teaspoons cornstarch
1 cup seedless green grapes
½ cup low-fat cream cheese or
    ½ cup grated low-fat cheddar

Each serving provides
• 306 calories • 8 g fat • 2 g
saturated fat • 12 g carbohydrates
• 31 g protein • 1 g fiber

ALTERNATIVE INGREDIENTS
• For a non-alcoholic meal, use
1¾ cups white grape juice instead
of wine.
• Make a fennel sauce to serve with
the fish. Trim and chop 1 small bulb
fennel and add it to the sauce instead
of the celery.
• Parsley, thyme, and lemon are a
good combination of ingredients for
flavoring white sauce. For a herb-
flavored fish recipe, add 2 fresh
thyme sprigs and the grated zest of
½ lemon with the wine in step 2. Add
2 tablespoons chopped fresh parsley
just before serving.

1 Dice the celery, and chop the leek. Heat the oil in a large frying pan over high heat. Add the bacon to the pan, reduce heat to medium and cook for 1 minute. Add the celery and leek and cook for 2 minutes, or until the leek has softened.

2 Pour the wine into the pan, turn up the heat, and return to a boil. Reduce heat to low, cover, and simmer for 3 minutes. Roll up the fish fillets, from head to tail end, and secure with wooden toothpicks.

3 Mix the cornstarch into a smooth paste with 1 tablespoon cold water, then stir this into the pan. Continue to stir the sauce until it begins to thicken. Add the fish rolls to the pan, return to a boil, reduce the heat, cover, and simmer for 10 minutes, or until the fish is cooked through. Stir once or twice during cooking.

4 Slice the grapes in half and place half of them on a serving plate. Add the fish rolls and remove the toothpicks. Whisk the cheese into the sauce and cook until just beginning to boil. Season to taste and spoon over the fish. Top with the remaining grape halves and a sprinkling of freshly ground black pepper before serving.

COOK'S TIPS
● Select a white wine for cooking that you would enjoy drinking with the meal, otherwise your sauce may taste acidic.
● Look for firm, creamy-colored fish fillets that are thin enough to be rolled. Avoid any that look old, gray, or discolored. Ask the fishmonger to skin the fish.

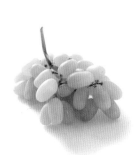

SUPER FOOD

GRAPES
The skins of grapes contain large quantities of flavonoids—the pigments that give grapes their color—and have beneficial antioxidant properties. Despite being higher in natural sugars than many other fruit, grapes have a low glycemic index (GI) which can help with appetite control.

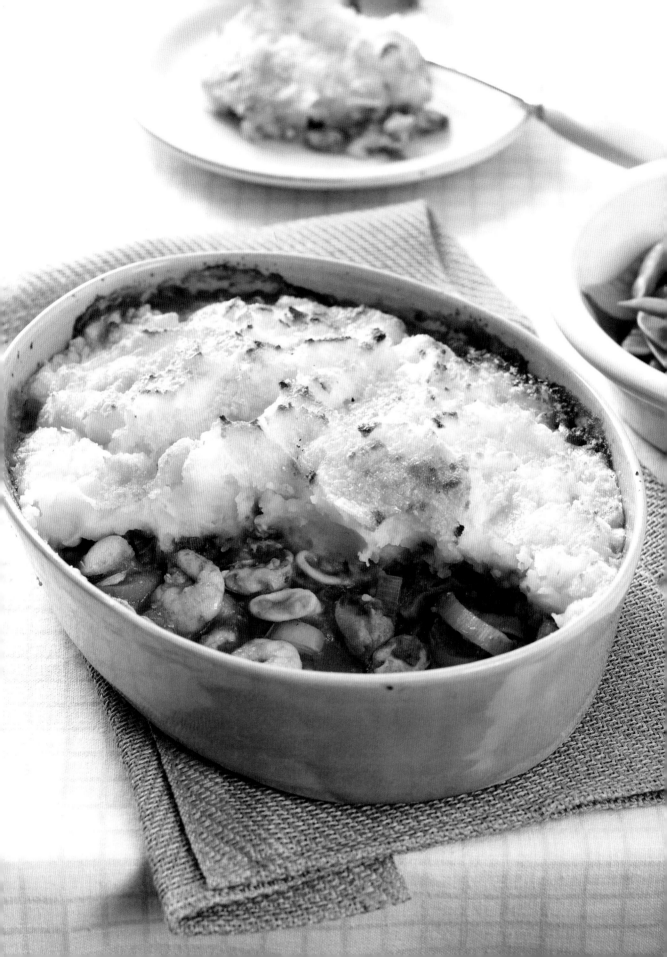

MEDITERRANEAN **SEAFOOD** PIE

For no-fuss healthy eating, it's hard to beat this luscious mix of shrimp, squid, and mussels. Here, oregano, tomatoes, and leeks combine temptingly with the seafood under a cheesy potato crust.

Serves 4
Preparation 10 minutes
Cooking 25 minutes

2 pounds potatoes
1 large leek
1 tablespoon olive oil
1 clove garlic, crushed
1 can (14½ ounces) chopped tomatoes
¼ teaspoon dried oregano
¾ pound frozen cooked mixed seafood, including mussels, shrimp, and squid
2 tablespoons grated parmesan

Each serving provides
• 378 calories • 8 g fat • 2 g saturated fat • 50 g carbohydrates • 29 g protein • 6 g fiber

ALTERNATIVE INGREDIENTS
• Add ¼ cup sliced pitted black olives to the seafood mixture and the grated zest of 1 lemon to the potatoes.
• For a 'meatier' dish, use ½ pound white fish, cut into chunks, and only half the seafood. Cook for 2–3 minutes at step 3 before adding the seafood.
• Mussels and boiled eggs are a good alternative to mixed seafood. Use ¾ pound cooked mussels and 4 hard-boiled eggs. Shell the eggs then cut into quarters. Arrange in the dish before pouring in the mussel mixture.

1 Peel the potatoes and cut into 1½–2-inch chunks. Transfer them to a large saucepan. Add boiling water, cover, and return them to a boil. Simmer for 10 minutes, or until they are tender.

2 Meanwhile, preheat the broiler to high. Slice the leek. Heat the oil in a saucepan and cook the leek and garlic over high heat for 2–3 minutes, stirring regularly, until the leek has softened. Stir in the tomatoes, rinsing out the can with 1 tablespoon of water. Add the oregano and return to a boil. Reduce the heat, cover, and simmer for 2 minutes.

3 Add the frozen cooked seafood to the pan with the tomatoes and return to a boil. Stir, cover, and simmer for another 2 minutes, or until the seafood is thoroughly heated through. Season to taste. Pour into a 6-cup or 10-inch ovenproof dish.

4 Drain the potatoes and mash them. Spoon the potatoes evenly over the seafood, using a fork to spread them up to the edge of the dish. Sprinkle with parmesan and broil for 12–13 minutes, or until the topping is golden.

COOK'S TIPS
● Cutting root vegetables into chunks and using boiling water from a kettle reduces cooking time and saves energy. Pour in just enough water to cover the vegetables and use a large pan that covers the heating element on your stove.
● The green parts of leeks add color, flavor, and nutritional value. Thinly slice the leek and separate into rings so that any grit can be washed away when rinsed in a colander under cold running water.
● Baking potatoes are ideal for this recipe as they tend to break down quickly when boiled, making them easy to mash.

SUPER FOOD

SEAFOOD
Low in fat, especially saturated fat, seafood is a good source of high-quality protein. It is also full of vital minerals and trace elements, including iron, zinc, and selenium, important for maintaining a healthy immune system.

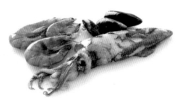

CHILE SHRIMP
AND PEA STIR-FRY

Rustle up a health-boosting meal in no time using shrimp and frozen peas, which are often higher in nutrients than some store-bought 'fresh' ones. Noodles make a satisfying accompaniment.

Serves 4
Preparation 10 minutes
Cooking 6 minutes

2 tablespoons finely grated
   fresh ginger
1 fresh red chile
⅔ pound white cabbage
1 tablespoon olive oil or canola oil
1 teaspoon sesame oil
1½ cups frozen peas
¾ pound peeled cooked large shrimp
4 tablespoons chopped fresh cilantro

Each serving provides
• 178 calories • 6 g fat • 1 g
saturated fat • 11 g carbohydrates
• 19 g protein • 6 g fiber

ALTERNATIVE INGREDIENTS
• If fresh shrimp are not available, use frozen ones instead. You can cook them frozen, adding them to the pan at the end of step 1, allowing an additional 1–2 minutes cooking time for them to thaw and heat through.
• Substitute fresh scallops for the shrimp. Use them whole if small or slice larger ones. Other cooked shellfish, such as baby clams or squid rings, work well in this dish.

1 Chop the chile into thin slivers (see Cook's Tips), discarding the seeds. Slice the cabbage into thin ⅛-inch-wide strips.

2 Heat the two oils in a large frying pan over a high heat. Stir-fry the ginger and chile for a few seconds, then add the peas and stir-fry for 2 minutes, or until they turn bright green and are completely thawed.

3 Add the cabbage to the pan. Stir-fry for another 3 minutes, then add the shrimp and cook for another minute to heat them through. Toss in the cilantro, stir, and serve immediately.

COOK'S TIPS
● Select chilies according to how hot you want the dish—their strength is usually stated on the package. Mild to medium are good with light ingredients. Remember that starchy accompaniments such as noodles or rice will 'absorb' the heat.
● When you are preparing chilies, be careful to avoid accidentally rubbing your eyes. Wash your hands immediately to remove the chile oils, or wear a pair of rubber gloves.
● Use the kind of frozen peas you prefer—baby peas are small and sweet, but this recipe also works well with ordinary green peas.

SUPER FOOD

PEAS
Frozen peas are frozen within hours of harvesting, locking in the nutrients, unlike some fresh peas that may have spent many days in transit. Peas are an excellent source of fiber, which promotes a healthy digestive system.

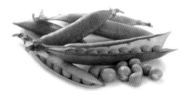

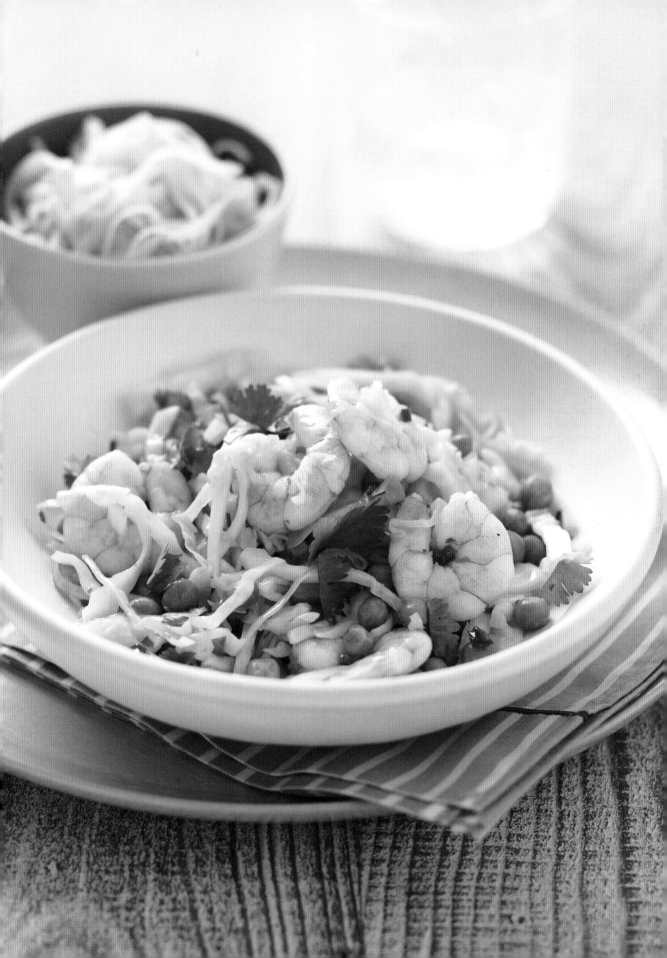

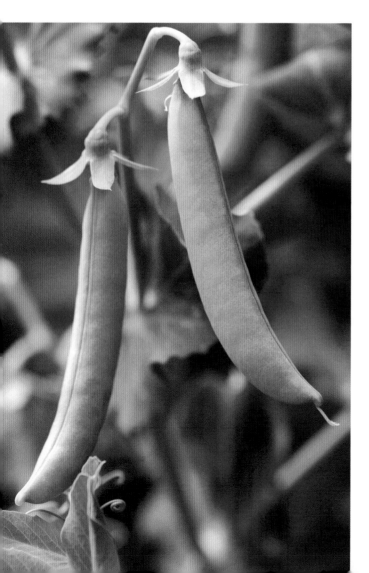

SUPER FOOD

PEAS

Rich in a range of vitamins and minerals, peas are an excellent source of vitamin C to boost the immune system, and potassium for healthy muscle and nerve function. Peas are also high in fiber, which is good for digestion and for the heart, and in lutein, a natural plant pigment that helps to protect eyesight.

FRENCH-STYLE PEAS

Serves 4
Preparation 10 minutes Cooking 25 minutes

Each serving provides • 168 calories • 7 g fat
• 2 g saturated fat • 19 g carbohydrates
• 10 g protein • 12 g fiber

Melt a **small pat of butter** in a saucepan over a medium heat with **1 tablespoon olive oil**. Add **16 small peeled shallots** and cook, stirring occasionally, for 5 minutes, or until lightly golden. Slice **a head of boston lettuce** into eight pieces and add to the pan with **2½ cups frozen peas, 1 cup hot vegetable stock** and **1 teaspoon superfine sugar**. Bring to a boil, cover and simmer over low heat for 20 minutes. Season to taste before serving.

COOK'S TIPS

● Use 2 sliced onions if you can't find shallots, and substitute fresh peas for frozen ones when in season. Note that shelling the fresh peas will increase your preparation time by 15 minutes.
● Chicken or lamb are ideal served with these peas.
● To add a minty twist, scatter a few fresh mint leaves, or spearmint if available, and a handful of chopped fresh chervil into the pan 5 minutes before the end of cooking. Remove the mint leaves before serving.

SPICY PUNJABI PEAS WITH LAMB

Serves 4
Preparation 10 minutes Cooking 30 minutes

Each serving provides • 352 calories • 20 g fat
• 6 g saturated fat • 15 g carbohydrates
• 29 g protein • 2 g fiber

Put **1 large chopped onion, a grated 1½-inch piece of fresh ginger, 2 finely chopped chilies** and **2 chopped cloves garlic** in a blender, or a bowl if you have a stick blender, and process to a coarse paste. Heat **2 tablespoons olive oil or canola oil** in a large frying pan over a medium heat. Add the paste and stir until fragrant. Add **1 pound ground lamb, 1 tablespoon garam masala,** and **2 teaspoons turmeric** and cook, stirring, for 5 minutes, or until the meat is lightly browned. Add **1 cup chopped peeled tomatoes,** cover, and cook over medium-low heat for 20 minutes. Add **1 cup frozen peas** and continue cooking for another 5 minutes. Add salt and pepper to taste. Stir a handful of **chopped fresh cilantro** into **1 cup low-fat plain yogurt** and serve it with the lamb.

● Serve with white or brown rice or chapatis (Indian flatbread).

LEMON AND PEA SAUCE

Serves 4
Preparation 5 minutes Cooking 4 minutes

Each serving provides • 197 calories • 13 g fat
• 2 g saturated fat • 12 g carbohydrates • 9 g protein
• 10 g fiber

Add **2 cups frozen peas** to a saucepan and pour boiling water to cover. Return to a boil, cover, and simmer over low heat for 4 minutes, or until tender. Drain and refresh under cold running water. Put the cooked peas in a blender, or a bowl if you have a stick blender, with **1 large chopped garlic clove, 1 tablespoon tahini, juice of ½ lemon, 1 teaspoon ground cumin, 1 teaspoon ground coriander, 2 tablespoons olive oil** and **1 teaspoon ground black pepper**. Blend for about 20 seconds, or until smooth. Season, spoon into a serving bowl and garnish with **1 tablespoon finely chopped fresh parsley**.

COOK'S TIPS
● Use this pea sauce as a dip, or as a refreshing starter or party dish served with fresh-cut crunchy raw vegetables.
● Serve as a refreshing accompaniment to grilled meats or fish.

CREAMY ITALIAN SNOW PEAS WITH PASTA

Serves 4
Preparation 5 minutes Cooking 10 minutes

Each serving provides • 347 calories • 6 g fat
• 3 g saturated fat • 56 g carbohydrates
• 17 g protein • 4 g fiber

Add **10 ounces dried pasta** such as penne or fusilli to a saucepan filled with boiling water. Cook the pasta for 10 minutes, or until tender but firm to the bite. Meanwhile, cook **1⅓ cups snow peas** in a pan of boiling water for 3 minutes, or until cooked. Drain and return the snow peas to the pan. Add **1 cup low-fat ricotta, 1 tablespoon snipped chives, 2 teaspoons finely chopped fresh mint** and **4 chopped scallions** and toss together gently. Drain the pasta and transfer it to the pan with the sauce and snow peas. Mix thoroughly and serve with **2 teaspoons grated parmesan** sprinkled over each portion.

● For contrasting flavor, add ½ cup lima beans to this dish, cooked with the snow peas.

MINTED PESTO WITH LEEKS AND PEAS

Serves 4
Preparation 5 minutes Cooking 5 minutes

Each serving provides • 167 calories • 12 g fat
• 2 g saturated fat • 10 g carbohydrates • 5 g protein
• 7 g fiber

First make the pesto by mixing **1 small handful of finely chopped fresh mint leaves, 1 tablespoon extra virgin olive oil, 2 teaspoons balsamic vinegar, ½ teaspoon superfine sugar**, and salt and pepper to taste in a small bowl. Thinly slice **2 small leeks**. Heat **2 tablespoons olive oil** over medium-low heat and add the leeks. Sauté for 5 minutes, or until softened. Meanwhile, simmer **1⅓ cups frozen peas** in a pan of boiling water for 4 minutes, or until cooked. Drain the cooked peas and add to the leeks in the pan, then stir in the minted pesto.

COOK'S TIPS
● Try this recipe as a side dish with lamb steaks.
● Mix the pesto, leeks, and peas with whole-wheat pasta and top with grated parmesan for a tasty supper.

POTATO AND ZUCCHINI MEDLEY WITH PICKLED HERRING

Toss hot new potatoes, crunchy zucchini, and gherkins in a dill and yogurt dressing, then heap them on a plate with tangy pickled herring. Here is a meal that will help to keep your body in shape.

Serves 4
Preparation 15 minutes
Cooking 15 minutes

1 pound new potatoes or
    waxy salad potatoes
4 small zucchini
4 large gherkins
2 tablespoons chopped fresh dill
2 tablespoons snipped fresh chives
1 tablespoon olive oil
⅓ cup plain yogurt
2 tablespoons whole-grain mustard
1 jar (9 ounces) pickled herring or
    rollmops, drained
1 large head of red or white endive

Each serving provides
• 326 calories • 15 g fat • 2 g
saturated fat • 32 g carbohydrates
• 19 g protein • 3 g fiber

ALTERNATIVE INGREDIENTS
• Use smoked mackerel, salmon, or
trout instead of herring.
• Substitute a small head of boston
lettuce or baby romaine lettuce for the
endive. These have a less bitter flavor
than endive, while still providing a
crunchy texture.

1 Cut the potatoes in half, place them in a saucepan, and cover with boiling water. Return to a boil over high heat, cover, and simmer for 15 minutes, or until tender.

2 Trim and slice the zucchini and slice the gherkins. Mix the raw zucchini and gherkins in a large bowl with the dill, chives, and oil. Drain the potatoes and add them to the bowl, tossing to coat them with the herbs and oil.

3 Mix the yogurt and mustard to make a dressing. Slice the herring in half or thirds. Arrange the endive leaves on four plates. Divide the potato salad among the plates, arrange the herring on top, and spoon a little dressing over each portion.

COOK'S TIPS
● Scissors are ideal for snipping chives. They are also great for finely shredding soft-leaf herbs, such as dill, fennel, mint, and sage.
● Pickled herring is sold canned or in jars in the supermarket cooler case. The name 'rollmops' refers to the way the fillets are rolled up and packed in a sweetened vinegar marinade.

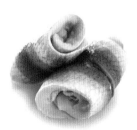

SUPER FOOD

HERRING
Oily fish, such as herring, is one of the few foods naturally high in vitamin D, which is great for bone health. Emerging evidence suggests that a lack of vitamin D may be linked to an increase in the risk of developing diabetes, osteoporosis, multiple sclerosis, and cancer.

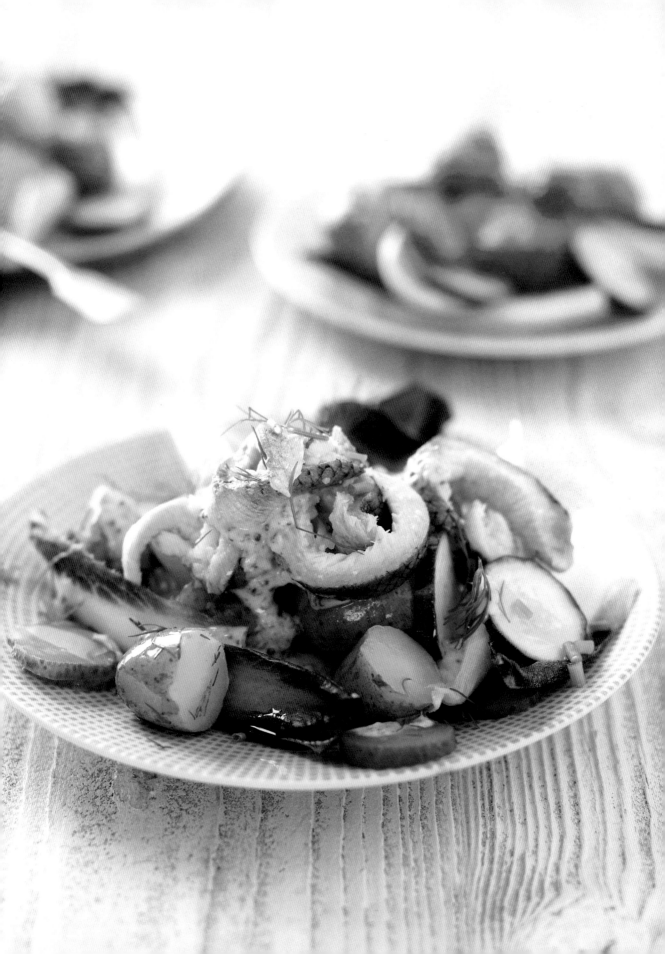

SHRIMP GOULASH WITH CAULIFLOWER AND BEANS

Smoky paprika and the anise flavor of caraway seeds transform juicy shrimp in this twist on a Hungarian classic. Cool yogurt and rice perfectly complement the rich spices.

Serves 4
Preparation 5 minutes
Cooking 13 minutes

1 onion
2 tablespoons olive oil
1 clove garlic, crushed
1 head cauliflower, about ¾ pound
1 tablespoon paprika
1 teaspoon caraway seeds
2 bay leaves
1 can (14½ ounces) chopped
    tomatoes
1½ cups frozen green beans
⅔ pound cooked large shrimp
¾ cup plain yogurt

Each serving provides
• 232 calories • 13 g fat • 4 g
saturated fat • 11 g carbohydrates
• 19 g protein • 3 g fiber

ALTERNATIVE INGREDIENTS
• Use frozen cooked shrimp if fresh
shrimp are not available. Bring the
sauce to a boil, add the frozen shrimp,
and simmer for 2–3 minutes until they
have thawed. Don't boil the shrimp or
they will be tough.
• Try skinless fresh salmon instead
of shrimp. Cut ¾–1 pound salmon fillet
into bite-sized chunks and add them
to the pan in step 4. Simmer for
3–4 minutes until cooked but still firm.

1 Finely chop the onion. Put the oil, onion, and garlic in a large saucepan over medium-high heat. Cook for 5 minutes, or until the onion is beginning to soften.

2 Break the cauliflower into bite-sized florets and add them to the pan. Stir in the paprika, caraway seeds, and bay leaves. Cover and cook for 2 minutes.

3 Stir in the chopped tomatoes and 4 tablespoons of boiling water. Return to a boil, reduce the heat slightly, cover, and simmer for 3 minutes, or until the cauliflower is just tender.

4 Stir in the frozen green beans. Return to a boil, cover, and cook for 2 minutes. Finally, add the shrimp and gently heat through for a minute. Serve topped with a large spoonful of yogurt.

COOK'S TIPS
● Tender young cauliflower leaves and stalks are mild and sweet, and are just as nutritious as the florets. Although not used in this recipe, reserve leftover leaves and stalks for another use.
● This dish also works well served with potato gnocchi, small dumplings sold fresh or in vacuum packs.

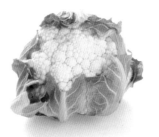

SUPER FOOD

CAULIFLOWER
A member of the brassica family of vegetables, along with brussels sprouts, broccoli, and cabbage, cauliflower has a range of antioxidants that can disarm potentially harmful free radicals and help to protect the body against cancer and heart disease.

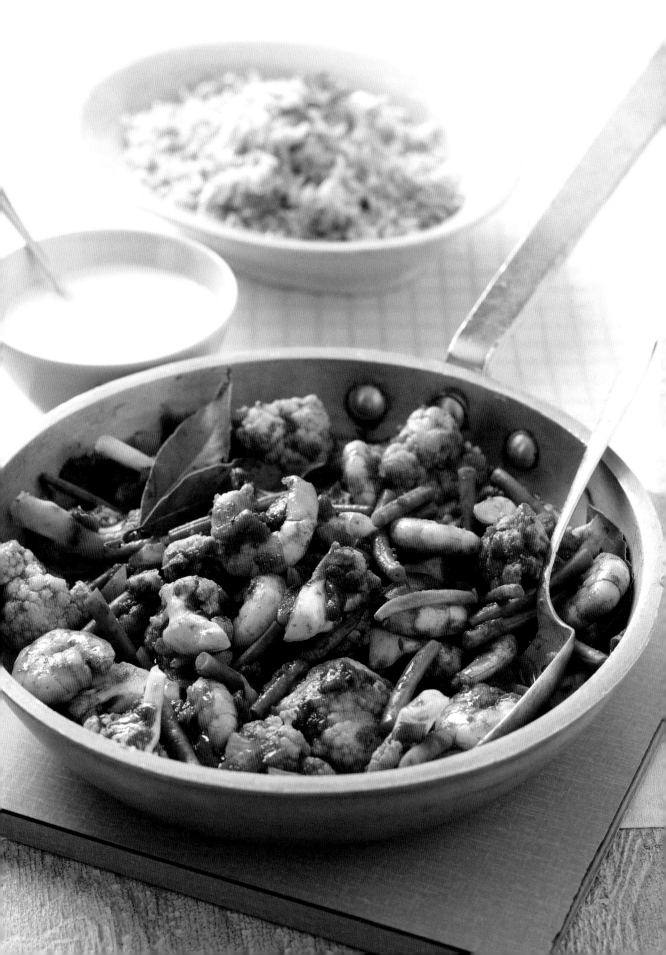

SESAME SQUID
WITH CRUNCHY VEGETABLES

Chile pepper, garlic, and sesame seeds lend their tempting aromas to protein-packed squid. A serving of soft noodles makes a great contrast to the crisp vegetables.

Serves 4
Preparation 15 minutes
Cooking 6 minutes

1 pound squid tubes
1 red chile
2 cloves garlic, crushed
grated zest of 1 lemon
1 leek
2 celery stalks
1 large yellow bell pepper
1 large zucchini
½ pound bok choy
3 tablespoons olive oil or canola oil
4 tablespoons toasted sesame seeds
4 lemon wedges, to garnish

Each serving provides
• 294 calories • 21 g fat • 3 g saturated fat • 5 g carbohydrates
• 22 g protein • 4 g fiber

ALTERNATIVE INGREDIENTS
• Instead of toasted sesame seeds, use 4 tablespoons pine nuts.
• For a stronger vegetable flavor, use red instead of yellow bell pepper and choy sum (mustard greens) instead of bok choy.

1 Slice the squid tubes into 1-inch-thick rings and place them in a bowl. Finely chop the chile and mix it with the squid. Stir in the garlic and lemon zest. Thinly slice the leek, celery, pepper, and zucchini. Slice the bok choy, discarding the tough base.

2 Heat 2 tablespoons of the oil in a large frying pan over high heat. Add the leek and celery and stir-fry for 2 minutes. Add the yellow bell pepper and zucchini and continue to stir-fry for 1 minute. Add the bok choy and cook for 2 minutes, or until it has wilted.

3 Heat another pan over high heat. Add the remaining tablespoon of oil. Add the squid and chile mixture. Stir-fry for 1 minute, turning once, until the squid is just firm. Divide the vegetables among four plates. Place the squid on top of the vegetables and sprinkle with sesame seeds. Garnish each portion with a lemon wedge and serve.

COOK'S TIPS
● Heat the pan before adding the oil to cook the squid—the pan will retain the heat and the squid will cook quickly. Cook it too slowly, and the squid will be chewy.
● Marinating the squid with garlic and chile at the end of step 1 will intensify the flavor. Use a mild chile for a hint of heat or a tiny birdseye chile for fiery flavor. If marinating the squid, mix 1 tablespoon oil with the seasoning, then cover and chill until needed.
● If you buy sesame seeds that are not already toasted, heat them in a large dry frying pan over medium heat for 3–5 minutes, stirring, until they begin to brown. Don't let them burn or they will be bitter.

SUPER FOOD

SESAME SEEDS
Even eaten in small amounts, sesame seeds are still highly nutritious. They are rich in unsaturated fats, particularly polyunsaturated fats, which help to lower harmful cholesterol, making them good for heart health. The seeds also contain fiber to boost digestive health and calcium to protect bones.

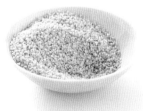

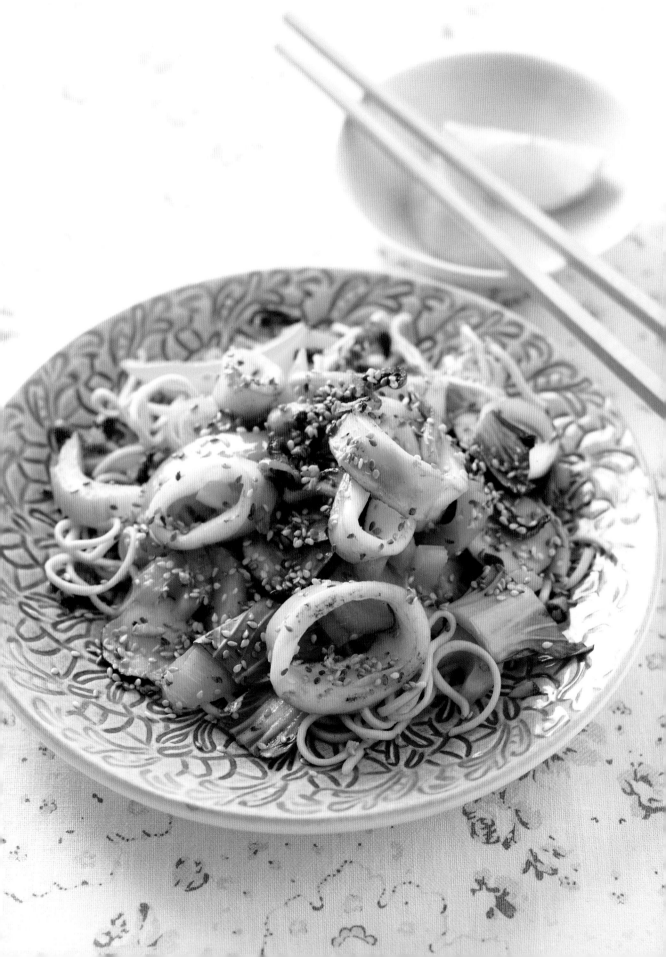

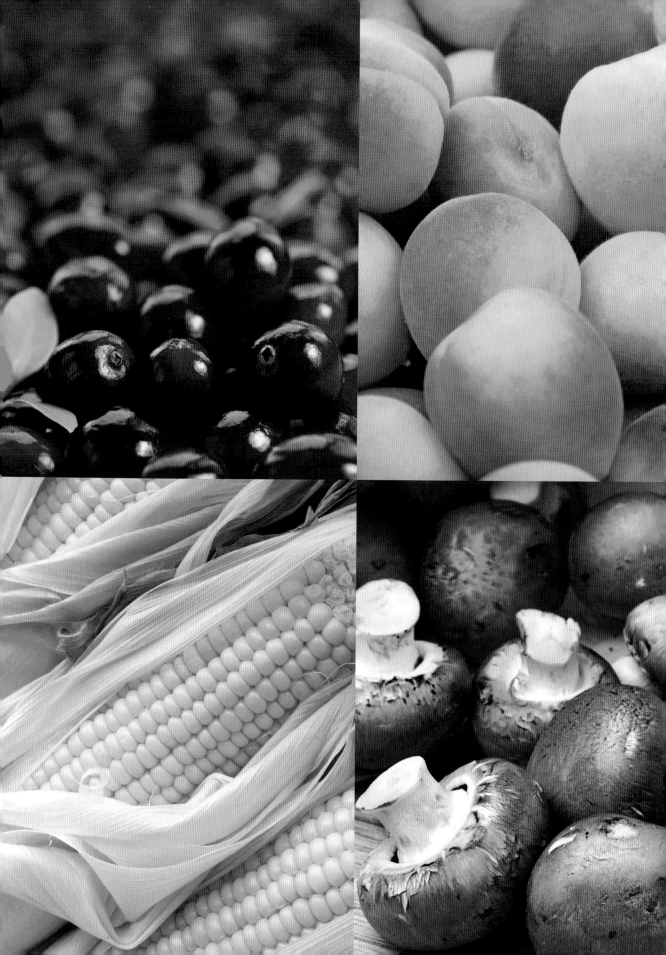

POULTRY *and* GAME

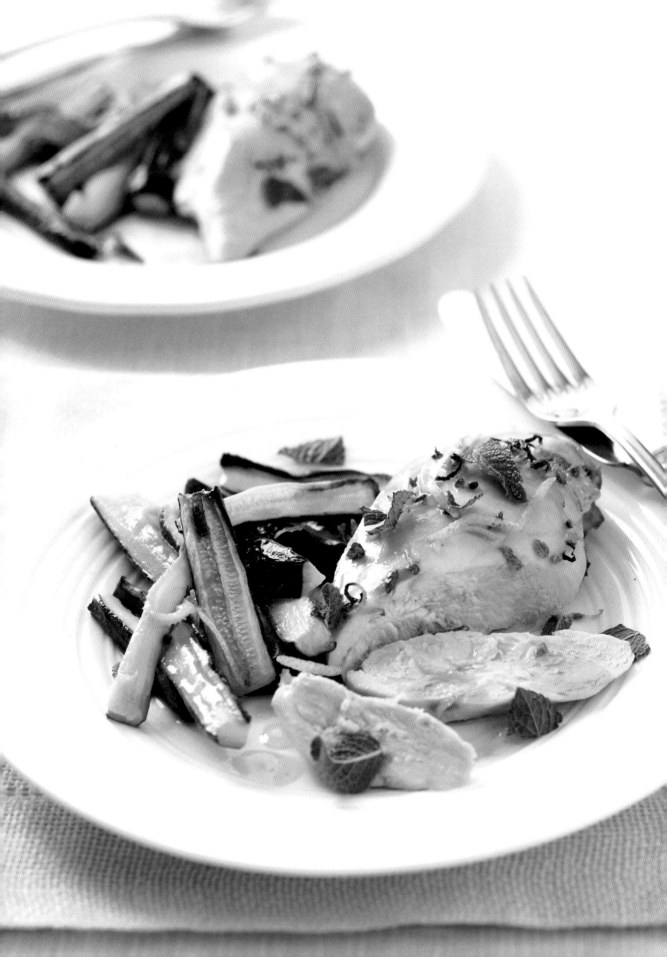

AROMATIC **CHICKEN** WITH GRILLED **VEGETABLES**

Cardamom and lemon lend exotic flavor and irresistible Indian aromas to simple low-fat ingredients. The zucchini are filling yet low in calories, so you can enjoy this tastebud-tingling dish without guilt.

Serves 4
Preparation 10 minutes
Cooking 15 minutes

8 green whole cardamom pods
grated zest of 2 lemons
2 tablespoons olive oil
12 baby zucchini
½ cucumber
4 boneless, skinless chicken breasts,
    about ¼ pound each
4 shredded fresh mint leaves

Each serving provides
• 268 calories • 13 g fat • 3 g saturated fat • 3 g carbohydrates
• 34 g protein • 2 g fiber

ALTERNATIVE INGREDIENTS
• Use any white meat, such as turkey or pork, instead of chicken.
• The seasonings and vegetables in this recipe work well with fish, too. Broil mackerel, sardines, or salmon fillets for 3–5 minutes on each side, depending on the thickness of the fish.
• Substitute 2 teaspoons fennel seeds for the cardamom pods.
• Leave out the cardamom and add 1 tablespoon chopped rosemary and 2 finely chopped garlic cloves.

1 Preheat the grill to high and line the grill pan with foil. Scrape the seeds from the cardamom pods into a small dish. Add the zest from 1 lemon and stir in the oil. Cut the zucchini in half lengthwise. Cut the cucumber in half widthwise, then in half lengthwise into pieces about the same size as the zucchini.

2 Place the chicken in the center of the grill pan and arrange the zucchini and cucumber around the edges. Brush the chicken, zucchini, and cucumber with the cardamom and lemon oil.

3 Grill everything for 5 minutes, then turn the chicken and vegetables over and grill for another 10 minutes, or until the chicken is cooked through and the vegetables begin to brown. Divide the chicken among four plates and sprinkle with the mint and remaining lemon zest. Transfer the zucchini and cucumber to the plates and spoon any cooking juices on top of each portion.

COOK'S TIPS
● To check that the chicken is done, turn one piece over and pierce the thickest part with the tip of a sharp knife. The meat should be white, not pink, and the juices should run clear. If necessary, cook a few minutes longer. Turn the fillet over to conceal the slit when serving.
● Serve the chicken and vegetables with brown rice or new potatoes.
● If you don't have a grill, you can also make this in the broiler.

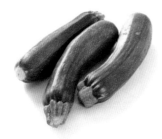

SUPER FOOD

ZUCCHINI
A water content of over 90 percent, makes zucchini a low-energy, low-calorie food. With potassium to regulate blood pressure, folate for heart health, and carotenes with antioxidant benefits, zucchini adds plenty of health boosters to a balanced diet.

CHICKEN STIR-FRY WITH MUSHROOMS AND CASHEWS

Mildly sweet and crunchy, cashews are crammed with fiber, antioxidants, vitamins, and minerals. Even better, when combined with chicken and vegetables, they make an easy, appetizing stir-fry.

Serves 4
Preparation 20 minutes
Cooking 10 minutes

2 teaspoons cornstarch
⅓ cup dry sherry
2 tablespoons soy sauce
2 teaspoons sesame oil
¾ cup snow peas
1 onion
4 celery stalks
⅓ cup shiitake mushrooms
2 carrots
⅓ cup unsalted cashews
2 tablespoons olive oil or canola oil
⅔ pound boneless chicken strips
1 clove garlic, crushed
1 cup bean sprouts

Each serving provides
• 257 calories • 11 g fat • 2 g saturated fat • 17 g carbohydrates • 23 g protein • 4 g fiber

ALTERNATIVE INGREDIENTS
• Try boneless steak cut into ¾-inch strips instead of the chicken. Use 1½ cups shiitake mushrooms and omit the bean sprouts.
• In this recipe, you could also use a 16-ounce package of mixed stir-fry vegetables. Add them in step 3, adding them all at once instead of in stages.
• Use oyster or cremini mushrooms instead of the shiitakes.

1 In a small bowl, mix the cornstarch with a tablespoon of cold water to form a smooth paste. Stir in the sherry, soy sauce, and sesame oil. Put the snow peas in a large saucepan. Add just enough boiling water to cover, return to a boil, and immediately drain and set aside. Thinly slice the onion, celery, and mushrooms. Cut the carrots into 2-inch sticks.

2 Dry roast the cashews in a large frying pan over medium-high heat for 2 minutes, shaking the pan until they begin to brown. Transfer to a plate. Add the oil and chicken strips to the pan. Stir-fry for 1 minute, increasing the heat to high, if necessary, so the chicken begins to brown. Add the onion, celery, carrots, and garlic and stir-fry for 2 minutes.

3 Return the cashews to the pan, add the mushrooms, and stir-fry for 2 minutes. Pour in ½ cup of boiling water and stir in the cornstarch paste. Bring to a boil and add the snow peas and bean sprouts. Simmer for 2 minutes, stirring, until the sauce thickens and the bean sprouts are heated through. Season to taste and serve with rice or noodles.

COOK'S TIP
● There are many kinds of soy sauce, but the choice in supermarkets is usually between dark and light varieties. Dark soy sauce is richer and thicker than light, with a lower salt content. If the amount of salt is a concern, use low-sodium soy sauce.

SUPER FOOD

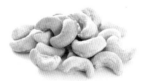

CASHEWS
High in nutritional value, cashews are a good source of fiber, vitamin E, B vitamins, and folate. Like other nuts, they satisfy hunger better than many other foods. Studies suggest nuts can help with weight management when eaten as part of a balanced diet.

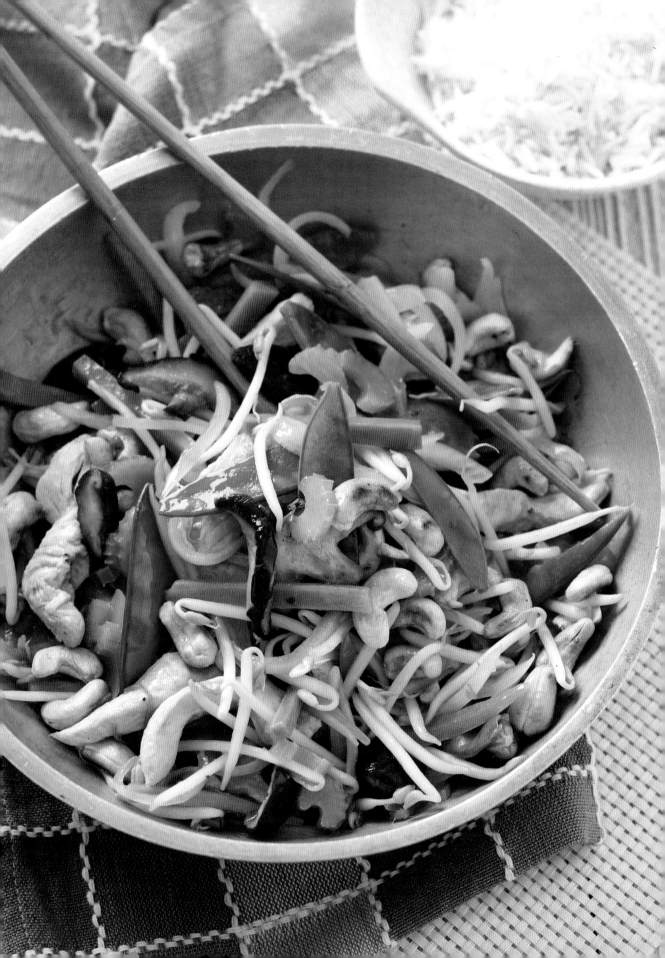

TARRAGON **CHICKEN** WITH **APRICOT** SAUCE

An energizing dish, with dried fruit, pine nuts, and fresh orange juice that complements the more traditional tarragon seasoning. Perfect served with green beans and smashed new potatoes.

Serves 4
Preparation 5 minutes
Cooking 20 minutes

4 boneless, skinless chicken breasts, about ¼ pound each
4 tablespoons dijon mustard
1 tablespoon olive oil or canola oil
½ cup sliced dried apricots
6 sprigs fresh tarragon
juice of 2 oranges
4 tablespoons pine nuts

Each serving provides
• 350 calories • 17 g fat • 2 g saturated fat • 16 g carbohydrates
• 34 g protein • 2 g fiber

ALTERNATIVE INGREDIENTS
• Use 1–2 sprigs rosemary instead of the tarragon, or try 1 teaspoon dried tarragon if fresh is not available.
• Substitute chopped walnuts or pecans for the pine nuts.
• Try pork chops or cutlets instead of the chicken breasts.

1 Preheat the broiler to high. Spread 2 tablespoons of the mustard on one side of the chicken breasts. Turn and spread with the remaining 2 tablespoons of mustard. Place the chicken, skin side down, in a flameproof baking dish and drizzle with oil. Broil on one side for 10 minutes.

2 Turn the chicken over and broil for another 5 minutes. Sprinkle with the apricots and tarragon. Pour the orange juice over all and broil for another 5 minutes, or until the chicken is browned and cooked through.

3 Sprinkle the pine nuts over the chicken and broil for 30 seconds to warm through. Serve the chicken with the apricots and pine nuts and spoon the pan juices on top of each portion.

COOK'S TIPS
● Salt and pepper are not used in this recipe because the mustard sufficiently seasons the chicken. Apricots and orange juice bring a sweet-tangy balance that would be compromised by adding salt.
● As an alternative to smashed potatoes, serve the chicken with broiled polenta slices. You can buy ready-made polenta (follow the package directions), or make your own (see page 95).

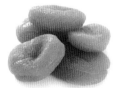

SUPER FOOD

DRIED APRICOTS
As a concentrated source of energy-boosting carbohydrate, dried apricots make great snacks. They are also rich in the antioxidant beta-carotene, and just a handful of apricots provides up to one-sixth of your daily vitamin A needs—good news for eye health.

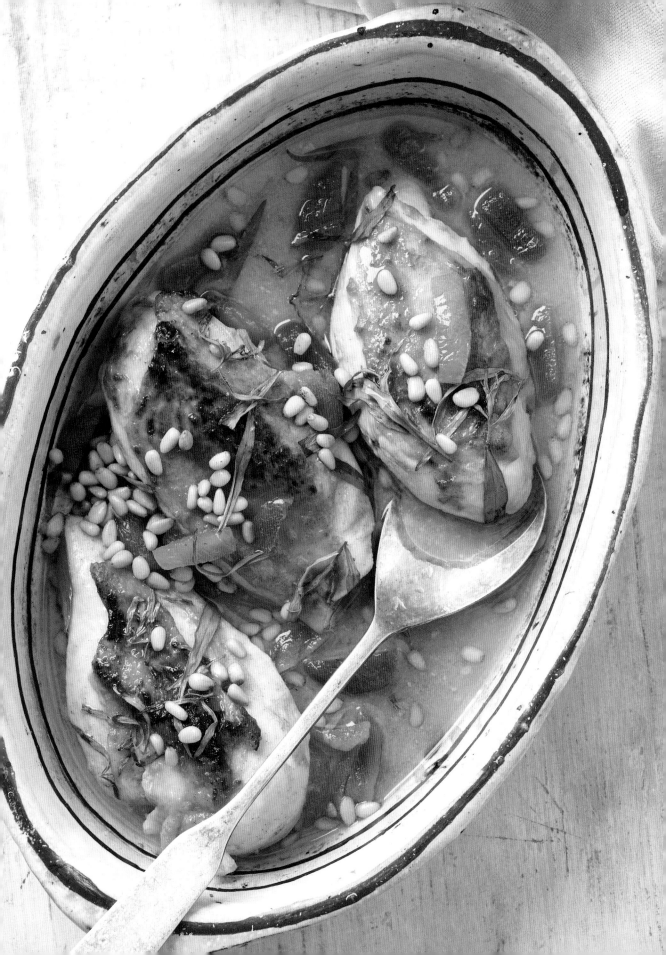

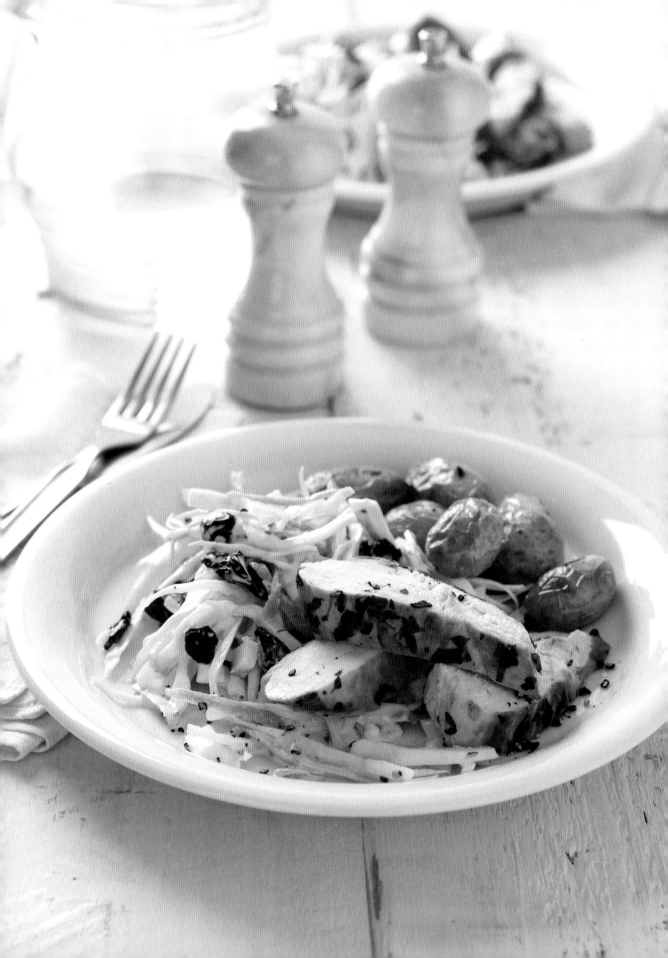

HERBED **CHICKEN** WITH **CRANBERRY** COLESLAW

Dried cranberries lend a rich intensity to a yogurty coleslaw, turning it into a light but distinctive accompaniment for thyme and sage-flavored chicken. Team it with golden roast potatoes.

Serves 4
Preparation 15 minutes
Cooking 12 minutes

8 sprigs fresh thyme
6 large fresh sage leaves
2 tablespoons olive oil or canola oil
1 pound boneless, skinless
  chicken breasts
1⅓ cups shredded white cabbage
1 carrot
1 onion
4 tablespoons low-fat mayonnaise
4 tablespoons low-fat plain yogurt
¼ cup dried cranberries

Each serving provides
• 335 calories • 16 g fat • 3 g saturated fat • 21 g carbohydrates
• 27 g protein • 7 g fiber

ALTERNATIVE INGREDIENTS
• This recipe is a great way to use up leftovers from a roast chicken. Remove the meat from the bones and sprinkle with 2 tablespoons fresh thyme before serving with the coleslaw.
• Try raisins, diced dried apricots, or chopped apple with its skin on instead of cranberries.

1 Put the leaves from the thyme sprigs into a large, shallow dish. Shred the sage leaves and add them to the dish with 1 tablespoon oil. Add the chicken breasts and turn them in the herb mixture to coat.

2 Coarsely grate the carrot, finely chop the onion, and mix them together with the cabbage in a large bowl. Blend the mayonnaise and yogurt and stir them into the vegetables. Season to taste and stir in the cranberries.

3 Heat a frying pan over high heat. Add the remaining 1 tablespoon oil and add the chicken, including any herb mixture from the dish. Reduce heat to medium and cook for 2 minutes on each side, or until browned. Reduce heat to low and cook for 8 minutes, turning once or twice, until the chicken is cooked through (see Cook's Tip).

4 Divide the cranberry coleslaw among four plates. Slice the chicken and divide the pieces evenly, arranging them on top of the slaw.

COOK'S TIP
● Chicken breast sizes vary so the cooking time will depend on how large and thick they are. Make a small slit in the side of one of the chicken breasts using a sharp knife to see if the center is done. If the meat is still pink, continue to cook for a few more minutes.

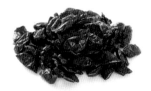

SUPER FOOD

CRANBERRIES
Dried cranberries, like other dried fruit, have more concentrated nutritional goodness than the fresh variety. There is some evidence that cranberries can reduce the risk of developing urinary tract infections.

SPANISH **CHICKEN** WITH **PEPPERS** AND **OLIVES**

Here's a complete meal-in-a-pan that makes the most of the flavor-drenched ingredients that give Mediterranean cooking its healthy reputation. For contrasting texture, serve with a crisp salad.

Serves 4
Preparation 15 minutes
Cooking 23 minutes

4 boneless, skinless chicken breasts, about ¼ pound each
1 large onion
3 bell peppers (2 red, 1 green)
2 tablespoons olive oil
2 large cloves garlic, crushed
1 cup long-grain rice
2½ cups hot chicken stock
1 can (14½ ounces) chopped tomatoes
½ cup pitted black olives
1 tablespoon chopped fresh parsley

Each serving provides
• 466 calories • 12 g fat • 2 g saturated fat • 59 g carbohydrates • 35 g protein • 3 g fiber

ALTERNATIVE INGREDIENTS
• Use sautéed strips of lamb or beef as a change from chicken. Allow 1 pound of meat for four people and cook it for just 1 minute in step 1.
• When you have slightly more time to spare, use brown rice instead of white. Cook the rice for an extra 10 minutes in step 2.

1 Cut each piece of chicken lengthwise into three thick strips. Chop the onion and dice the peppers. Heat the oil in a large covered frying pan and cook the chicken for 3 minutes over medium heat or until browned and partly cooked. Transfer the chicken to a plate.

2 Fry the onion, peppers, and garlic for 5 minutes over a medium heat, stirring until slightly softened. Return the chicken to the pan with any juices and sprinkle in the rice. Add the hot stock, then pour in the tomatoes. Return to a boil over a high heat. Stir, cover, and simmer for 15 minutes, or until the rice is tender, stirring occasionally to prevent the rice from sticking to the bottom of the pan.

3 Roughly chop the olives and sprinkle them over the dish together with the parsley. Remove the pan from the heat, season to taste, cover, and let stand for 1–2 minutes before serving.

COOK'S TIP
● If pitted olives are not available, buy olives with their pits and use a cherry pitter to remove the pits before chopping. Or on a cutting board, press down on an olive with the flat side of a chef's knife to loosen the pit and then you can remove it with your fingers.

SUPER FOOD

CHICKEN
Lean chicken is a good source of the amino acid tyrosine, which can help to promote mental alertness. It also contains the energy-releasing B vitamin niacin, which can help to boost energy levels, especially when you eat chicken with starchy foods such as rice.

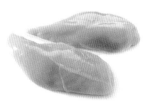

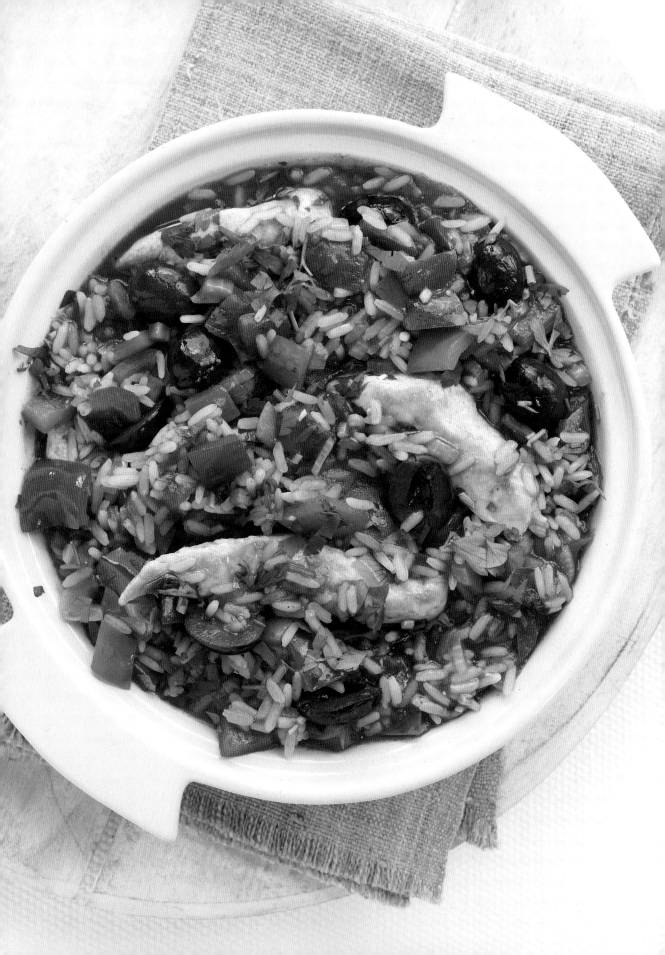

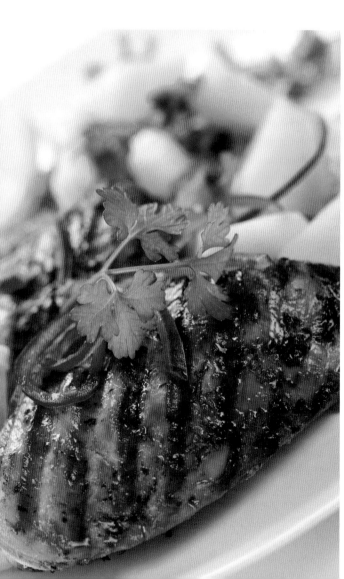

CHICKEN

High in protein and low in cholesterol-raising saturated fat, succulent chicken is a good meat to eat regularly. It contains all the essential amino acids, including tryptophan, which boosts levels of serotonin in the body, helping to combat emotional fatigue.

CHICKEN AND TOMATO SALAD

Serves 4
Preparation 35 minutes Marinating 30 minutes
Cooking 15 minutes

Each serving provides • 333 calories • 22 g fat • 3 g saturated fat • 8 g carbohydrates • 25 g protein • 1 g fiber

Preheat broiler to medium-high. In a large bowl, mix **3 tablespoons olive oil, juice of ½ lemon, 2 crushed cloves garlic**, and salt and pepper to taste. Cut **3 boneless, skinless chicken breasts**, about ¼ pound each, into three diagonal slices each and add them to the bowl. Turn the chicken in the oil mixture and let marinate for about 30 minutes. Meanwhile, make a dressing by mixing **2 tablespoons olive oil, 1 tablespoon balsamic vinegar, 1 tablespoon oil from a jar of sun-dried tomatoes, a pinch of sugar** and **ground black pepper**. Transfer the chicken pieces to a nonstick baking pan and broil for 8 minutes. Turn, baste with the marinade, and cook for 7 minutes, or until the juices run clear when the chicken is pierced with the tip of a sharp knife. In another large bowl, mix **½ cup watercress, ½ cup arugula leaves, 10 halved cherry tomatoes, 6 chopped sun-dried tomatoes** and **¼ sliced cucumber**. Divide the salad among four plates and arrange the grilled chicken on top. Drizzle with the dressing and scatter **1 teaspoon finely chopped sun-dried tomatoes** over each serving.

COOK'S TIP
● Serve with warmed focaccia or olive bread.

LAZY DAY BAKE

Serves 4
Preparation 10 minutes Cooking 45 minutes

Each serving provides • 359 calories • 15 g fat • 2 g saturated fat • 37 g carbohydrates • 22 g protein • 5 g fiber

Preheat the oven to 350°F. Heat **1 tablespoon olive oil** in a frying pan over a medium heat. Add **8 boneless, skinless chicken thighs** and fry for 10 minutes to brown all over. Cut **1 pound of sweet potatoes** into ¾-inch slices and put them in a large bowl. Add **3 large red onions**, cut into quarters, and **2 tablespoons olive oil**. Coat the vegetables with oil, then transfer to a large roasting pan. Place the browned chicken in the roasting pan then add **8 unpeeled whole cloves garlic, 1 tablespoon finely chopped fresh thyme, 1 teaspoon finely chopped**

fresh rosemary, and salt and pepper to taste. Roast for 15 minutes, then turn and sprinkle with the **juice of 1 lemon** and **1 cup hot chicken stock**. Roast for another 20 minutes, or until the chicken is cooked through and the vegetables are tender. Serve with the pan juices poured over.

COOK'S TIPS

● If the pan juices in the roasting pan begin to look dry near the end of cooking, add 4 tablespoons hot chicken stock or water.

● Steamed kale or spring greens add bite and plenty of beneficial iron when served as a side vegetable with this dish.

TEX-MEX CHICKEN WRAPS

Serves 4
Preparation 10 minutes Cooking 8 minutes

Each serving provides • 574 calories • 17 g fat • 3 g saturated fat • 75 g carbohydrates • 35 g protein • 5 g fiber

Cook **½ cup frozen sweet corn** in a saucepan of boiling water for 3 minutes, then drain and set aside. Slice **4 boneless, skinless chicken breasts**, about ¼ pound each, into ½-inch strips. Heat **1 tablespoon olive oil** in a frying pan over a medium heat. Add the chicken fillets, **1 crushed clove garlic, 1 teaspoon paprika**, and salt and pepper to taste. Sauté for 5 minutes, or until the chicken is cooked through. In a bowl, mash **1 sliced large ripe avocado** with **4 tablespoons store-bought tomato salsa**. Stir in the corn and chicken, divide the mixture among **8 warmed whole-wheat flour tortillas** (see Cook's Tip) and top with **1 heaping teaspoon reduced-fat crème fraîche**. Fold each tortilla up at the bottom and in at each side to make a packet.

COOK'S TIP

● Warm the tortillas in a microwave or oven, according to the package directions.

CHICKEN PASTA SALAD

Serves 4
Preparation 5 minutes Cooking 13 minutes

Each serving provides • 363 calories • 6 g fat • 1 g saturated fat • 50 g carbohydrates • 30 g protein • 2 g fiber

Cook **¾ cup whole-wheat pasta spirals** in a pan of boiling water for 10 minutes, or according to the package directions. In a small bowl, make the dressing by combining **½ cup plain yogurt, 1 tablespoon lemon juice, ½ teaspoon dijon mustard, a pinch of sugar**, and salt and pepper to taste. Add **1 cup small broccoli florets** to the pasta, cook for 3 minutes then drain and let cool for 5 minutes. Transfer the pasta and broccoli to a serving bowl, add 4 tablespoons of the dressing and toss to coat. Cut **⅔ pound cooked boneless, skinless chicken breasts** into 1-inch chunks and add them to the pasta with **1 chopped green bell pepper, 1 chopped red apple** with the skin left on, **3 tablespoons golden raisins** and **2 tablespoons walnut pieces**. Mix all the salad ingredients together and serve.

COOK'S TIPS

● Replace the broccoli with green beans—cook them for 3 minutes, or until tender but firm to the bite.

● Add sliced almonds instead of walnut pieces for a slightly sweeter, more delicate flavor.

WINTER BARLEY SOUP

Serves 4
Preparation 10 minutes Cooking 43 minutes

Each serving provides • 321 calories • 12 g fat • 1 g saturated fat • 31 g carbohydrates • 26 g protein • 6 g fiber

Heat **2 tablespoons olive oil or canola oil** in a large saucepan over a medium-low heat. Add **1 large chopped onion, 2 sliced celery stalks** and **2 sliced carrots**. Cook for 10 minutes, stirring occasionally. Slice **⅔ cup mushrooms** and add them to the pan with **2 crushed cloves garlic**, then stir-fry for 1 minute. Slice **¾ pound boneless, skinless chicken breasts** into ½-inch strips and add them to the pan with **⅓ cup pearl barley**. Pour in **4 cups hot chicken stock**, cover and bring to a boil. Reduce the heat to low and simmer for 30 minutes, or until the barley is tender. Season to taste. Just before serving, toast **4 teaspoons sliced almonds** in a dry frying pan over medium heat for 2 minutes. Ladle the soup into bowls and garnish with **1 teaspoon chopped fresh parsley** and 1 teaspoon of the toasted sliced almonds per portion.

COOK'S TIP

● Use leftover roast chicken instead of raw chicken and reduce the cooking time by 10 minutes.

SHERRY-INFUSED **CHICKEN LIVERS** WITH **MUSHROOMS** AND **BEANS**

Rich chicken livers are invigorated with a splash of sherry and served with soft mushrooms and crisp green beans in this iron-rich dish. Velvety mashed potatoes makes the perfect accompaniment.

Serves 4
Preparation 10 minutes
Cooking 15 minutes

½ pound chicken livers
1 onion
3 tablespoons olive oil
2 cloves garlic, crushed
5 sage leaves, shredded
1⅓ cups small mushrooms
1⅓ cups frozen green beans
2 tablespoons dry or medium sherry
grated zest of 1 lemon
4 tablespoons chopped fresh parsley
4 lemon wedges, to garnish

Each serving provides
• 211 calories • 14 g fat • 2 g saturated fat • 6 g carbohydrates
• 14 g protein • 4 g fiber

ALTERNATIVE INGREDIENTS
• To use fresh green beans instead of frozen, trim the ends and cook in boiling water for 3–4 minutes, or until tender. Drain and toss into the chicken livers in step 3 just before serving.
• For fans of liver and bacon, add ¼ cup diced bacon to the onion, garlic, and sage in step 1.
• For a non-alcoholic meal, substitute white wine vinegar for the sherry.

1 Remove any tough white parts from the chicken livers and cut them into bite-sized pieces. Slice the onion. Heat 1 tablespoon of the oil in a large frying pan over high heat. Add the onion, garlic, and sage, reduce heat to medium and cook for 5 minutes, or until softened.

2 Cut the mushrooms in half and add them to the frying pan. Cook for 3 minutes, then add the frozen beans and cook, stirring, for another 3 minutes, or until the beans are hot and most of the juice from the mushrooms has evaporated.

3 Push the vegetables to one side of the pan and add the remaining 2 tablespoons of oil. Add the chicken livers and cook over medium heat for 2–3 minutes, turning until they are firm and cooked. Stir in the sherry and lemon zest and simmer for 1 minute. Sprinkle with parsley and garnish with lemon wedges.

COOK'S TIP
● The best way to prepare chicken livers is to place them on a plate and snip away the tough white sinews with a pair of scissors.

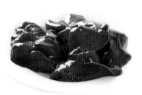

SUPER FOOD

CHICKEN LIVER
A rich source of easily absorbed iron and low in fat, chicken livers are packed with vitamin A, needed for healthy skin and to promote good vision. In addition, they contain some zinc and B vitamins, including B_{12}, and heart-protecting folate.

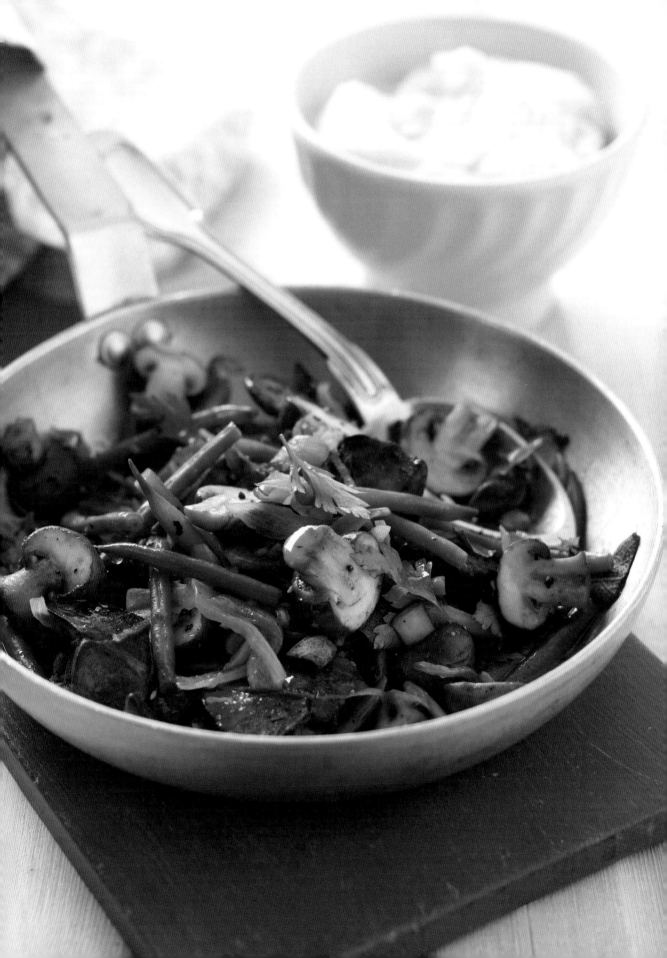

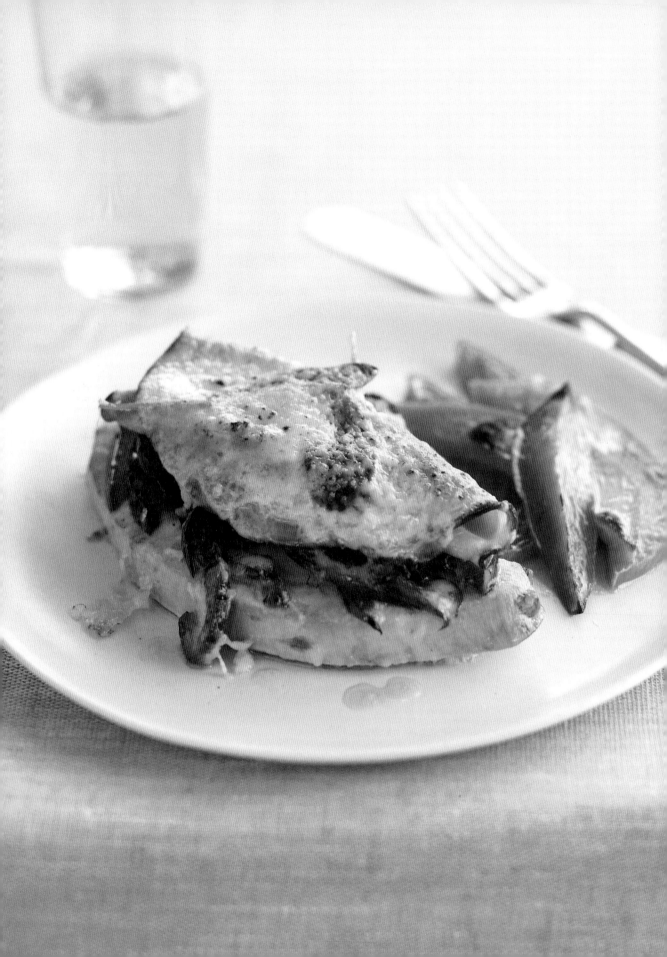

SWEET **PEPPERS** AND **TURKEY CUTLETS** WITH GLAZED **MANGO**

The classic combo of turkey, ham, and cheese is made lighter and healthier by adding broiled fruit and vegetables. Plenty of protein and fiber will satisfy your hunger and help to keep you lean.

Serves 4
Preparation 10 minutes
Cooking 15 minutes

4 turkey breast cutlets, about
    ¼ pound each
2 tablespoons olive oil or canola oil
1 ripe mango
2 red bell peppers
1 teaspoon sugar
1 tablespoon cider vinegar
4 thin slices cooked ham
4 large fresh sage leaves
¼ cup grated sharp cheddar

Each serving provides
• 278 calories • 13 g fat • 4 g saturated fat • 12 g carbohydrates
• 27 g protein • 2 g fiber

ALTERNATIVE INGREDIENTS
• Boneless, skinless chicken breasts or thighs, or pork cutlets make good alternatives to turkey.
• Thinly sliced pears work just as well as mango. Use green bell pepper strips instead of red, and use a blue cheese instead of the cheddar.

1 Preheat the broiler to high. Place the turkey cutlets on a broiler pan and brush with 1 tablespoon of the oil. Broil for 6 minutes, or until lightly browned. Peel and thinly slice the mango. Cut the peppers into ½-inch strips.

2 Turn the turkey cutlets over. Arrange the mango around the turkey, top the cutlets with the pepper strips, and brush with the remaining oil. Broil for another 6 minutes, or until the turkey is cooked—pierce it with a knife, and when the juices run clear, it's done.

3 Stir the sugar and cider vinegar together until the sugar dissolves and spoon it over the peppers and mango. Top each turkey cutlet with a folded ham slice, a sage leaf, and some of the cheese. Broil for 3 minutes, or until the cheese has melted to a golden crispness. Serve drizzled with any cooking juices.

COOK'S TIPS
● Reduce the total fat content of this recipe by using reduced-fat cheddar and lean slices of ham, trimming any excess fat.
● Serve the turkey cutlets with couscous or bulgur for added fiber and B vitamins, or use them to make a turkey melt on whole-grain bread.

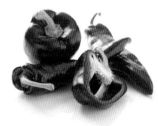

SUPER FOOD

RED BELL PEPPERS
Red bell peppers are low in saturated fat and are a good source of fiber. They are rich in antioxidants and packed with several essential nutrients including vitamin C and beta-carotene.

LIGHT AND SPICY **TURKEY CHILI**

Cholesterol-lowering turkey brings guilt-free eating to this variation on traditional chili. Mushrooms and kidney beans add low-fat flavor. Serve with rice and a salad for a complete main meal.

Serves 4
Preparation 10 minutes
Cooking 30 minutes

1 tablespoon olive oil or canola oil
1 pound ground turkey
2 teaspoons cumin seeds
½–2 teaspoons red pepper flakes
   (see Cook's Tips)
1 large onion
1 red bell pepper
2 carrots
⅓ cup small mushrooms, quartered
2 cloves garlic, crushed
1 can (14½ ounces) chopped
   tomatoes
1 can (15 ounces) red kidney beans,
   rinsed and drained
1 cup frozen peas

Each serving provides
• 459 calories • 15 g fat • 4 g
saturated fat • 24 g carbohydrates
• 57 g protein • 8 g fiber

ALTERNATIVE INGREDIENTS
• For a vegetarian chili, replace
the turkey with soy protein crumbles
or tofu.
• An equal quantity of ground pork or
chicken makes a tasty alternative.
• Replace the peas with 1 cup sliced
zucchini and cook for another
2–3 minutes, or until the zucchini
is tender.
• Try cannellini beans or chickpeas
instead of red kidney beans, and add
frozen sweet corn instead of peas.
• Okra is a good addition to this
recipe. Thickly slice 1 cup okra,
discarding the stalk ends. Add to
the chili 5 minutes before the end
of cooking in step 3.

1 Heat the oil in a large saucepan over medium-high heat for a few seconds. Add the ground turkey, cumin seeds, and red pepper flakes and cook for 5 minutes, stirring occasionally, until the turkey is lightly browned. If necessary, increase the heat to high for the final minute to boil away any juices from the turkey.

2 Prepare the vegetables. Coarsely chop the onion, seed and dice the pepper, and coarsely dice the carrots. Add the garlic, onion, pepper, carrots, and mushrooms to the pan. Continue to cook over medium-high heat for another 5 minutes, stirring frequently, until the vegetables soften.

3 Stir in the tomatoes and ½ cup of boiling water. Return to a boil, reduce heat slightly, and cover the pan. Cook at a rapid simmer for 15 minutes, stirring once or twice. Stir in the kidney beans and peas. Simmer for 1 minute, or until the beans and peas are heated through.

COOK'S TIPS
● You can make your own ground turkey by processing 1 pound of lean turkey meat in a meat grinder or food processor, in batches, until the turkey has an even consistency.
● Add red pepper flakes according to your taste—½ teaspoon will give a slight piquancy, 1 teaspoon will create a medium-hot chili, while 2 teaspoons will produce a hot result.

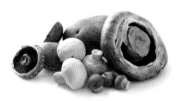

SUPER FOOD

MUSHROOMS
Low in fat and calories, mushrooms are an ideal addition to any weight-control diet plan. They offer B vitamins that encourage energy release from foods, and are a useful source of selenium, an important antioxidant.

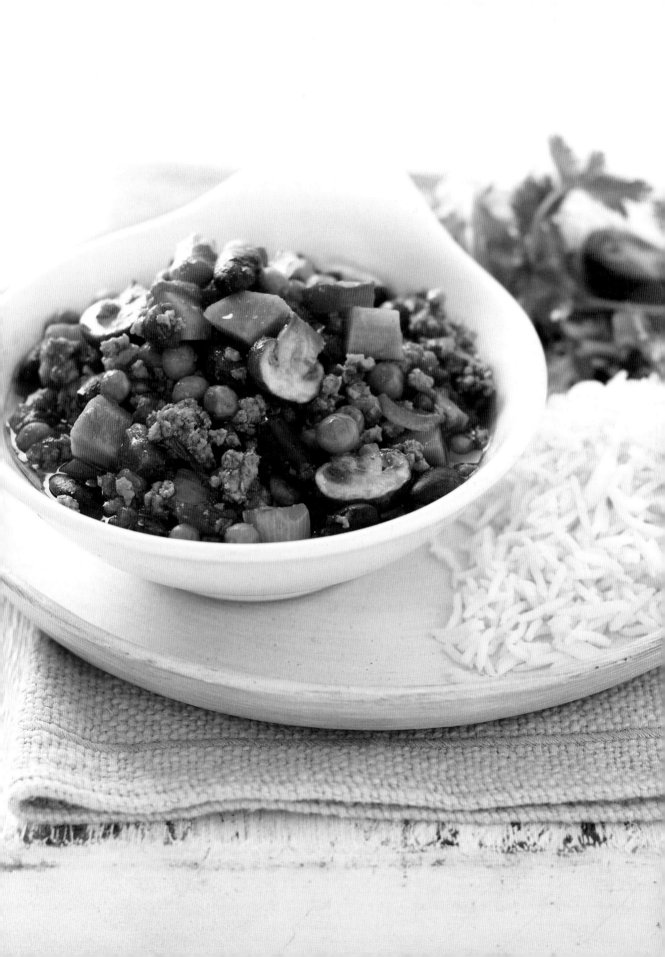

TURKEY SOUVLAKI WITH GRILLED VEGETABLES

Take a popular Greek fast food, combine it with sweet red bell peppers, punchy garlic, and onions, and you have a mouthwatering, easy-to-prepare meal. Serve it with brown rice.

Serves 4
Preparation 10 minutes
Cooking 10 minutes

1 cup quick-cooking brown rice
½ teaspoon red pepper flakes
3 teaspoons dried oregano
½ teaspoon ground nutmeg
4 cloves garlic, crushed
3 tablespoons olive oil or canola oil
4 thin boneless, skinless turkey breasts, about 1 pound
3 onions
2 red bell peppers
½ cucumber
1 cup plain yogurt
8–10 large fresh mint leaves, shredded for garnish
4 lemon wedges for garnish

Each serving provides
• 495 calories • 15 g fat • 2 g saturated fat • 61 g carbohydrates
• 34 g protein • 5 g fiber

ALTERNATIVE INGREDIENTS
• Use chopped fresh green or red chilies instead of red pepper flakes, selecting the variety according to your taste for fiery food.
• For a meat-free alternative, use 2 large eggplants instead of the turkey. Trim the ends and slice the eggplant lengthwise before broiling.
• Serve an iceberg lettuce salad instead of the cucumber and yogurt. Allow 1 large tomato, 1 scallion, and a wedge of lettuce per portion.

1 Cook brown rice according to the package directions. Preheat the broiler to high.

2 Meanwhile, cover the broiler pan with foil. Mix the red pepper flakes, oregano, nutmeg, garlic, and oil in a large shallow dish. Add the turkey breasts to the dish, turning them to coat.

3 Cut the onions into wedges and cut the peppers into thick strips. Transfer the turkey breasts to the broiler pan. Put the onions and peppers in the shallow dish. Using a spatula, scrape the remaining herb mixture over the vegetables and transfer them to the pan. Broil the turkey and vegetables for 8 minutes, turning them frequently so they don't burn.

4 Slice the cucumber and cut each slice in half. Divide the cooked rice among four plates. Top with the vegetables and turkey and add a spoonful of yogurt to each portion. Sprinkle with mint and garnish with lemon wedges to serve.

COOK'S TIP
● Thicker turkey breast portions that contain unevenly cut breast meat are more economical than turkey breast fillets. For even cooking, slice the turkey pieces into similar thicknesses before broiling.

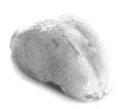

SUPER FOOD

TURKEY
Lower in fat than red meats, turkey is a healthy choice when watching your weight. Rich in high-quality protein, needed for the growth and repair of body tissues, turkey makes a nutritious contribution to a well-balanced diet.

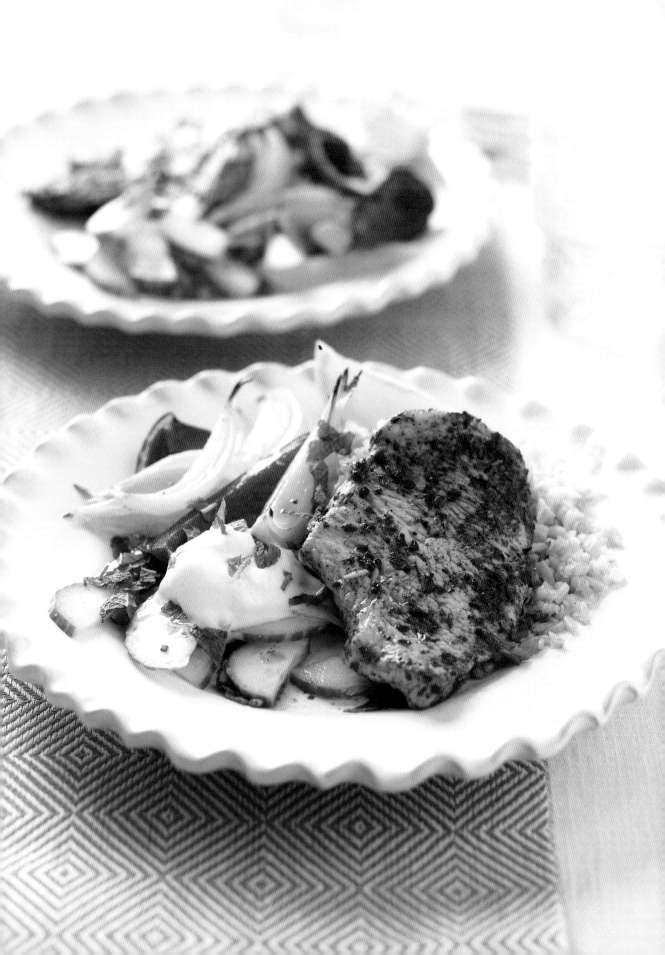

DUCK BREAST WITH CHESTNUTS AND PRUNES

Red wine and prunes bring out the richness of duck, seasoned with robust rosemary and juniper, while chestnuts and a hint of orange add extra flavor. This dish is particularly good served with zucchini and mashed potatoes.

Serves 4
Preparation 10 minutes
Cooking 15 minutes

1 onion
6 juniper berries
1 tablespoon olive oil or canola oil
4 boneless, skinless duck breasts, about ¼ pound each
2 sprigs fresh rosemary
16 pitted prunes
⅔ cup peeled cooked chestnuts
pared zest of 1 orange
1½ cups red wine
8 orange slices, to garnish

Each serving provides
• 338 calories • 13 g fat • 3 g saturated fat • 32 g carbohydrates
• 26 g protein • 5 g fiber

ALTERNATIVE INGREDIENTS
• Try venison leg steaks or pork loin steaks instead of duck.
• Use dried peaches as a change from prunes. Cut the peaches in half and again widthwise to form chunks.
• Substitute cranberry juice or pomegranate juice for the red wine.
• Replace the chestnuts with small button mushrooms.

1 Slice the onion and crush the juniper berries. Heat a frying pan over high heat. Add the oil and the duck breasts and pan-fry for 1 minute on each side, pressing the duck on the hot pan to brown evenly. Reduce heat to medium, add the onion and rosemary, and cook for 2 minutes. Turn the duck and onions, cover, and cook for another 2 minutes. Transfer them to a plate.

2 Add the crushed juniper berries, prunes, chestnuts, and orange zest to the pan. Pour in the wine and bring to a boil over high heat. Boil for 3 minutes to reduce the wine.

3 Return the duck and onions to the pan with any juices and reduce heat to low. Cover and simmer for 3 minutes, stirring now and then. Divide the duck, chestnuts, and prunes among four plates. Spoon the sauce on top of each portion and garnish with orange slices.

COOK'S TIPS
● Juniper berries are one of the flavoring ingredients in gin. They are dark purple-black, tender, and easily crushed into small pieces with a mortar and pestle. You will find them in the herb and spice aisle in most large supermarkets.
● Cooked chestnuts are usually sold vacuum-packed or in cans.

SUPER FOOD

PRUNES
Prunes have the highest antioxidant score of all fruit, helping to protect the body against cancer. They also provide a concentrated source of valuable nutrients, including fiber, carbohydrates, vitamins, minerals, and phytonutrients—essential nutrients found in plants that help to keep us healthy.

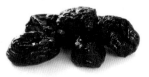

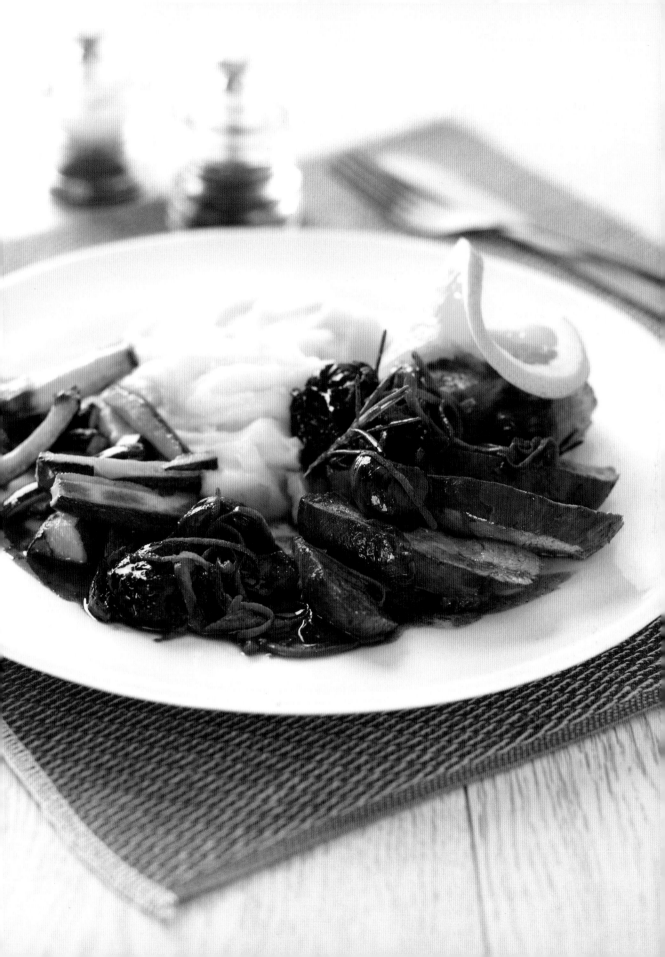

CHINESE **DUCK** WITH **PANCAKES**

A lower-fat version of crispy-skin duck, this recipe uses skinless duck breast, balancing the richness of the hoisin sauce with green bell peppers and a simple ginger marinade.

Serves 4
Preparation 15 minutes
Marinating 30–60 minutes
Cooking 8 minutes

¼ cup fresh grated ginger
1 clove garlic, crushed
1 tablespoon soy sauce
1 tablespoon sesame oil
⅓ cup dry sherry
4 boneless, skinless duck breasts, about ¼ pound each
1 green bell pepper
½ cucumber
8 scallions
2 tablespoons olive oil or canola oil
20 Chinese pancakes
4 tablespoons hoisin sauce

Each serving provides
• 459 calories • 18 g fat • 4 g saturated fat • 37 g carbohydrates • 29 g protein • 3 g fiber

ALTERNATIVE INGREDIENTS
• Instead of using whole duck breasts, try more economical stir-fry duck breasts. Stir-fry in hot oil for 3–5 minutes, then add the marinade and stir in the hoisin sauce. Bring to a boil, reduce the heat, and simmer for 1 minute.
• Pork or lamb steaks make a good alternative to duck.
• If you can't find Chinese pancakes, you can purchase ready-made crêpes at the supermarket and serve 2 large crêpes per portion.

1 Add the ginger to a large shallow dish. Stir in the garlic, soy sauce, sesame oil, and sherry. Add the duck and turn to coat in the marinade. Cover and marinate for 30–60 minutes. Cut the pepper and cucumber into sticks. Trim and slice the scallions into fine strips. Arrange the vegetables on a serving dish.

2 Heat the oil in a frying pan over high heat. Transfer the duck to the pan, reserving the marinade. Fry the duck for 1 minute on each side. Reduce heat to low, cover, and cook for 5 minutes, turning twice, until the duck is browned but still pink inside. Warm the pancakes according to the package directions.

3 Slice the duck and transfer it to a warmed serving dish. Add the marinade to the pan and boil the pan juices for 1 minute to thicken. Scrape the browned bits from the bottom of the pan and stir in the hoisin sauce before removing from the heat. Serve each pancake with vegetables, a few slices of duck, and the sauce.

COOK'S TIPS
● Marinate the duck breasts in a ziplock bag in the fridge for up to 24 hours to intensify the garlic flavor.
● To check whether the duck is cooked, pierce one breast with a small knife—if the meat is bloody, continue cooking; if it's pink but firm, it's done. If you prefer your duck well-done, cook the duck for 9–10 minutes, until the inside is brown.

SUPER FOOD

GINGER
Some studies have linked ginger to relief from arthritis and joint pain. Compounds in ginger called gingerols may have antioxidant properties, helping to protect against heart disease and some cancers.

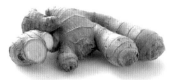

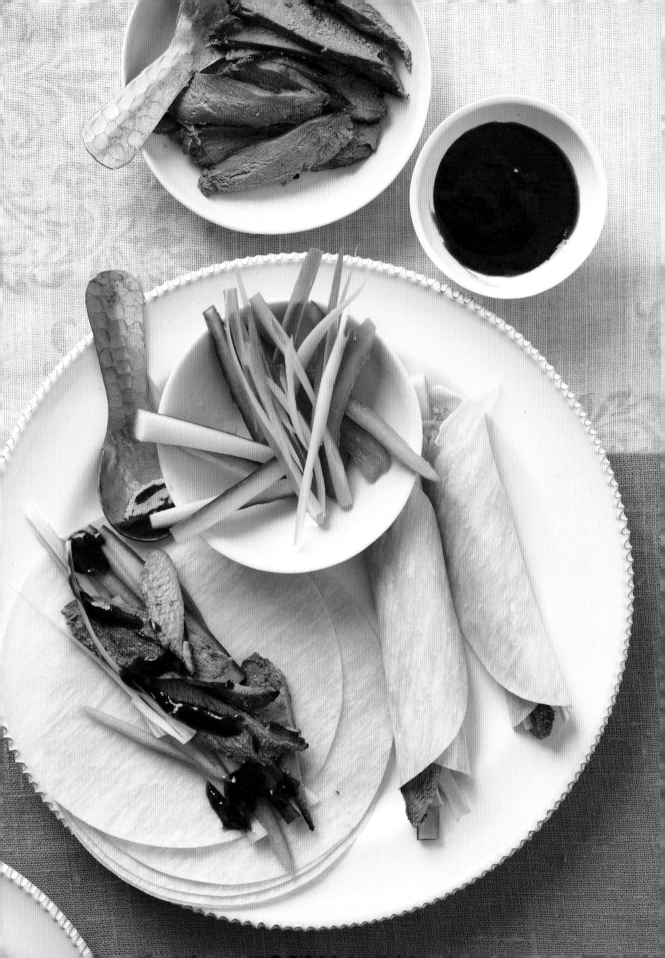

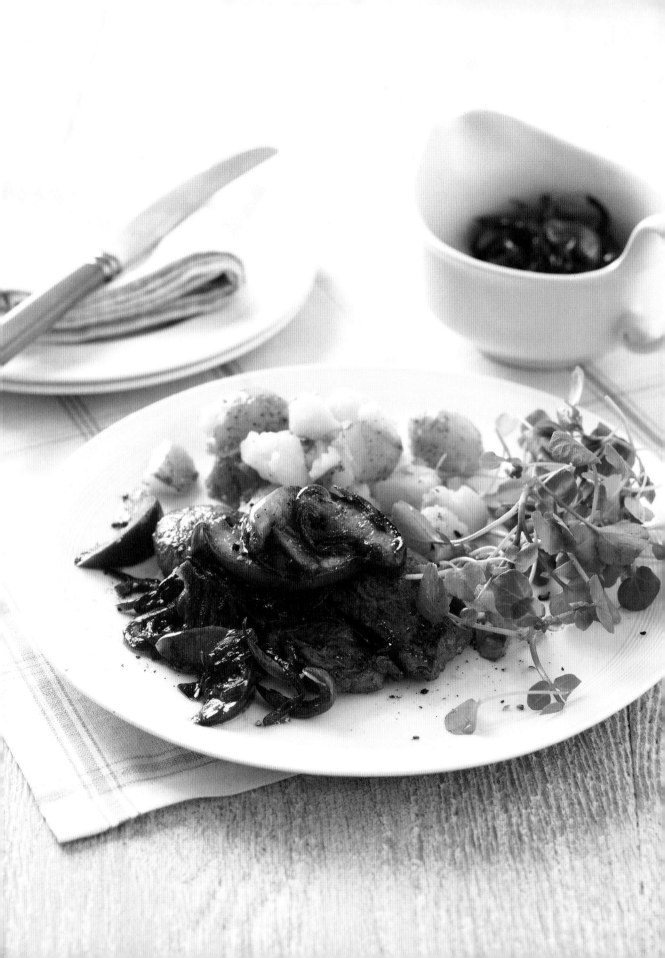

PAN-FRIED **VENISON** WITH **NECTARINE** CHUTNEY

Venison has about one-third the fat of beef, and is lower in saturated fat and calories, too. Dress it up with a fruity chutney, and serve with smashed potatoes and watercress for a mouthwatering, guilt-free steak dinner.

Serves 4
Preparation 15 minutes
Cooking 15 minutes

2 red onions
4 ripe nectarines
2 tablespoons olive oil or canola oil
2 tablespoons light brown sugar
2 tablespoons red wine vinegar
¼ teaspoon ground allspice
4 venison steaks,
   about ¼ pound each

Each serving provides
• 282 calories • 11 g fat • 2 g saturated fat • 20 g carbohydrates
• 30 g protein • 2 g fiber

ALTERNATIVE INGREDIENTS
• Use duck breasts, which also go well with fruit chutney, instead of venison.
• A pinch each of ground cinnamon and nutmeg, instead of allspice, gives warmth to the chutney.
• Try peaches, plums, or firm mangoes as a change from nectarines.

1 Thinly slice the onions and cut the nectarines into ½-inch slices. Heat 1 tablespoon of oil in a saucepan over a medium heat. Add the onions and cook for 5 minutes, or until beginning to brown. Stir in the sugar and vinegar and reduce heat to low. Stir in the allspice and nectarines. Cook for 3 minutes, or until the onions and nectarines soften.

2 Meanwhile, use scissors to snip off any membrane around the edge of the venison steaks as it will shrink during cooking causing the steaks to curl. Heat a large frying pan over high heat until very hot. Pour in the remaining tablespoon of oil and add the steaks. Cook for 2 minutes on each side, or until browned. Use a spatula to press them gently against the pan so that they brown evenly.

3 Reduce heat to medium-low and cook the steaks for another 2 minutes, turning once, until the meat is done to your liking (see Cook's Tips). Transfer the steaks to four warmed plates, season with freshly ground black pepper, and serve with the chutney.

COOK'S TIPS
● Cook the venison for 5 minutes, turning once, for a steak that is pink in the middle. Cook up to 8 minutes, turning twice, for a steak that is well-done throughout.
● Venison steaks vary in thickness, which will affect cooking time. Place the steaks between two sheet of plastic wrap, and pound them with a meat mallet or rolling pin until they are evenly thick. For this recipe, a steak ½- to ¾-inch thick is best.

SUPER FOOD

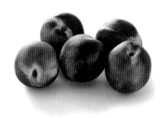

NECTARINES
As a good source of potassium, which lowers blood pressure, nectarines may help to protect against strokes. They also contain insoluble fiber for a healthy digestive system, plus soluble fiber to help lower blood cholesterol.

SAUSAGES WITH SWEET CORN RELISH

A honey and vinegar relish full of colorful vegetables makes an eye-catching accompaniment to meaty sausages. Serve with a green salad and crispy roasted potatoes for a satisfying meal.

Serves 4
Preparation 10 minutes
Cooking 20 minutes

2 bell peppers (1 red, 1 orange)
1 carrot
1 onion
8 meaty sausages, such as pork, bratwurst, or Italian style
2 tablespoons olive oil or canola oil
1 clove garlic, crushed
⅔ cup frozen sweet corn
1 teaspoon cornstarch
3 tablespoons cider vinegar
3 tablespoons honey
1 tablespoon whole-grain mustard

Each serving provides
• 474 calories • 26 g fat • 7 g saturated fat • 34 g carbohydrates • 28 g protein • 5 g fiber

ALTERNATIVE INGREDIENTS
• Transform the relish into a cold accompaniment by reducing the vinegar and honey to 1 tablespoon each. Add ⅓ cup frozen fava beans with the corn. Stir in the vinegar and honey but leave out the cornstarch and mustard. Allow the relish to cool before serving.
• Serve sliced sausages on top of large baked potatoes with the relish. Add a spoonful of crème fraîche or Greek yogurt.
• Try some of the delicious low-fat varieties of sausage, such as turkey or chicken.

1 Preheat the broiler to high. Finely dice the peppers and carrot, and chop the onion. Broil the sausages for 20 minutes, turning, until they are evenly browned.

2 Meanwhile, heat the oil in a saucepan over high heat. Add the pepper, carrot, onion, and garlic. Mix well, reduce heat to medium, and cook for 5 minutes, stirring occasionally, until the vegetables soften. Stir in the corn, cover, and cook for 1 minute, or until the corn has thawed.

3 Mix the cornstarch with the vinegar to form a paste. Stir the honey, mustard, and vinegar paste into the pan. Bring the relish to a boil and simmer for 1 minute. Transfer the cooked sausages to four plates and serve with the relish.

COOK'S TIP
● If the oven is already hot for roasting potatoes, save energy by also roasting the sausages in a shallow ovenproof dish or pan. Allow about 30 minutes at 350°F, until the skins are browned and the sausages are done, turning them halfway through cooking.

SUPER FOOD

SWEET CORN
The distinctive yellow color of corn is due to the pigment lutein, a compound with an important role in eye health. Lutein can help protect eyes from age-related macular degeneration, an increasingly common form of blindness.

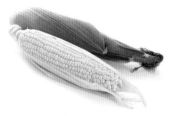

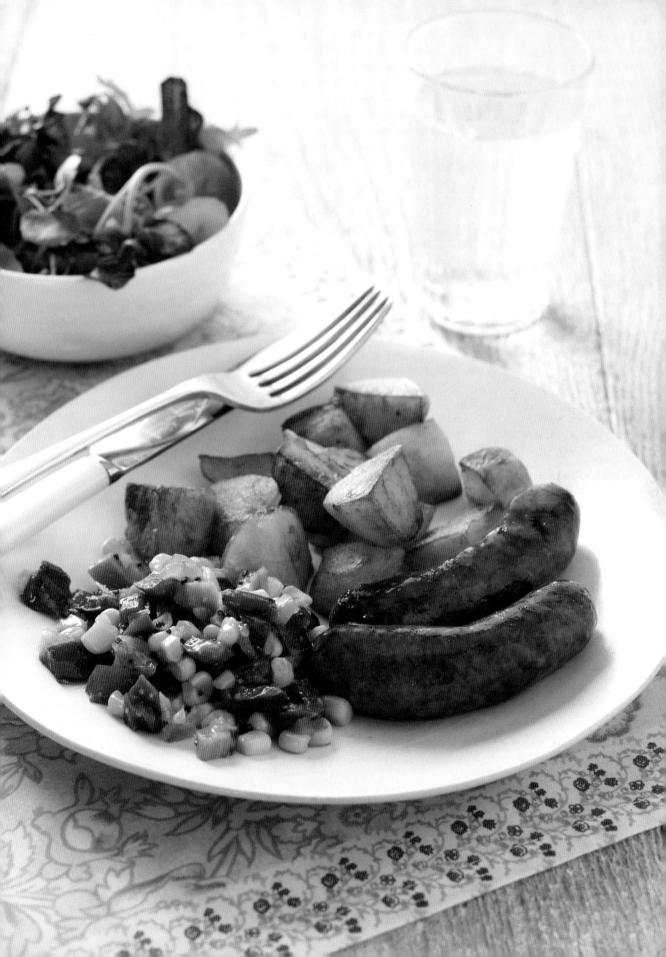

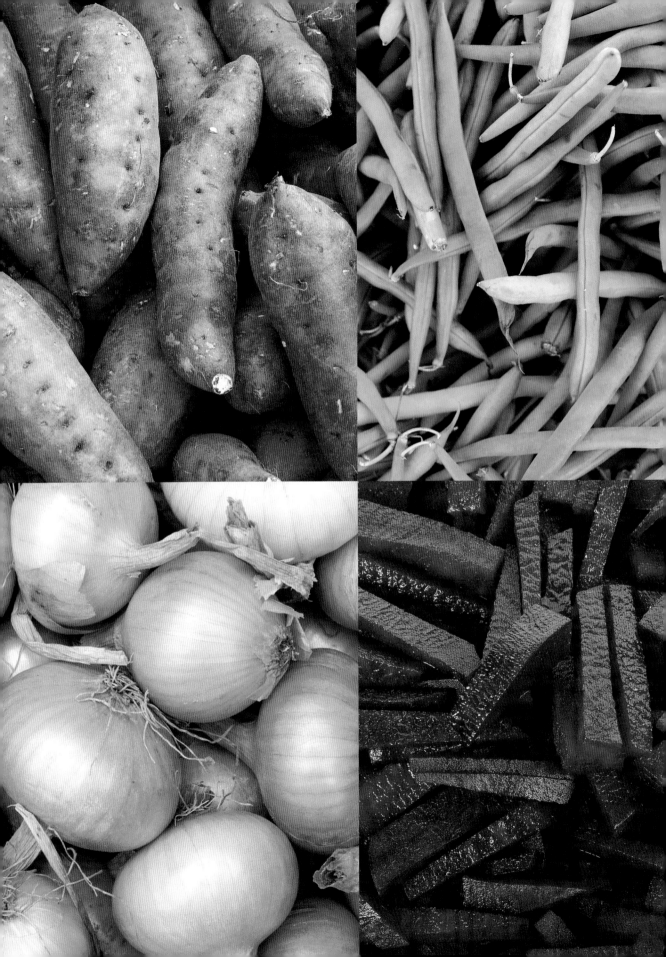

MEAT

LAMB MEDALLIONS WITH RED CURRANT JUS

This quick, lower-fat version of a slow-roasted country classic has lost none of its flavor or goodness. Team it with smashed new potatoes for a hearty, comforting meal.

Serves 4
Preparation 10 minutes
Cooking 15 minutes

½ pound new potatoes
2 leeks
1 pound lamb loin fillet
3 tablespoons olive oil
1 cup small broccoli florets
1 can (**15 ounces**) cannellini beans, drained
2 chopped fresh rosemary sprigs
⅓ cup balsamic vinegar
2 tablespoons red currant jelly

Each serving provides
• 437 calories • 28 g fat • 9 g saturated fat • 20 g carbohydrates
• 26 g protein • 2 g fiber

ALTERNATIVE INGREDIENTS
• As a less expensive alternative to fillet, slice lean lamb steaks at an angle into thick slices across the grain of the meat.
• Sliced pork tenderloin or pork strips make good alternatives to lamb.
• Try chickpeas, borlotti beans, or navy beans instead of cannellini beans.
• Red currant jelly has a sharp-sweet flavor. Other suitable fruit preserves include crabapple jelly and orange marmalade.

1 Boil the potatoes in a pan of water for 15 minutes, or until cooked. Meanwhile, slice the leeks, cut each slice in half, and rinse in a colander. Cut the lamb fillet into ¾-inch-thick slices. Heat 2 tablespoons oil in a large frying pan over high heat. Add the leeks, reduce heat to medium, and cook, stirring, for 3 minutes, or until tender.

2 Add the broccoli and cook, stirring, for another 3 minutes. Stir in the cannellini beans and heat through for 1 minute. Put the vegetables and beans in a dish, cover, and keep warm.

3 Add the remaining tablespoon oil, lamb slices, and rosemary to the pan. Cook over medium-high heat for 2 minutes, pressing the lamb slices into the pan to brown quickly and evenly. Turn the slices and cook for another 3 minutes, or until browned. Transfer the lamb to the dish with the vegetables and keep warm.

4 Reheat the pan over high heat. Pour in 4 tablespoons of water and the balsamic vinegar. Add the red currant jelly, stirring until melted. Boil the sauce rapidly, stirring continuously, for 1 minute. Drain the potatoes and gently crush them with a fork. Divide the lamb, beans, and potatoes among four plates and spoon the sauce over each portion.

COOK'S TIP
● Fillet of lamb is a lean cut from the neck or loin. It is sometimes sold as tenderloin or pre-sliced medallions. This recipe uses loin fillet because it cooks relatively quickly without becoming tough.

SUPER FOOD

CANNELLINI BEANS
As with other beans, cannellini beans score low on the glycemic index (GI), which makes them a longer-lasting energy source than many other foods. These beans also contain high levels of fiber—good news for heart and digestive health.

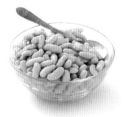

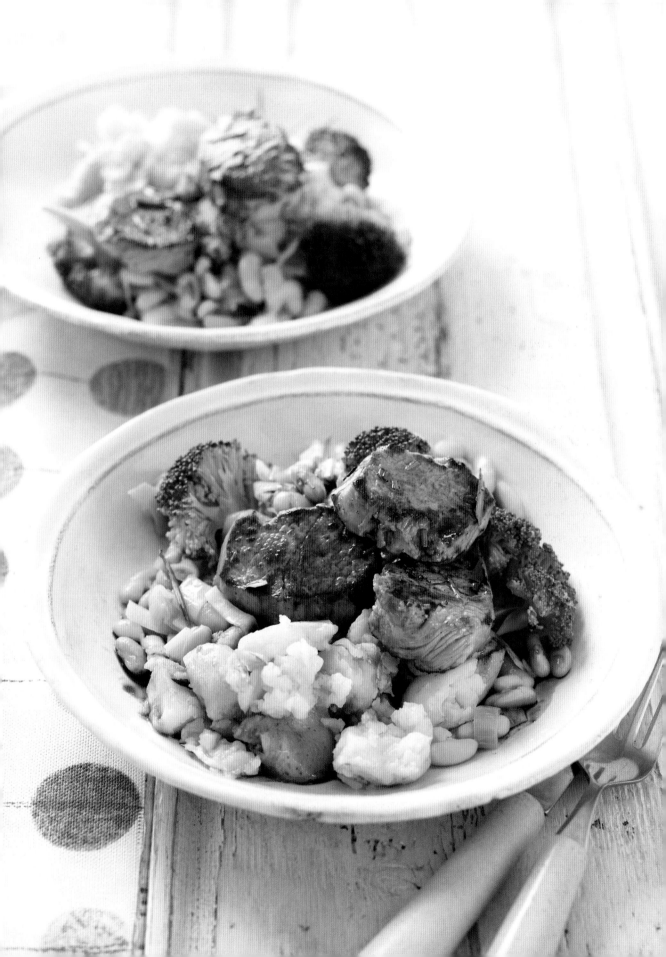

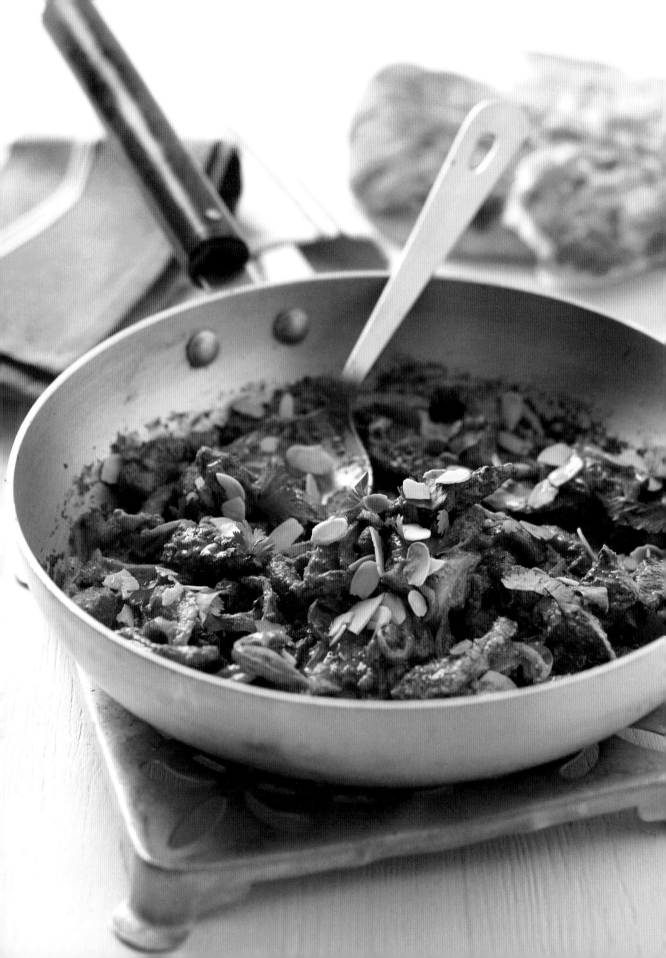

INDIAN **LAMB** WITH **APRICOTS**

Everyone enjoys a no-fuss meal on the weekend and this korma-style curry is both quick and nutritious. Serve the tender strips of lamb and succulent apricots with warmed naan.

Serves 4
Preparation 15 minutes
Cooking 12 minutes

4 tablespoons sliced almonds
¾ pound lean lamb
1 onion
½ cup sliced dried apricots
1 tablespoon olive oil or canola oil
1 large clove garlic, crushed
4 tablespoons ground almonds
1 tablespoon tandoori spice mix
1 cup plain yogurt
2 tablespoons chopped fresh
   cilantro leaves

Each serving provides
• 294 calories • 15 g fat • 4 g saturated fat • 17 g carbohydrates • 23 g protein • 7 g fiber

ALTERNATIVE INGREDIENTS
• For a change, use pork or chicken instead of lamb.
• For a full-flavored alternative, try ostrich or bison, now sold in many supermarkets—lean meats that are great for stir-frying.
• If you can't find tandoori spice mix, good-quality curry powder works well.
• Try pistachios instead of almonds, toasting them very lightly.
• Reduce the apricots to ⅓ cup and add 2 tablespoons dried cranberries.

1 Toast the almonds in a large, dry frying pan over medium heat, shaking the pan occasionally, until they are browned. Remove from the pan and set aside. Cut the lamb into bite-sized strips and halve and thinly slice the onion.

2 Increase heat to high, add the oil, and cook the lamb for about 4 minutes, or until the meat is browned. Add the onion and garlic to the pan. Cook for 2 minutes, or until the onion begins to soften.

3 Stir the apricots, ground almonds, and spice mix into the lamb and continue to cook for 2–3 minutes, reducing the heat slightly so the mixture doesn't burn.

4 Add the yogurt carefully, so the hot liquid won't spit. Let the sauce bubble for 1–2 minutes, stirring, until it is thick and creamy. Add the cilantro leaves and toasted almonds just before serving.

COOK'S TIPS
● Scissors work better than a knife for cutting apricots into strips.
● Leg steaks or fillet are the best cuts of lamb for this recipe. You can use pre-cut stir-fry strips, too.
● Getting the pan hot before adding the meat is the key to a tasty result. This lets the meat brown and cook quickly, becoming tender and succulent, instead of stewing—and toughening—in its own juices.

SUPER FOOD

DRIED APRICOTS
Good for eye, heart, and digestive health, just three dried apricots count as one of your seven-a-day servings of fruit and vegetables. Unusual for a fruit, dried apricots are a useful source of calcium, which is good for keeping bones strong.

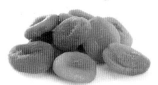

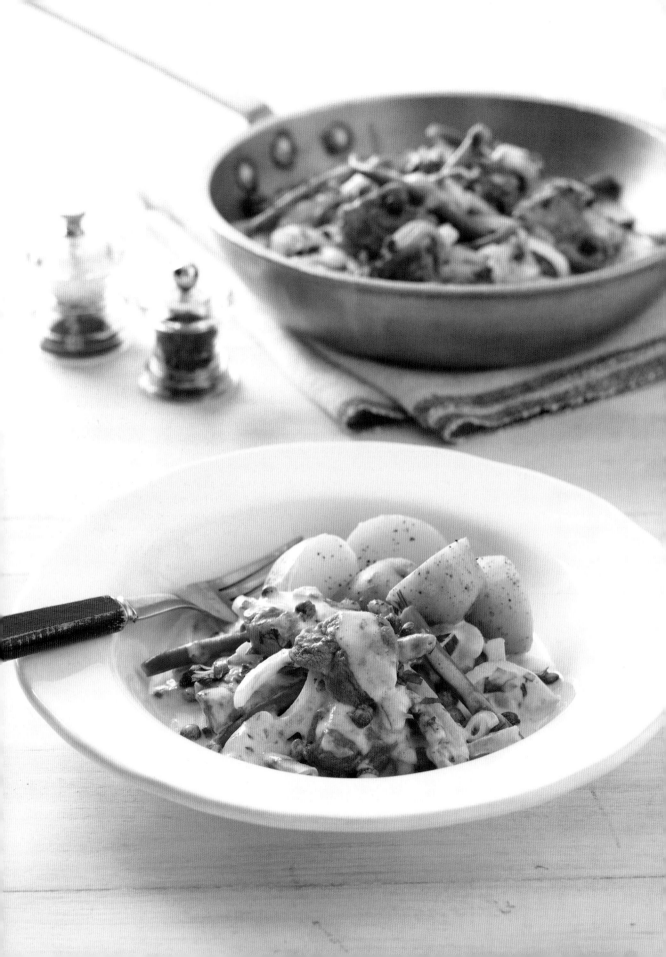

SAUTÉED **LAMB** AND **GREEN BEANS** WITH CREAMY **CAPER** SAUCE

A seemingly self-indulgent dish cleverly deceives your tastebuds by using low-fat cream cheese instead of cream. Salty capers work brilliantly with lamb and give a real flavor kick. Serve with boiled new potatoes.

Serves 4
Preparation 10 minutes
Cooking 20 minutes

1 onion
1 pound lamb fillet, trimmed of fat
2 tablespoons capers
1 tablespoon olive oil or canola oil
1 cup frozen green beans
1 teaspoon cornstarch
2 tablespoons low-fat (1%) milk
½ cup low-fat cream cheese or
    ½ cup grated low-fat cheddar
3 tablespoons chopped fresh parsley

Each serving provides
· 252 calories · 12 g fat · 3 g saturated fat · 6 g carbohydrates · 27 g protein · 3 g fiber

ALTERNATIVE INGREDIENTS
· Fresh green beans work just as well as frozen ones. Trim them and cook in boiling water for 2–3 minutes until just tender. Drain and continue as for the frozen beans.
· Use frozen fava beans instead of green beans.
· Try thin veal or pork scallops instead of lamb. Cook the meat as is, frying it on each side, or cut it into thin strips and stir-fry.

1 Slice the onion, then slice the lamb into ½-inch-thick pieces. Drain and rinse the capers. Heat the oil in a large frying pan over high heat. Add the onion, reduce heat to medium, and cook for 5 minutes, or until the onion begins to soften and brown.

2 Push the onion to one side of the pan and add the lamb. Cook for 6 minutes, turning the meat occasionally and pressing on the pieces in the hot pan so they brown evenly. Add the green beans and onion and cook, stirring, for another 2 minutes. In a small dish, stir the cornstarch and milk together to form a smooth paste. Use tongs or a slotted spoon to transfer the meat, beans, and onion to a dish and keep warm.

3 Add 6 tablespoons of boiling water to the pan and boil over high heat, stirring with a whisk. Reduce heat to low, whisk in the milk and cornstarch paste, and return to a boil. Beat the cream cheese lightly with a fork to soften it and gradually whisk it into the sauce until smooth and hot. Stir in the capers and parsley. Transfer the lamb and beans to four plates and spoon a little sauce over each portion.

COOK'S TIP
● When adding boiling water to the pan in step 3, scrape up any browned bits from the bottom of the pan with the whisk. This will add extra flavor to the creamy caper sauce.

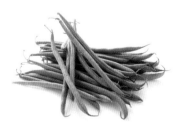

SUPER FOOD

GREEN BEANS
This versatile vegetable is a good source of both vitamins and minerals, including some calcium and folate. Just 4 tablespoons of green beans count as one of your seven-a-day, and with virtually no fat, they are a low-calorie bonus to any weight-management program.

DEVILED **STEAK** AND **PEPPERS**

A hot tomato-and-mustard coating gives plenty of 'devilish' flavor to lean beef. Sun-ripened peppers and onions soak up the delicious pan juices. Serve with oven-roasted potato wedges.

Serves 4
Preparation 15 minutes
Cooking 10 minutes

1 tablespoon tomato paste
2 tablespoons whole-grain mustard
4 thin beef scallopini, about
   ¼ pound each
4 tablespoons rolled oats
4 bell peppers (2 red, 2 yellow)
2 onions
2 tablespoons olive oil or canola oil

Each serving provides
• 260 calories • 13 g fat • 3 g
saturated fat • 16 g carbohydrates
• 21 g protein • 5 g fiber

ALTERNATIVE INGREDIENTS
• When time is short, serve the steaks in hamburger buns with a side salad.
• For a spicier topping, add 1 crushed clove garlic and a pinch of red pepper flakes to the tomato mixture.
• Use pork, veal, chicken, or turkey scallopini instead of beef.
• To make a rich mushroom glaze for this dish, sauté 1 cup sliced or whole button mushrooms for 2–3 minutes in the pan after cooking the meat. Add 2 tablespoons brandy and boil rapidly to reduce the sauce to a thick consistency. Remove from the heat and serve over the steak.

1 Mix the tomato paste and whole-grain mustard and spread a thin layer of the mixture on one side of the beef. Sprinkle with the oats and press to make the coating. Turn and repeat on the other sides to make coated steaks. Slice the peppers and onions into long strips.

2 Heat a large nonstick frying pan over high heat. Add 1 tablespoon oil, reduce heat to medium and add the steaks. Press down on the steaks gently but firmly with a spatula for 3 minutes, or until the oat topping is crisp and golden. Turn the steaks and cook for 2 minutes, or until browned. Transfer to four plates and keep warm.

3 Reheat the pan over high heat and add the remaining oil, peppers, and onions. Cook for 2 minutes, stirring the juices in the pan. Reduce the heat and cook for another 3 minutes, or until the vegetables slightly soften. Transfer the peppers and onions to the plates and serve.

COOK'S TIP
● Scallopini is an Italian term for thinly sliced meat. Be sure that you buy beef scallopini rather than thin frying steaks. Beef scallopini are lean and not marbled with fat, making them ideal for coating. In addition, they don't have the chewy connective tissue that some thin steaks have, which needs to be removed before cooking.

SUPER FOOD

OATS
Because they help to stabilize blood glucose levels, oats, if eaten regularly, can lower the risk of developing type 2 diabetes. As part of a low-fat diet, oats can also help to lower blood cholesterol levels, which may lessen the risk of developing heart disease.

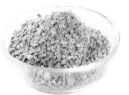

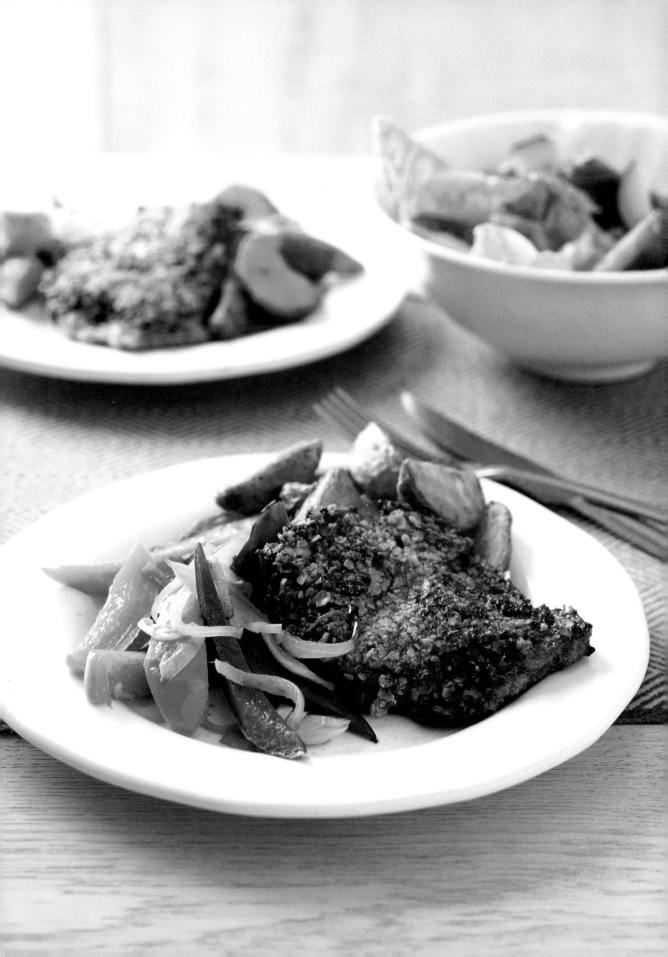

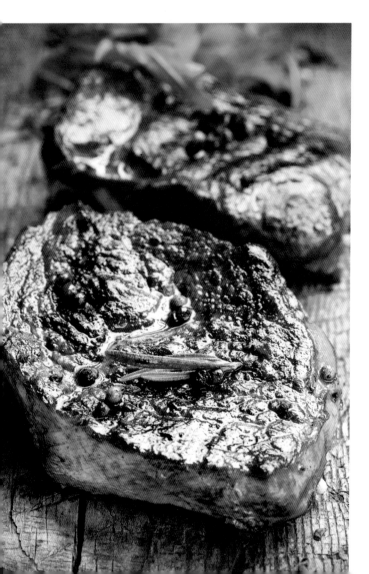

SUPER FOOD

BEEF

Lean beef is an excellent source of high-quality protein—just one 2-ounce serving provides up to a third of your daily needs. It also contains only about 5 percent fat, almost half of which is the healthier monounsaturated type. Rich in iron, zinc, and B vitamins, beef helps to boost the immune system and improves the health of your blood.

ITALIAN SUMMER CASSEROLE

Serves 4
Preparation 10 minutes Cooking 40 minutes

Each serving provides • 243 calories • 12 g fat • 3 g saturated fat • 8 g carbohydrates • 27 g protein • 2 g fiber

Heat **1 tablespoon olive oil or canola oil** in a ovenproof baking dish over medium heat. Slice **1 onion** and **1 yellow bell pepper** and add them to the dish. Cook for 5 minutes, stirring occasionally. Add **1 chopped clove garlic** and **1 pound thinly sliced lean beef steak**. Sauté for 2 minutes or until the meat is lightly browned. Add **1 can (14½ ounces) chopped tomatoes, 1 tablespoon red pepper pesto, 1 beef stock cube, ½ cup boiling water,** and **2 tablespoons chopped fresh parsley**. Bring to a boil, reduce heat to low, cover, and simmer for 20 minutes, stirring halfway through. Uncover and cook for another 5–10 minutes, or until the liquid is reduced but not dry. Scatter **¼ cup sliced pitted green olives** over each portion and serve.

COOK'S TIPS

● For quick cooking, a cut of beef such as rump or sirloin is best, but less expensive chuck steak is fine. Trim any excess fat and increase cooking time to 1 hour, adding more water to the pan as needed to prevent the meat from drying out.
● Serve the casserole with new potatoes and a green vegetable, or with whole-wheat penne pasta.

BEEF AND VEGETABLE BOLOGNESE SAUCE

Serves 4
Preparation 10 minutes Cooking 1 hour 10 minutes

Each serving provides • 201 calories • 8 g fat • 2 g saturated fat • 10 g carbohydrates • 23 g protein • 3 g fiber

Heat **1 tablespoon olive oil** in a large frying pan and add **1 large onion, 1 large carrot** and **1 large celery stalk**, all finely chopped. Sauté over medium-high heat, stirring occasionally, for 5 minutes, or until the onion softens. Push the vegetables to the side of the pan and add **¾ pound lean ground beef**. Increase heat and fry the meat for 2 minutes to brown slightly. Stir in **1 cup canned chopped tomatoes, 1 tablespoon tomato purée, 1 beef stock cube, ½ cup boiling** water and **2 teaspoons mixed dried herbs**. Season to taste. Bring to a boil, reduce heat to low, cover, and simmer for 1 hour, adding a little water if needed to prevent the sauce from drying out.

COOK'S TIP
● Serve the bolognese sauce over whole-wheat spaghetti or brown rice and top with grated parmesan and some extra ground black pepper.

SPINACH, BEEF, AND BEAN SPROUT STIR-FRY

Serves 4
Preparation 10 minutes Cooking 7 minutes

Each serving provides • 192 calories • 9 g fat
• 3 g saturated fat • 3 g carbohydrates • 26 g protein
• 2 g fiber

Heat **1 tablespoon olive oil or canola oil** in a wok or large frying pan over high heat. Add **1 pound lean beef steak strips** and cook, stirring occasionally, for 1–2 minutes, or until browned. Reduce heat to medium-high and stir in **1 finely chopped red chile** and **2 teaspoons grated fresh ginger**. Add **6 chopped scallions, 6 ounces baby spinach** and **½ cup fresh bean sprouts**. Stir-fry for 2 minutes, or until the spinach has wilted and the bean sprouts are thoroughly cooked. Stir in **2 teaspoons soy sauce, 1 beef stock cube** and **½ cup boiling water** and cook 1–2 minutes. Transfer the stir-fry to four plates and garnish with **2 tablespoons chopped fresh cilantro**.

SWEET POTATO AND MUSHROOM COTTAGE PIE

Serves 4
Preparation 10 minutes Cooking 1 hour 10 minutes

Each serving provides • 408 calories • 17 g fat
• 4 g saturated fat • 43 g carbohydrates • 26 g protein
• 7 g fiber

Preheat the oven to 350°F. Bake **1¼ pounds unpeeled sweet potatoes** for about 45 minutes, or until tender. Meanwhile, heat **1 tablespoon olive oil or canola oil** in a large saucepan and add **1 finely chopped onion** and **1 diced carrot**. Cook over a medium heat, stirring, for 5 minutes, then add **¾ pound lean ground beef**. Cook for 2–3 minutes until lightly browned. Stir in **⅔ cup roughly chopped mushrooms, 1 can (14½ ounces) chopped tomatoes**, **2 teaspoons mixed dried herbs**,

and **2 tablespoons tomato paste**. Add **1 cup hot beef stock**. Bring to a boil, reduce heat to low, cover, and simmer for 30 minutes, stirring occasionally. When the potatoes are cooked, remove from the oven and increase oven temperature to 375°F. Carefully scoop the sweet potato flesh into a bowl and mash with **2 tablespoons olive oil** and **¼ cup low-fat (1%) milk**. Season to taste. Transfer the beef mixture to an ovenproof dish and spread the mashed sweet potatoes on top. Bake for 25 minutes and serve.

COOK'S TIP
● Instead of baking the sweet potatoes in the oven, microwave on high for 8 minutes, or until cooked.

PAPRIKA BEEF FAJITAS

Serves 4
Preparation 5 minutes Cooking 8 minutes

Each serving provides • 192 calories • 9 g fat
• 3 g saturated fat • 3 g carbohydrates • 26 g protein
• 2 g fiber

Thinly cut **¾ pound lean beef steak** into ¾-inch-thick strips and place in a shallow bowl. Sprinkle with **2 teaspoons paprika** and toss well to coat. Thinly slice **1 red onion** and **2 red bell peppers**. Heat **1 tablespoon olive oil or canola oil** in a large frying pan over medium-high heat and sauté the onion and pepper for 5 minutes, stirring until softened. Add **2 finely chopped jalapeños** or other **mild chilies** for the last 2 minutes of cooking. Season to taste, transfer vegetables to a plate, and keep warm. Heat **1 tablespoon olive oil or canola oil** in the pan and add the beef strips. Cook over high heat for 2 minutes. Gently warm **4 flour tortillas** in the microwave for 30 seconds on high. Divide the beef and cooked vegetables among the tortillas. Add **1 tablespoon mild tomato salsa** and **1 tablespoon reduced-fat sour cream** to each fajita, roll up, and serve.

COOK'S TIPS
● To save time, look for pre-sliced stir-fry strips of beef in the supermarket.
● Add slices of peeled ripe avocado to the tortillas, before rolling up, for a creamy texture.
● Serve with shredded lettuce.

BEEF AND PEPPER BURGERS

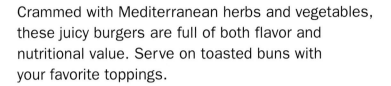

Crammed with Mediterranean herbs and vegetables, these juicy burgers are full of both flavor and nutritional value. Serve on toasted buns with your favorite toppings.

Serves 4
Preparation 15 minutes
Cooking 14 minutes

2 large carrots
2 scallions
1 small red bell pepper
1 egg
1 slice whole-grain bread
2 cloves garlic, crushed
1 teaspoon dried oregano
2 tablespoons tomato paste
¼ cup rolled oats
½ pound lean ground beef
1 tablespoon sunflower oil
4 medium burger buns
arugula, lettuce leaves, and
   tomato slices, to serve

Each serving provides
• 412 calories • 14 g fat • 3 g
saturated fat • 44 g carbohydrates
• 24 g protein • 7 g fiber

ALTERNATIVE INGREDIENTS
• You can use ground lamb instead of beef, although lamb has a much higher fat content.
• Try ground venison or bison instead of ground beef for a richly flavored low-fat alternative.

1 Preheat the broiler to medium-high. Finely grate the carrots, thinly slice the scallions, and finely chop the pepper. Beat the egg in a large bowl. Add the bread and turn in the egg a couple of times. Add the carrots, scallions, pepper, and garlic, but don't mix them in.

2 Stir in the oregano and tomato paste, breaking up the bread. Mix in the oats, ground beef, and a little salt and pepper. Use your hands to thoroughly mix the ingredients.

3 Line a broiler pan with foil. Shape meat mixture into four 4-inch burgers by first rolling into balls, then patting them flat. Place the burgers on the foil and brush with ½ tablespoon oil. Broil for 7 minutes, or until sizzling and browned.

4 Carefully turn the burgers using a large spatula, brush with the remaining ½ tablespoon oil, and cook for another 7 minutes. Let stand for 2–3 minutes before serving.

COOK'S TIPS
● Make a big batch of burgers and freeze them for future use. They will keep for at least 6 months wrapped tightly in plastic wrap and aluminum foil. They can be cooked from frozen by broiling slowly for 20–25 minutes.
● To make your own fresh ground beef, add ½ pound of lean steak to a meat grinder or food processor and process until crumbly.

SUPER FOOD

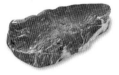

RED MEAT
Lean cuts are the healthiest choice for red meat, with any visible fat removed before cooking. Red meat is a key source of heme iron—the iron within the blood pigment hemoglobin—that is easily absorbed by the body and essential for healthy blood. Red meat also contains zinc to boost the immune system.

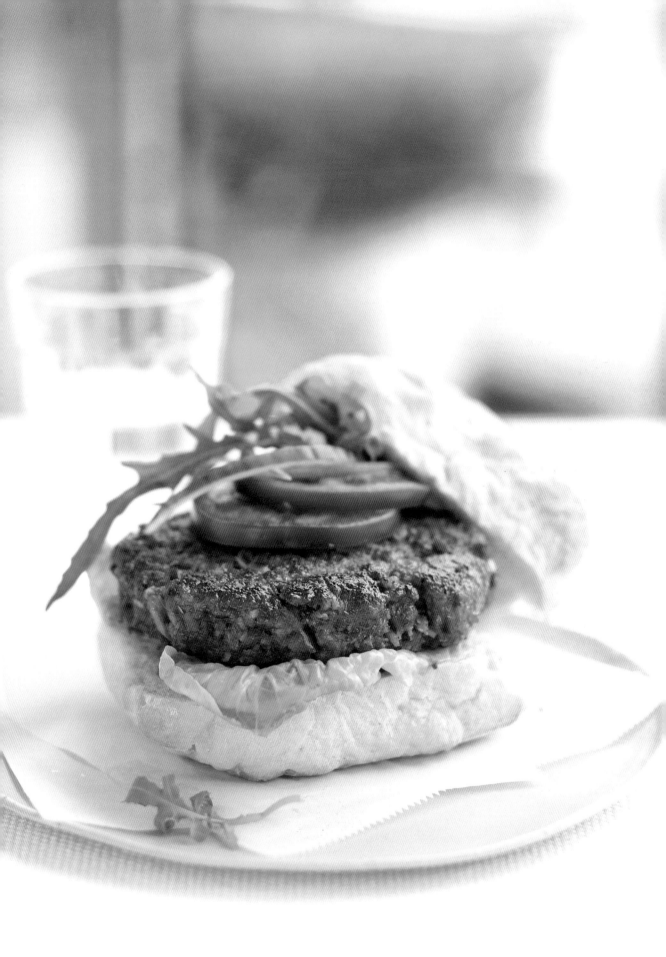

STEAK AND BEET STROGANOFF

A clever way to lighten classic stroganoff is to use another Russian favorite—beets—with yogurt instead of sour cream to reduce fat and add calcium. Noodles are traditional, but rice would also be nice.

Serves 4
Preparation 15 minutes
Cooking 17 minutes

1 large onion
¾ pound white mushrooms
1 pound lean top round steak
1 cup cooked beets, cut in
   ¾-inch strips
2 tablespoons sunflower oil
1 tablespoon whole-grain mustard
½ cup plain yogurt
2 tablespoons fresh thyme
   or oregano leaves

Each serving provides
• 290 calories • 14 g fat • 4 g saturated fat • 13 g carbohydrates
• 29 g protein • 4 g fiber

ALTERNATIVE INGREDIENTS
• Lamb is delicious cooked this way as an alternative to beef. Select lamb fillets or thin leg steaks.
• Lightly cooked carrot strips are tasty with beef in place of beets.
• Add tarragon instead of thyme or oregano.

1 Finely slice the onion and mushrooms and cut the steak into ¾-inch strips. Heat 1 tablespoon of the oil in a large frying pan over high heat. Sauté the onion for 5 minutes, or until it begins to brown. Add the mushrooms and cook for another 5 minutes, or until softened. Transfer the onion and mushrooms to a bowl and stir in the mustard.

2 Add the remaining tablespoon of oil to the pan and fry the steak over high heat for 3 minutes. Reduce heat slightly, if the steak is starting to burn, and continue to cook for 3 minutes until browned. Any juices should have evaporated, leaving the meat moist.

3 Stir in the beets and cook for 1 minute. Season to taste and gently fold in the onions and mushrooms. Add half the yogurt and remove the pan from the heat. Stir the mixture, sprinkle with thyme or oregano leaves, and divide among four plates. Drizzle each portion with a little of the remaining yogurt before serving.

COOK'S TIPS
● To save time, buy pre-sliced stir-fry beef strips, available at the supermarket meat counter.
● When buying cooked beets, make sure that you choose ones packed in their natural juices, not preserved in vinegar or your dish will have an unpleasant sour taste.

SUPER FOOD

BEETS
Fat-free, low-calorie, and a source of fiber, beets are good for maintaining a healthy digestive system. They also contain plenty of folate for heart, circulation, and pregnancy benefits, plus potassium to help regulate blood pressure.

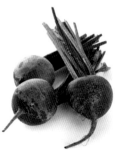

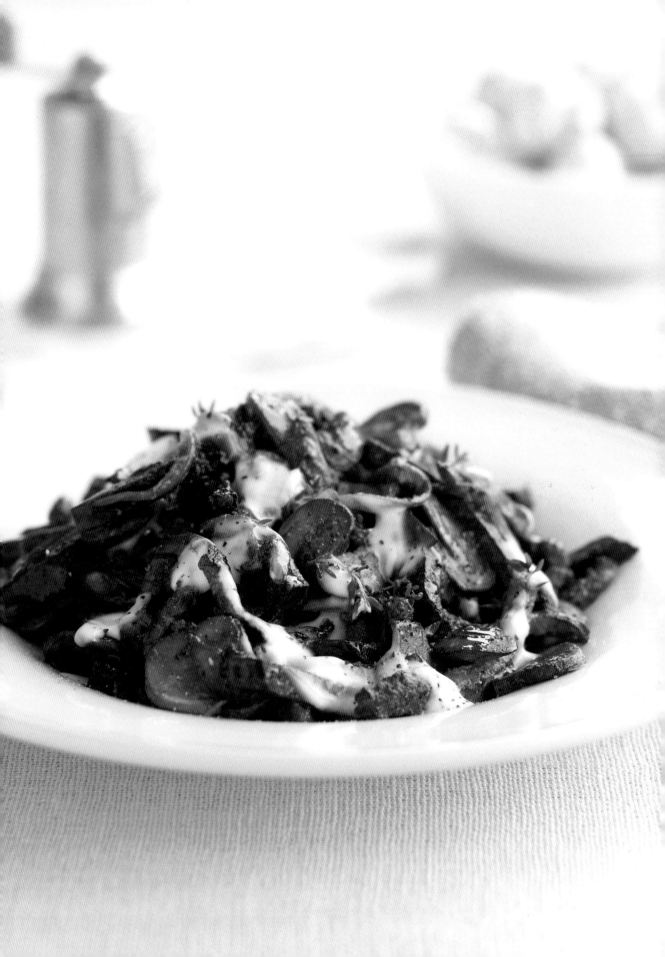

VEAL SCALLOPINI IN BRANDY SAUCE WITH SOUR CHERRIES

The bittersweet flavor of dried sour cherries is superb with lean, tender veal and a tantalizing brandy sauce satisfies even the most discerning palate. Serve with mashed potatoes.

Serves 4
Preparation 10 minutes
Cooking 10 minutes

1 onion
2 tablespoons olive oil or canola oil
1 clove garlic, crushed
1 cup small cremini mushrooms
4 veal scallopini, about ¼ pound
   each
⅓ cup dried sour cherries
4 tablespoons brandy
5 tablespoons hot chicken
   or vegetable stock
4 tablespoons chopped fresh parsley,
   to garnish

Each serving provides
• 252 calories • 3 g fat • 1 g
saturated fat • 23 g carbohydrates
• 34 g protein • 3 g fiber

ALTERNATIVE INGREDIENTS
• Use beef or pork scallopini instead
of veal. Lamb steaks or cutlets would
also go nicely with mushrooms. Cook
the lamb for 2–4 minutes on each side
after browning, depending on how
well-done you like your meat.
• Try sliced pitted prunes instead of
dried sour cherries.
• Unsweetened apple juice can be
used instead of brandy.

1 Thinly slice the onion. Heat the oil in a large frying pan over high heat. Add the sliced onion and garlic and cook, stirring frequently, for 2 minutes, or until softened.

2 Add the mushrooms and continue to cook for 2 minutes, or until the onion begins to turn golden. Use a slotted spoon to transfer the mushroom and onion mixture to a dish and set aside.

3 Add the veal to the pan and cook over high heat for 1 minute on each side, using a spatula to press the meat gently against the hot pan to brown both sides evenly. Reduce heat to medium or medium-low and cook for another 2 minutes, or until the meat is done.

4 Transfer the veal to four warmed plates. Return the mushroom and onion mixture to the pan and add the cherries and brandy. Increase heat to high and boil, stirring, for 1 minute. Add the hot stock and boil for another minute. Divide among the plates. Garnish each serving with a tablespoon of parsley.

COOK'S TIPS
● Veal scallopini are thin, tender, and quick to cook in a frying pan. Browning the meat, as done here, enhances the flavor and minimizes the amount of oil used in cooking.
● Dried sour cherries are usually stocked in the baking section or dried fruit aisle in the supermarket.

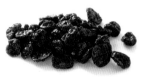

SUPER FOOD

DRIED CHERRIES
Rich in the plant-based antioxidants known as anthocyanins, dried cherries are good for protecting against heart disease. They are also fat-free, a good source of fiber, and provide an energy boost any time of day.

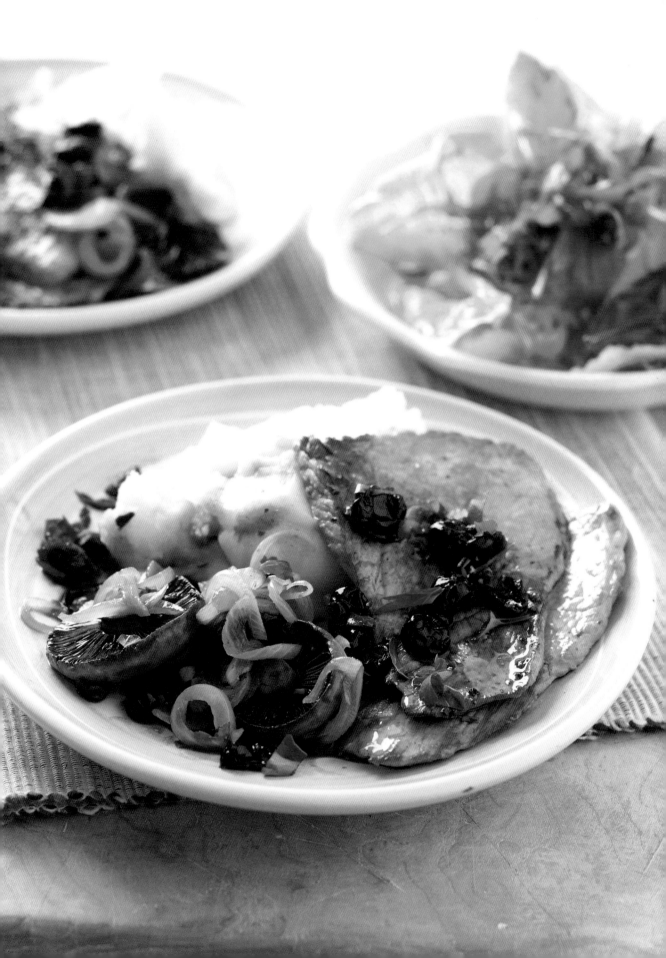

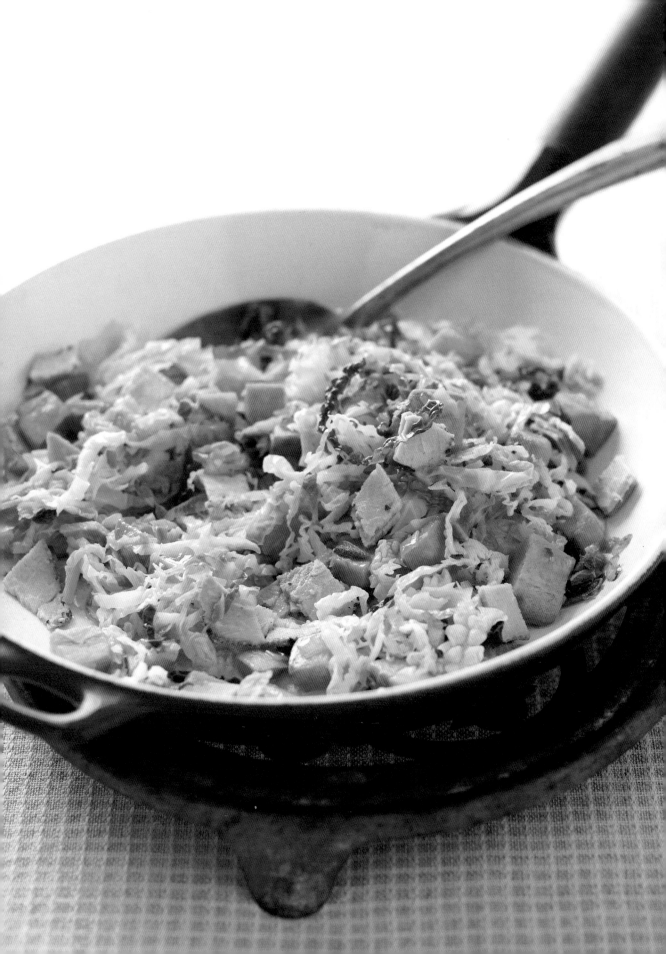

HAM AND SWEET POTATO
BUBBLE AND SQUEAK

Bubble and squeak is a traditional English dish, usually made with potatoes and cabbage, and so named because it makes bubbling and squeaking noises during cooking. Here, creamy sweet potatoes and juicy ham increase both the nutrient and flavor quotient of this family favorite.

Serves 4
Preparation 15 minutes
Cooking 15 minutes

1 leek
¾ pound sweet potatoes
½ pound lean cooked ham
½ pound cabbage, such as savoy
2 tablespoons olive oil
4 large shredded fresh sage leaves

Each serving provides
• 267 calories • 14 g fat • 3 g saturated fat • 22 g carbohydrates • 15 g protein • 5 g fiber

ALTERNATIVE INGREDIENTS
• Try a mix of parsnips, turnips, or potatoes instead of sweet potatoes.
• As a change from ham, use any cooked poultry or meat, such as corned beef, chicken, or leftover roast pork.
• Add diced chorizo in step 2 with the sweet potatoes for a spicy flavor or try diced salami, garlic sausage, or hot dogs.
• Bubble and squeak is a great recipe using up leftover cooked vegetables, such as carrot, beans, broccoli, or cauliflower. Dice the vegetables and add them with—or instead of—the cabbage.

1 Thinly slice the leek, dice the sweet potatoes and ham into ½-inch pieces, and finely shred the cabbage. Heat the oil in a large frying pan over high heat. Add the leek and stir-fry the mixture for 2 minutes, or until softened.

2 Stir in the sweet potatoes and sage leaves. Reduce heat to medium, add 3 tablespoons of boiling water, and cover the pan. Cook for 8 minutes, shaking the pan occasionally, or until the potatoes are tender and cooked through.

3 Stir in the shredded cabbage and ham. Cover the pan and cook for 5 minutes over medium heat, stirring occasionally. Reduce heat to medium-low if the ingredients are sticking to the bottom of the pan. Season to taste and serve.

COOK'S TIP
● When buying sweet potatoes, make sure that they are smooth, plump, dry, and free of bruises.

SUPER FOOD

SWEET POTATO
This colorful root vegetable is nutrient-packed with alpha- and beta-carotene—the antioxidant pigments that give sweet potato its bright orange flesh and helps protect against cancer. It also contains vitamin E for heart health and fiber to promote digestive well-being.

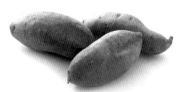

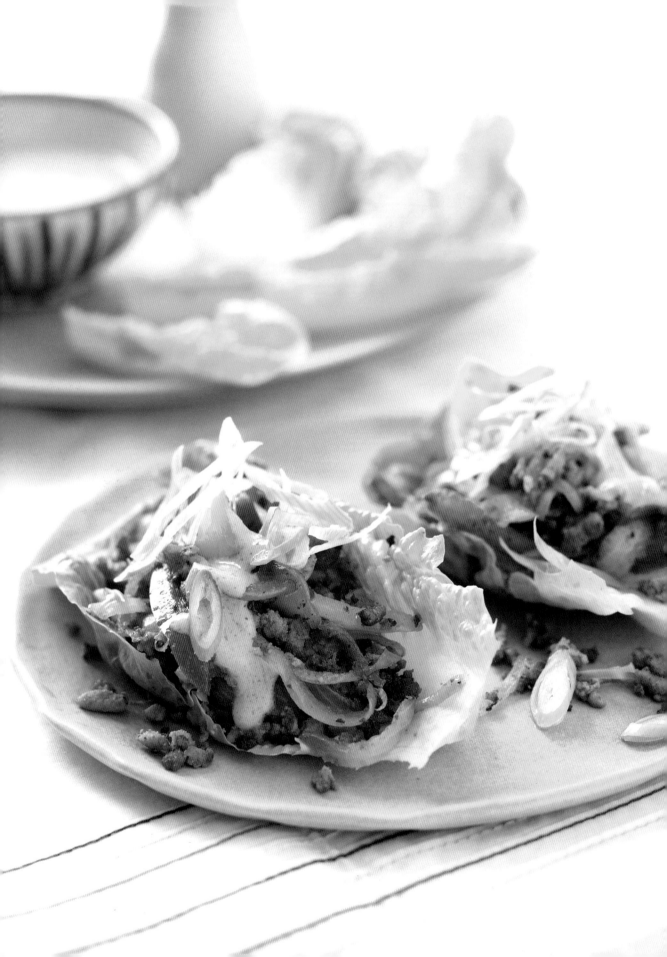

INDONESIAN SATAY **PORK** WITH **PEPPERS**

There's a juicy mouthful in every bite of this tempting combination of ground pork, crisp lettuce, and peanut sauce. Peppers and onions help to boost mental alertness.

Serves 4
Preparation 15 minutes
Cooking 12 minutes

2 onions
2 large bell peppers (1 red, 1 yellow)
2 tablespoons olive oil or canola oil
1 pound lean ground pork
3 cloves garlic
1 tablespoon ground coriander
2 tablespoons soy sauce
4 scallions
1 head of crisp lettuce, such as romaine, separated into leaves, to serve

For the satay sauce
4 tablespoons creamy peanut butter
1 clove garlic, crushed
1 teaspoon sesame oil
1 teaspoon soy sauce

Each serving provides
• 414 calories • 25 g fat • 5 g saturated fat • 18 g carbohydrates • 31 g protein • 6 g fiber

ALTERNATIVE INGREDIENTS
• Use a green bell pepper instead of the red bell pepper. Shred a quarter of a napa cabbage and add to the ground pork mixture in step 3 after stir-frying the pepper for 2 minutes. Finish as above.
• Shred the lettuce instead of using the leaves whole and serve with 2 warmed flour tortillas or similar flatbread or wraps per portion. Spread the sauce over the wraps, divide the pork and peppers among them, then roll up and serve with the lettuce and scallions on the side.

1 Start by making the satay sauce. Combine the peanut butter, 1 crushed clove garlic, and the sesame oil in a small bowl. Gradually whisk in 4 tablespoons of boiling water. The mixture will start thick and glossy, then soften after about 1 minute and become pale. Stir in the soy sauce and set aside.

2 Halve and slice the onions, then quarter and slice the peppers. Heat 1 tablespoon of the oil in a large frying pan over high heat. Add the ground pork and sauté, stirring occasionally, for about 5 minutes, or until the meat is crumbly and browned, and the excess cooking liquid has evaporated.

3 Add the remaining tablespoon of oil, the onions and the remaining 2 crushed cloves of garlic to the frying pan and stir-fry them for 2 minutes. Stir in the peppers and coriander and stir-fry for another 4–5 minutes, or until the peppers are tender. Remove from the heat and stir in the soy sauce.

4 Trim and slice the scallions diagonally. Arrange 2–3 lettuce leaves on each plate and divide the pork mixture among them. Spoon some of the satay sauce on each portion and garnish with the scallion slices.

COOK'S TIPS
● To prepare large peppers, hold them upright by the stem on a cutting board, and slice down to remove the flesh from the core. Slice three sides, then cut the stem and remaining seeds away from the fourth side.
● If ground pork is not available, you can make your own. Add 1 pound of lean boneless pork, for example, pork shoulder or steak, in a food processor or meat grinder and process to a consistent grind.

SUPER FOOD

ONION FAMILY
Rich in plant-based substances called phytochemicals that help to prevent and protect against disease, onions and shallots are also a great source of the flavonoid quercetin, a strong antioxidant. Some studies have linked quercetin to a lower risk of developing lung cancer.

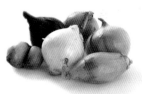

AROMATIC **PORK** KEBABS

Juicy pieces of pork flavored with orange zest and coriander make a brilliant match with broiled red bell peppers and a crunchy carrot salad. Serve with some warmed pita bread on the side.

Serves 4
Preparation 10 minutes
Cooking 10 minutes

1 pound lean pork cubes
2 large red bell peppers
2 large onions
2 tablespoons olive oil or canola oil
grated zest and juice of 1 orange
1 tablespoon finely crushed
   coriander seeds
6 carrots

Each serving provides
• 267 calories • 11 g fat • 2 g
saturated fat • 16 g carbohydrates
• 4 g fiber

ALTERNATIVE INGREDIENTS
• Lamb, turkey, or chicken breast all work well instead of pork.
• A meaty fish, such as swordfish or tuna, would be a good alternative to the pork.
• Coarsely grated zucchini makes a quick and easy salad accompaniment. Toss with a little olive oil and a handful of shredded basil leaves.

1 Preheat the broiler to high. Line the broiler pan with foil. Thread the pork onto metal skewers, leaving a little space between the cubes of meat, and place them on the broiler pan. Cut the peppers into ¾-inch-wide strips and thinly slice the onions. Arrange the vegetables around the the kebabs.

2 Brush the pork and vegetables with oil. Sprinkle the orange zest and crushed coriander seeds over the pork. Broil for 5 minutes. Grate the carrots, then add the orange juice and mix well.

3 Using an oven glove, carefully turn the pork skewers. Turn and rearrange the vegetables so that they cook evenly. Broil for another 5 minutes, until the meat is browned and cooked through and the vegetables are tender.

4 Transfer the kebabs to warmed plates, add a portion of broiled vegetables to each and serve with bowls of carrot salad.

COOK'S TIPS
● If using wooden skewers, soak them in water for 15 minutes before threading the pork to prevent them from burning under the broiler.
● Use a mortar and pestle to crush the coriander seeds. To prevent the seeds from escaping, put the mortar in a plastic bag, gather the edges around the pestle, and close the bag as you pound the seeds. If you don't have a mortar and pestle, put the seeds in a bowl and crush them with the end of a rolling pin.
● If you prefer, you can grill the pork kebabs and peppers instead of broiling them.

SUPER FOOD

RED BELL PEPPERS
Half a fresh red bell pepper will provide your total daily vitamin C requirement. Like all vegetables, bell peppers are low in calories, making them a good choice for weight control.

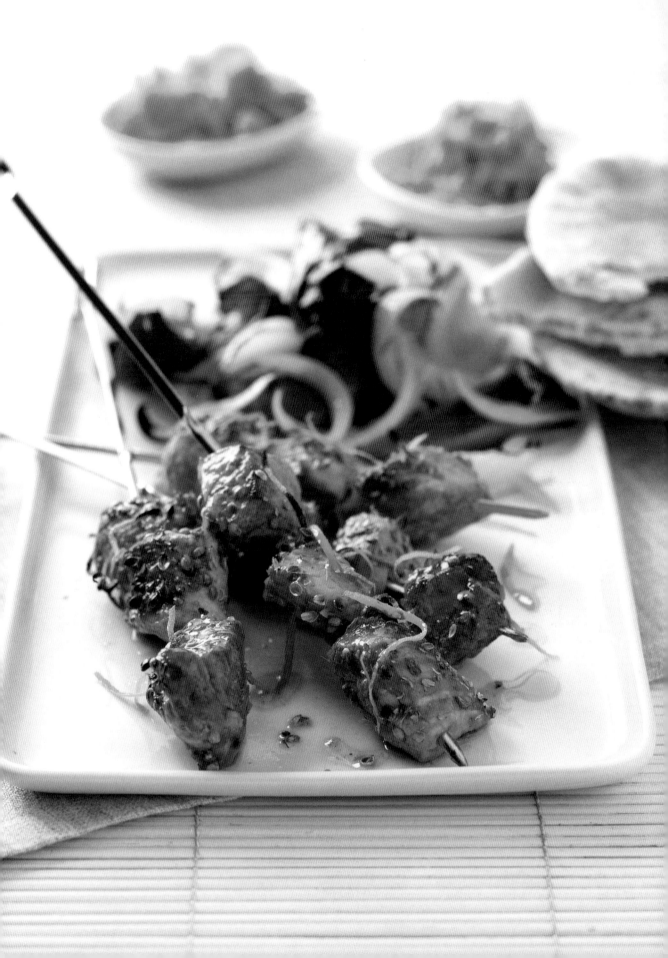

CITRUS FRUIT

You need vitamin C for healthy bones and skin, and few foods give you more of that vital nutrient than citrus fruit such as limes, lemons, oranges, grapefruit, and tangerines. Vitamin C also acts as an antioxidant, which helps to prevent cell damage, reducing the risk of cancer and other chronic diseases.

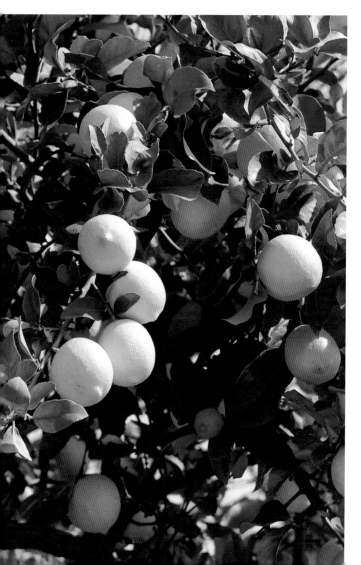

FRUIT SALAD

Serves 4
Preparation 20 minutes

Each serving provides • 172 calories • 1 g fat • 0 g saturated fat • 41 g carbohydrates • 3 g protein • 4 g fiber

Peel **2 blood oranges** and **1 ruby grapefruit**, cut them into segments, and add them to a bowl with any juice. Peel **½ pound watermelon**, removing all the seeds, and cut into ¾- to 1¼-inch cubes. Add the watermelon to the bowl, together with **⅓ cup seedless red grapes**, cutting any large grapes in half. Sprinkle **4 teaspoons superfine sugar** over the fruit and add **3½ cups unsweetened orange juice** or **orange-raspberry juice**. Stir and chill in the fridge until serving.

COOK'S TIPS

● The easiest way to peel citrus fruit is to remove the top and stem ends with a serrated knife, then place the flat base on a cutting board that has a channel around the edge to catch the juices. Hold the fruit at the top while slicing down between peel and flesh, from top to bottom. Turn the fruit a little after each cut and continue slicing down until all the peel is removed.
● This fruit salad makes a refreshing starter to a main course that features fish.

CITRUS PANCAKES

Serves 4
Preparation 10 minutes Cooking 12 minutes

Each serving provides • 228 calories • 5 g fat • 1 g saturated fat • 40 g carbohydrates • 9 g protein • 5 g fiber

Peel **2 large oranges** and slice them into segments, removing all the pith. Put the segments and any juice into a small saucepan with the **juice of 1 lemon** and **2 tablespoons honey**. Place the pan over low heat, stir the mixture, and warm through. Add **½ cup all-purpose whole-wheat flour** and a pinch of salt to the bowl. Add **1 egg** and **1 cup low-fat (1%) milk** and beat until the mixture becomes a smooth batter. Brush a non-stick frying pan with a little **olive oil or canola oil** and set over high heat. When the pan is very hot, spoon one-eighth of the batter into the center of the pan. Swirl it around to coat the pan and cook for 1 minute, or until the underside is flecked with brown. Turn the pancake with a spatula and cook for another 30 seconds. Transfer to a plate and keep warm. Repeat with the remaining mixture to make another seven pancakes. Serve with warm orange sauce spooned over each pancake.

COOK'S TIP

- For a sweeter pancake dish, use 1 cup canned mandarin oranges instead of orange segments and dust with confectioners' sugar just before serving.

PINK GRAPEFRUIT AND POMEGRANATE SALAD

Serves 4
Preparation 10 minutes

Each serving provides • 238 calories • 23 g fat
- 3 g saturated fat • 7 g carbohydrates • 1 g protein
- 2 g fiber

Arrange **frisée or other lettuce leaves**, washed and torn, in a large salad bowl. Peel and segment **1 large pink grapefruit**, then halve the segments and arrange them over the leaves. Remove the seeds from **1 pomegranate** using a small spoon to pry them out. Make a dressing by combining **⅓ cup olive oil** with **1 tablespoon red wine vinegar**, **1 teaspoon balsamic vinegar** and any juice from the grapefruit. Drizzle the dressing over the salad and toss to combine. Sprinkle the pomegranate seeds over the salad and serve.

COOK'S TIPS

- Frisée lettuce (also known as curly endive) has thin, green, curly leaves that are very decorative. Other attractive salad leaves include sweet lamb's lettuce (mâche) or peppery arugula.
- Use raspberry vinegar instead of red wine vinegar for a fruitier flavor.

PORK FILLETS WITH LIME GREMOLATA

Serves 4
Preparation 10 minutes Marinating 30 minutes
Cooking 10 minutes

Each serving provides • 244 calories • 13 g fat
- 3 g saturated fat • 2 g carbohydrates • 27 g protein
- 1 g fiber

In a shallow non-metallic dish, mix **2 tablespoons olive oil, juice of 1 lime, 2 tablespoons dry white wine,** and **2 crushed cloves garlic**. Cut **4 pork fillets, about 1 pound total**, diagonally in half. Coat with the

marinade and let marinate for 30 minutes. To make the gremolata, first zest **1 unwaxed lime**. Peel and remove the pith, then cut the lime into small chunks. Combine the lime zest with **1 tablespoon finely chopped fresh parsley** and **2 large finely chopped cloves garlic**. Cook the pieces of pork together with the marinade in a large frying pan over medium heat for 10 minutes, or until golden and cooked through. Stir in the lime chunks and add **2 tablespoons low-fat sour cream** and let warm through. Serve the pork with the creamy lime sauce and gremolata sprinkled on the top.

COOK'S TIPS

- Serve the pork with pan-fried potato slices and sautéed green beans for a taste of summer.
- Other white meat, such as chicken and turkey, also taste great sprinkled with gremolata. Substitute a lemon for the lime for a sharper flavor.

ORANGE AND RED ONION CHUTNEY

Serves 4
Preparation 10 minutes Cooking 10 minutes

Each serving provides • 156 calories • 10 g fat
- 1 g saturated fat • 14 g carbohydrates • 2 g protein
- 3 g fiber

Preheat the oven to 350°F. Peel **6 small oranges** and cut each across the grain into 4 slices. Transfer the slices to an ovenproof dish, lightly brushed with **1 teaspoon olive oil**. Finely chop **1 red onion** and scatter it over the oranges. Drizzle **2 tablespoons olive oil** and **3 teaspoons red wine vinegar** over the mixture, then add **1 teaspoon soft dark brown sugar**. Bake for 10 minutes and serve warm with a little extra virgin olive oil drizzled over the top.

COOK'S TIP

- This chutney goes well with grilled chicken, venison sausage, or duck breast fillets. Serve with a hearty green salad, as well.

PORK STEAKS WITH BLUEBERRY AND APPLE SAUCE

Brimming with protective antioxidants, blueberries also bring color and sweetness to this quick and easy dish. Serve the pork with stir-fried cabbage and leeks, along with tender baby carrots.

Serves 4
Preparation 10 minutes
Cooking 18 minutes

2 apples, about ½ pound
1 large leek
1¾ cups finely shredded cabbage
1 tablespoon sugar
⅔ cup blueberries
2 tablespoons olive oil or canola oil
4 lean pork steaks

Each serving provides
- 308 calories • 13 g fat • 3 g saturated fat • 18 g carbohydrates
- 30 g protein • 6 g fiber

ALTERNATIVE INGREDIENTS
- Blackberries or sliced plums also taste great with pork. Halve, pit, and slice the plums and cook them with the apples for 1 minute.
- For a cranberry and apple sauce, cook the cranberries and apples with 3 tablespoons of water until the cranberries have softened. Add 2 tablespoons sugar and cook gently for a minute.
- This fruity sauce also makes a wonderful accompaniment to venison, lamb, turkey, and pheasant.

1 Peel and coarsely grate the apples. Trim, thinly slice, and rinse the leeks. Place the apples in a saucepan over high heat. Add the sugar and a tablespoon of water and bring to a boil, stirring. Reduce heat to low, cover, and cook for 1–2 minutes, or until the apples soften. Stir in the blueberries to warm through and transfer to a serving bowl.

2 Heat a large frying pan over high heat until very hot. To the pan, add 1 tablespoon of the oil and the pork steaks. Brown for 1 minute on each side, reduce heat to medium-low, and fry for 4 minutes on each side. Transfer the pork to a plate and keep warm.

3 Add the remaining tablespoon of oil to the frying pan, increase heat to high, and cook the leeks for 3 minutes, or until softened. Add the cabbage and cook for another 2 minutes, or until the cabbage is tender. Transfer the pork and vegetables to four warmed plates and add a large spoonful of blueberry and apple sauce before serving.

COOK'S TIPS
- Make light work of preparing the apples by peeling them whole, hold them by the core ends, and grate them directly into the pan.
- The leeks and cabbage reduce rapidly as they soften and cook, so add the cabbage in batches if your pan is small.

SUPER FOOD

CABBAGE
Bursting with nourishment, cabbages of all colors contain high levels of antioxidants that work to protect cell membranes from damage by free radicals. As a result, there are studies that link eating cabbage with a lower risk of developing cancer, especially of the digestive tract.

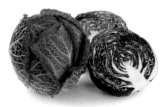

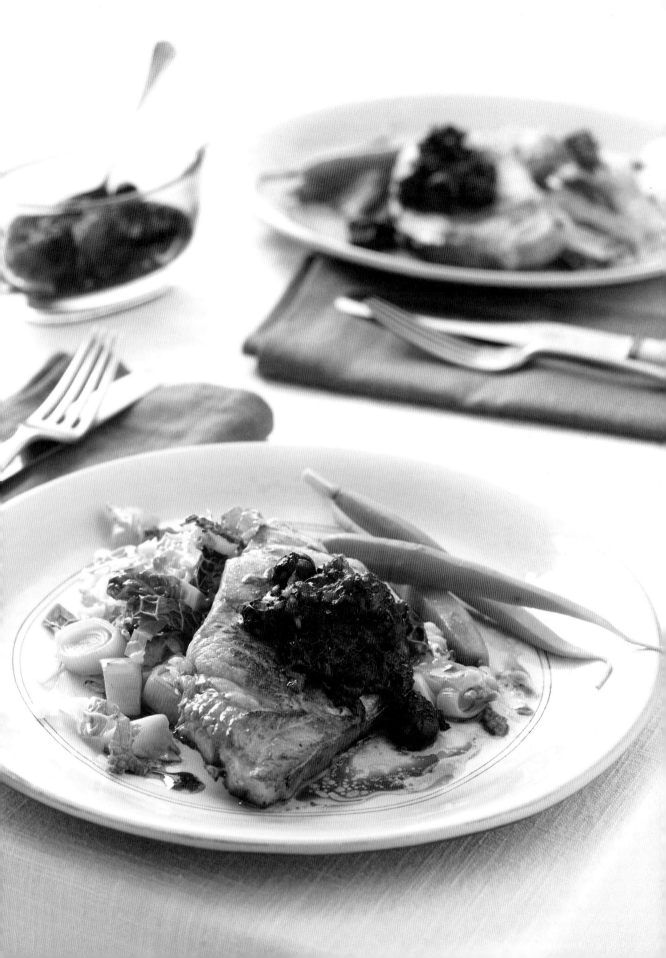

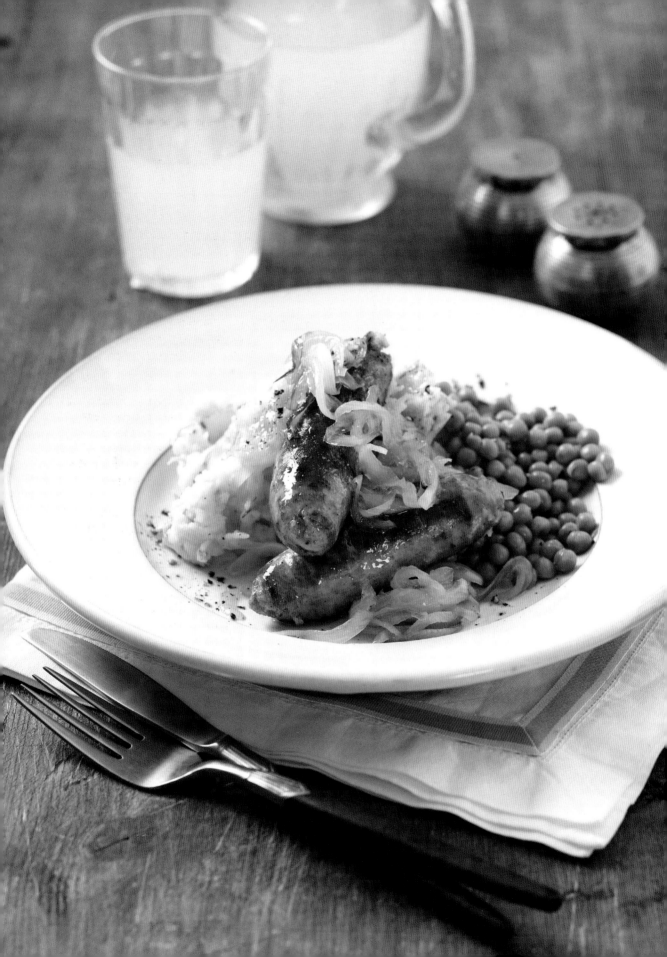

SAUSAGES AND SUPERMASH WITH ONION RELISH

Creamy mashed potatoes hit new heights with an addition of vitamin-packed carrot and zucchini. Add an easy onion relish and you have the perfect match for juicy poached sausages. Serve with peas for a splash of color.

Serves 4
Preparation 15 minutes
Cooking 35 minutes

8 meaty pork sausages,
  about 1 pound
2 pounds potatoes
1 zucchini
1 large carrot
4 onions
4 tablespoons olive oil or canola oil
2 tablespoons raw or brown sugar
2 tablespoons cider vinegar
4 tablespoons low-fat (1%) milk

Each serving provides
• 630 calories • 34 g fat • 9 g saturated fat • 63 g carbohydrates • 21 g protein • 6 g fiber

ALTERNATIVE INGREDIENTS
• Grated celeriac or butternut squash make good alternatives to zucchini.
• Chopped celery, grated carrot, and chopped walnuts are another excellent mixture of complementary flavors for livening up mashed potatoes.
• Serve broiled, good-quality burgers or grilled chicken instead of sausages.

1 Place the sausages in a saucepan with water, and cover. Bring the water to the boil, reduce the heat to low, and poach the sausages for 30 minutes. Meanwhile, peel the potatoes and cut into 1¼-inch chunks. Transfer to a saucepan, cover with boiling water, and simmer for 10 minutes, or until tender. Coarsely grate the zucchini and carrot. Thinly slice the onions.

2 Heat 2 tablespoons of the oil in a saucepan over medium heat. Add the onions and cook for 5 minutes, stirring once or twice, until softened. Add the sugar and cook for 5–6 minutes, reducing the heat if the onions begin to burn. When the sausages are cooked, carefully remove them with a slotted spoon and dry on paper towels. Fry them in a dry non-stick frying pan for 3–5 minutes, or until browned all over.

3 Stir the vinegar into the onions, increase the heat, and boil for 1 minute. Reduce heat to low and simmer for 3–5 minutes, or until the liquid has evaporated and the onions are glazed.

4 Drain the potatoes in a colander. Add the remaining 2 tablespoons of oil, plus the zucchini and carrot, to the empty potato pan and cook over low heat for 1 minute. Remove from the heat, add the potatoes and the milk, and mash until smooth. Stir in the zucchini and carrot, season to taste, and serve with the sausages and onion relish.

COOK'S TIPS
● You can make the onion relish up to several hours in advance, transfer it to a dish, and cover it until needed.
● If you prefer, cook the sausages by broiling them on high heat for 20 minutes, turning until browned all over and cooked through.

SUPER FOOD

ONIONS
Research indicates that onions, along with other members of the allium family, may protect against stomach cancer. This is because natural phytochemicals in the onions may stimulate enzymes that get rid of harmful chemicals in the body.

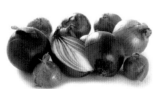

FRUITY **PORK STEAKS** WITH GLAZED **PLUMS** AND **RED CABBAGE**

The tangy, sweet-and-sour flavors of ripe plums and red wine vinegar work well with pork and cabbage. Serve with fiber-rich mashed rutabaga and carrots for a real treat.

Serves 4
Preparation 10 minutes
Cooking 25 minutes

2 red onions
14 ounces red cabbage
8 ripe plums
2 tablespoons olive oil or canola oil
4 lean boneless pork loin chops, about 5 ounces each
pinch of ground cloves or allspice
3½ ounces pomegranate juice drink
3 tablespoons raw or brown sugar
3 tablespoons red wine vinegar

Each serving provides
• 405 calories • 17 g fat • 4 g saturated fat • 34 g carbohydrates • 31 g protein • 6 g fiber

ALTERNATIVE INGREDIENTS
• Grind 6 juniper berries in a mortar and pestle and use instead of the ground cloves or allspice.
• This recipe also works well with venison or lamb steaks.
• Instead of using fresh fruit, add 5½ ounces thickly sliced pitted prunes or dried apricots in step 2. Stir the dried fruit into the cabbage before replacing the meat. Omit the extra tablespoon sugar and vinegar used to glaze the fruit in step 5.

1 Slice the onions, shred the red cabbage, and cut the plums in half. Heat the oil in a large frying pan over high heat. Add the pork steaks and cook for 3 minutes on each side, or until browned. Reduce heat to medium, add the onions, and cook for another 5 minutes, stirring occasionally, until the meat is cooked through. Transfer the steaks to a shallow dish, leaving the onions in the pan.

2 Add the cabbage and cloves or allspice to the pan and fry, stirring, for 5 minutes. Pour in the pomegranate juice drink and bring to a boil. Return the pork to the pan with any juices from the dish. Reduce heat to medium, cover, and cook for 3 minutes. Transfer the pork to four plates. Add 1 tablespoon each of sugar and vinegar to the cabbage and boil for 30 seconds, stirring, to glaze the cabbage. Divide among the plates of pork.

3 Add the plums to the pan, cut sides down. Sprinkle in the remaining 2 tablespoons each of sugar and vinegar and cook over high heat for 4 minutes, shaking the pan so that the sugar dissolves. Season to taste and divide the plums and their glaze among the plates and serve.

COOK'S TIP
● To halve the plums, cut around the dimple in the fruit and twist the halves apart, leaving the pit in one half. Use a small pointed knife to cut out the pit.

SUPER FOOD

PLUMS
The goodness of plums, as with most fruit, is found in or around the skin— so don't peel them. Their nutritional benefits include potassium to help regulate blood pressure and fiber for keeping the digestive system healthy. Plums also contain antioxidants to help fight the signs of ageing.

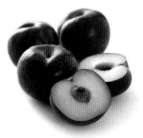

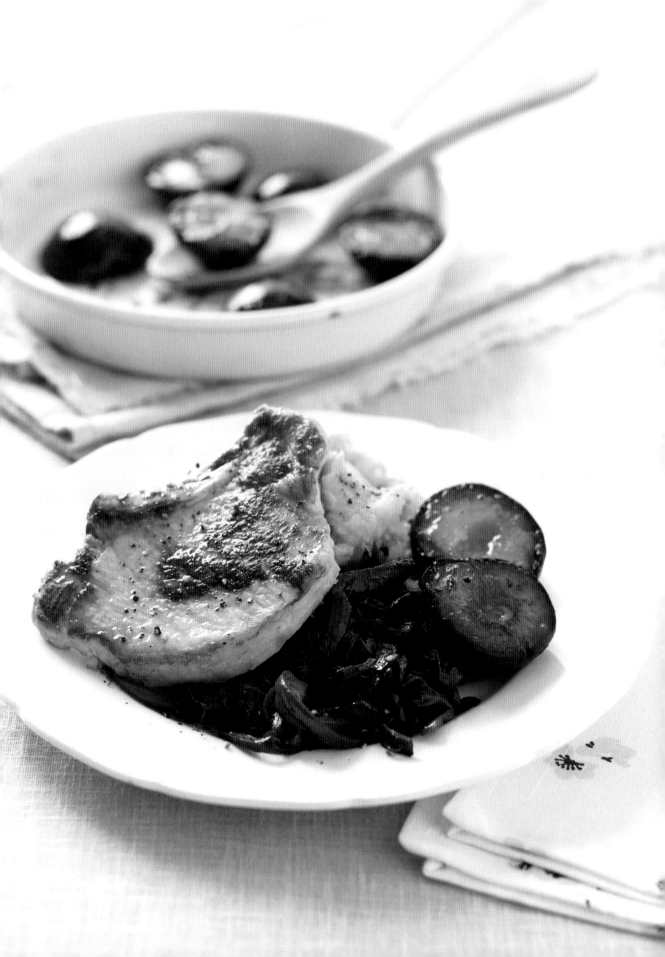

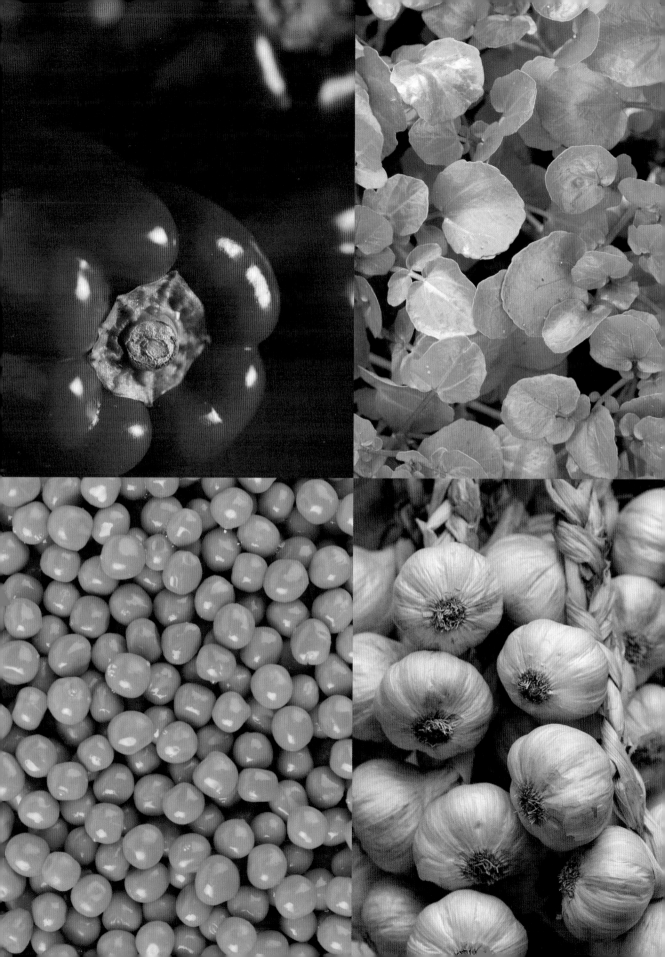

PASTA, LEGUMES *and* GRAINS

ITALIAN SPIRALS WITH **WATERCRESS** AND **OLIVE** DRESSING

Peppery watercress provides a zingy bite to pasta spirals tossed in a gremolata dressing. Crunchy pistachio nuts and a little parmesan add to the flavor. Serve with cherry tomatoes.

Serves 4
Preparation 10 minutes
Cooking 10 minutes

10 ounces pasta spirals or fusilli
2 small leeks
1 medium bunch watercress
¼ cup shelled pistachios
⅓ cup pimento-stuffed olives, halved
4 tablespoons olive oil
3 cloves garlic, crushed
2 tablespoons chopped fresh parsley
grated zest of 1 lemon
⅓ cup grated parmesan

Each serving provides
• 588 calories • 31 g fat • 7 g saturated fat • 61 g carbohydrates • 20 g protein • 7 g fiber

ALTERNATIVE INGREDIENTS
• Boost the nutty flavor by using a mixture of olive oil and walnut oil. Cook the leeks in 2 tablespoons olive oil, then add 2 tablespoons walnut oil to the pan when the leeks are cooked. Add walnuts instead of pistachios.
• For herb-flavored pasta, add tarragon or basil to the recipe in addition to the parsley. Chop 2 fresh tarragon sprigs with the parsley. Basil loses its flavor when chopped, so it's best to add 2–3 tender shredded leaves just before adding the olives in step 3.
• Try other cheeses, such as gruyère, manchego, pecorino romano, or a sharp cheddar, instead of parmesan.

1 Bring a large saucepan of water to a boil. Add the pasta, return to a boil, and partly cover the pan. Reduce heat and cook for 10 minutes, or according to package directions, until pasta is tender but still firm to the bite. Slice the leeks into rings, cut the rings into quarters, and rinse. Chop the watercress and pistachios.

2 Halfway through cooking the pasta, heat the oil in a saucepan over high heat. Add the garlic and leeks and reduce heat to medium-low. Cover and cook for 5 minutes, stirring once, until the leeks soften.

3 Pour the pasta into a colander and quickly return it to the hot pan without draining all the cooking liquid. This will keep the pasta moist and hot. Add the leeks, watercress, parsley, pistachios, lemon zest, and stuffed olives. Toss to mix well and divide among four plates. Serve topped with grated parmesan.

COOK'S TIP
● For faster preparation—though the final dish won't look quite as attractive—finely chop the watercress, parsley, and pistachios together in a food processor.

SUPER FOOD

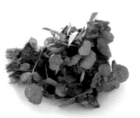

WATERCRESS
Packed with essential nutrients, watercress contains calcium to help maintain bone strength, iron for preventing anemia, and folate to promote heart health. It's also a good source of antioxidants, which may have anti-cancer effects that protect the body against harmful free radicals.

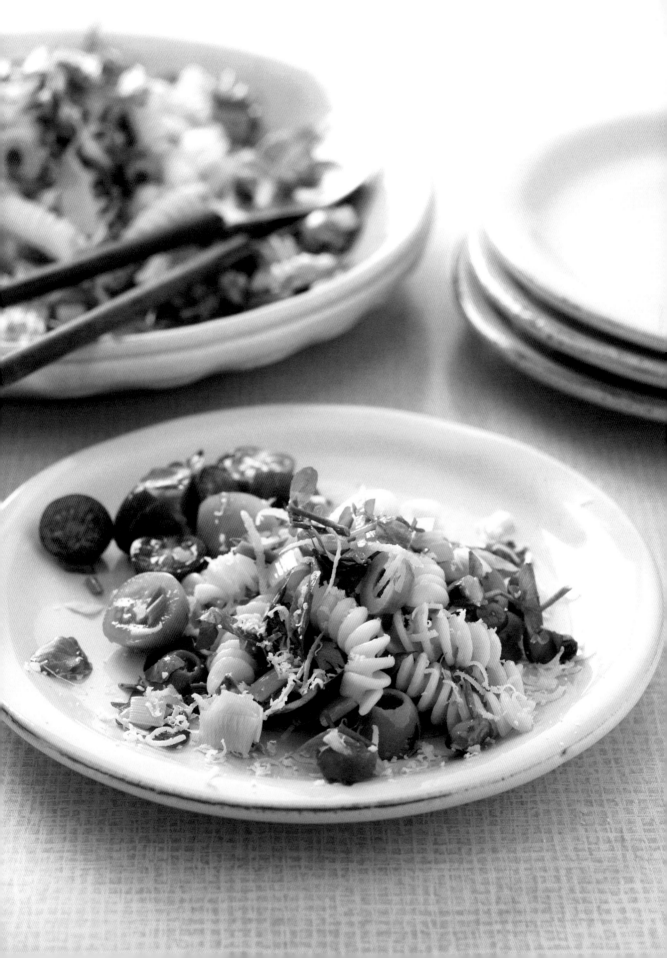

CREAMY **MUSHROOMS** WITH **TAGLIATELLE**

An indulgent but nutritious sauce coats a fusion of succulent, earthy mushrooms and heart-healthy, antioxidant-packed walnuts, turning a simple bowl of pasta into a hearty meal.

Serves 4
Preparation 10 minutes
Cooking 15 minutes

½ pound tagliatelle pasta
1⅓ cups sliced cremini mushrooms
⅓ cup chopped walnuts
2 tablespoons olive oil
3 teaspoons cornstarch
1¾ cups low-fat (1%) milk
½ cup low-fat cream cheese or
   ½ cup grated low-fat cheddar
4 tablespoons finely chopped
   fresh parsley
½ pound oyster mushrooms
3 tablespoons snipped fresh chives

Each serving provides
• 575 calories • 29 g fat • 3 g
saturated fat • 55 g carbohydrates
• 23 g protein • 7 g fiber

ALTERNATIVE INGREDIENTS
• Replace the oyster mushrooms with other mushrooms such as shiitakes or chanterelles. These can be found in the vegetable or salad section in most large supermarkets.
• Use 1⅓ cups low-fat (1%) milk and ⅓ cup dry sherry instead of all milk. Boil the milk sauce first, then stir in the sherry and simmer.
• Cook 2 sliced scallions and a crushed clove of garlic with the mushrooms in step 2.

1 Bring a large saucepan of water to a boil. Add the tagliatelle, return to a boil, and partly cover the pan. Reduce heat and cook for 12 minutes, or according to package directions, until the pasta is tender but still firm to the bite. Set aside 1 tablespoon of the walnuts. Heat 1 tablespoon of oil in another pan and add the creminis. Cook over high heat for 5 minutes, or until softened.

2 Whisk the cornstarch with milk and add to the mushroom mixture in the pan. Bring to a boil, stirring, then reduce the heat and simmer for 3 minutes. Stir in the cheese, walnuts, and parsley, and season to taste.

3 Drain the tagliatelle and add it to the sauce. Cover and remove from the heat without mixing. Add the remaining tablespoon of oil and oyster mushrooms to the pan used for the pasta. Cook over high heat for 1 minute, or until hot and beginning to brown. Divide the pasta among four bowls and top with the oyster mushrooms and reserved walnuts. Sprinkle with chives and serve.

COOK'S TIP
● If you are using fresh tagliatelle, reduce the cooking time as fresh pasta cooks much more quickly than dried—usually 2–4 minutes. Follow the package for cooking directions.

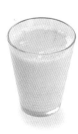

SUPER FOOD

LOW-FAT MILK
Studies show that a diet rich in low-fat dairy foods, along with other healthy lifestyle choices such as reducing salt intake and exercising regularly, can lower blood pressure in people with hypertension. Low-fat milk may also offer protection against colon cancer.

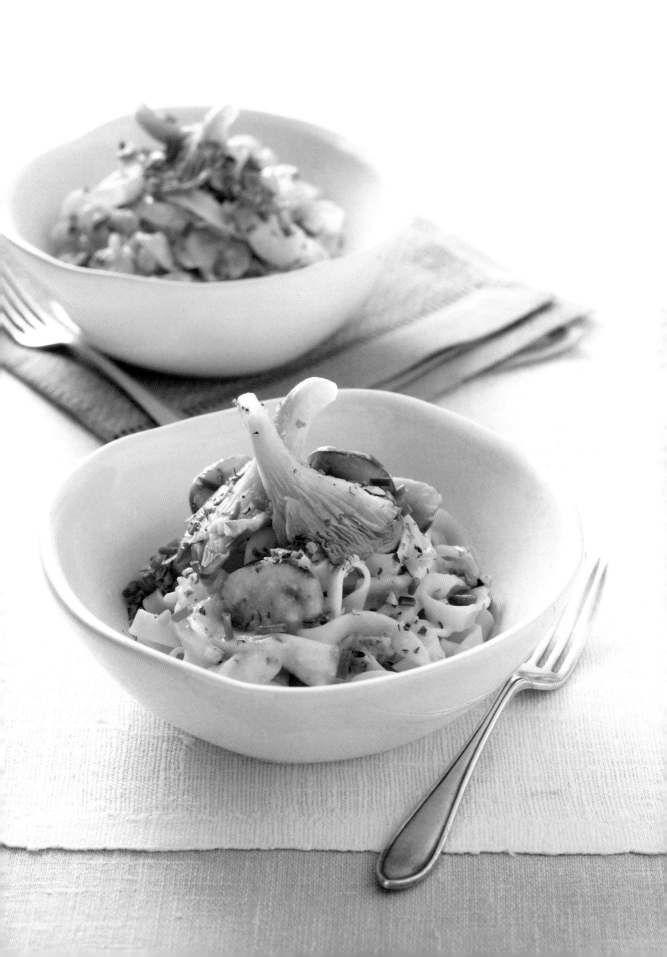

FIERY ITALIAN **VEGETABLE** PASTA

Pasta is wonderful at absorbing and enhancing flavors. Combine pasta with colorful vegetables and a little spicy chile pepper for a zesty meal.

Serves 4
Preparation 10 minutes
Cooking 20 minutes

10 ounces pasta, such as shells, bows, spirals or tubes
1 onion
1 red chile
2 cloves garlic
¼ cup pitted black olives
6 sun-dried tomato halves
2 celery stalks
1¼ pounds ripe plum tomatoes
3 tablespoons olive oil
2 tablespoons chopped fresh parsley
finely grated zest of 1 lemon
¼ cup parmesan, shaved

Each serving provides
• 486 calories • 18 g fat • 5 g saturated fat • 68 g carbohydrates
• 17 g protein • 7 g fiber

ALTERNATIVE INGREDIENTS
• Instead of using chopped sun-dried tomatoes, use sun-dried tomato purée. Add 1–2 tablespoons purée in step 2, stirring it into the cooked onion mixture before adding the fresh tomatoes.
• Add ¼ cup chopped anchovy fillets in olive oil with the tomatoes and reduce the oil for cooking the onion to 1 tablespoon.

1 Bring a large saucepan of water to a boil. Add the pasta, return to a boil, and stir once. Reduce heat and partly cover the pan. Boil for 12 minutes, or according to package directions, until tender but still firm to the bite. Drain the pasta in a colander.

2 Meanwhile, finely chop the onion, chile, and garlic. Halve the olives, quarter the sun-dried tomatoes, and dice the celery. Chop the fresh tomatoes. Heat the olive oil in a pan and add the onion, chile, half of the garlic, and the celery. Cook over high heat for 5 minutes, stirring frequently.

3 Stir in the fresh tomatoes, sun-dried tomatoes, and olives. Cook the sauce for 3 minutes and return the pasta to the pan. Toss together and season to taste.

4 Mix the remaining chopped garlic with the parsley and lemon zest. Divide the pasta among four bowls and serve topped with the parsley mixture and shaved parmesan.

COOK'S TIPS
● Plum tomatoes are ideal for this recipe because they have firmer flesh with fewer seeds than other varieties.
● Whether this dish is piquant with a little heat or fiery in flavor depends on your choice of chile. A mild chile will give a gentle warmth to the pasta and vegetables, but if you like it hot, use 2 hot chilies.

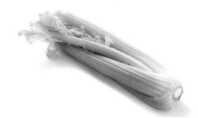

SUPER FOOD

CELERY
Crunchy celery helps to maintain a healthy digestive system thanks to the soluble and insoluble fiber it contains. With its folate and potassium, celery is also great for heart health and for regulating blood pressure.

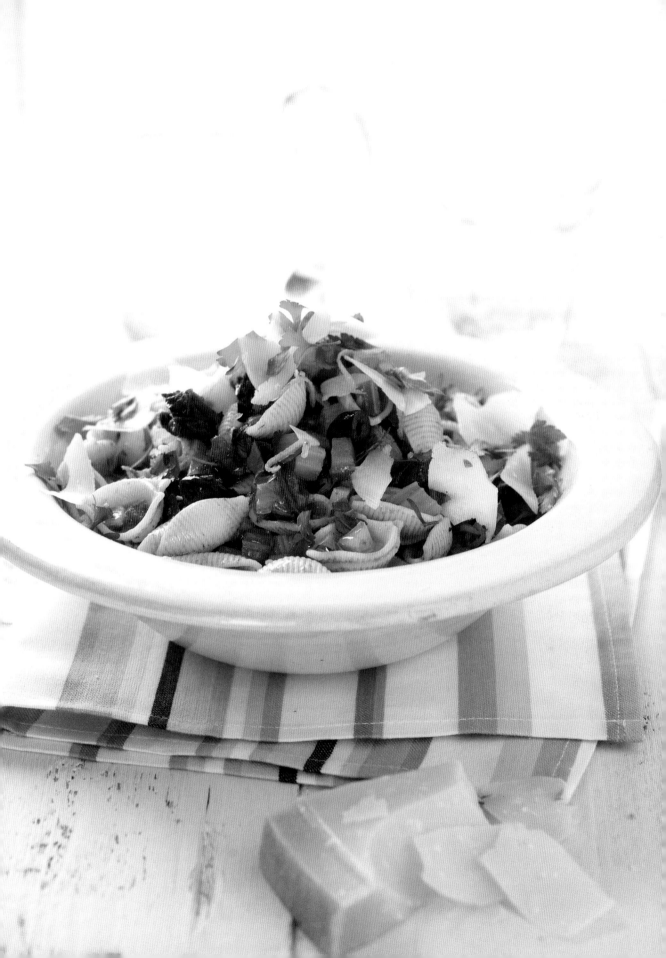

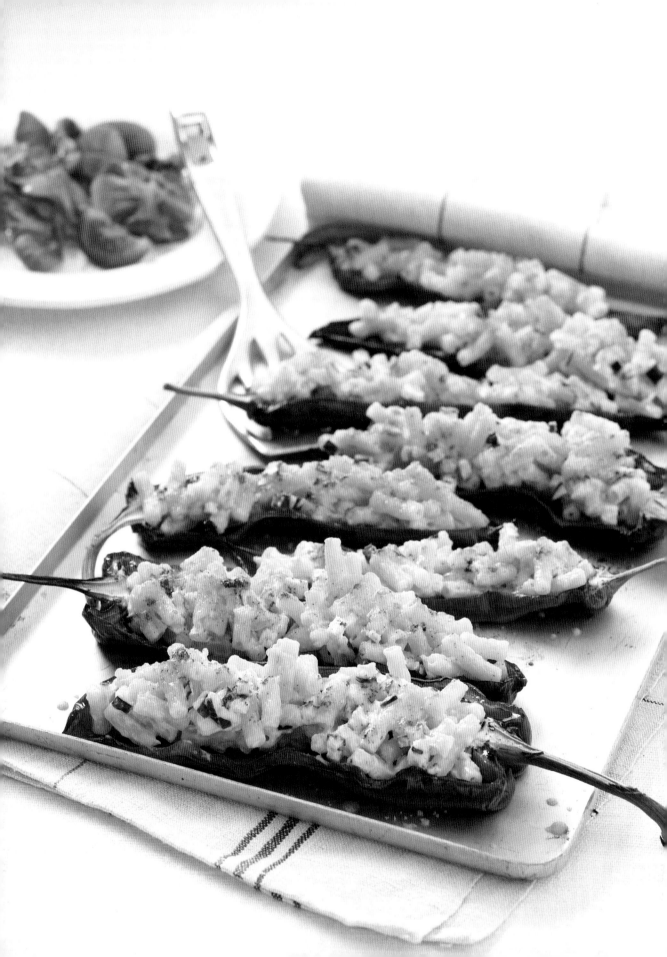

BANANA PEPPERS WITH CHEESY PASTA

Enjoy hearty elbow macaroni with a twist—served in lightly grilled red banana peppers. Although they're red in color, they're not hot—their sweetness cuts through the full-bodied savory sauce.

Serves 4
Preparation 15 minutes
Cooking 17 minutes

6 ounces elbow macaroni
1 small zucchini
4 large red banana peppers
¾ cup low-fat cream cheese
  or ricotta
2 tablespoons snipped fresh chives
¼ cup grated parmesan
1 tablespoon olive oil
1 teaspoon paprika

Each serving provides
• 281 calories • 11 g fat • 5 g saturated fat • 29 g carbohydrates • 15 g protein • 2 g fiber

ALTERNATIVE INGREDIENTS
• Use yellow or orange banana peppers instead of red ones. If you can't get banana peppers, use sweet bell peppers and cut them into four pieces.
• Try other pasta shapes instead of elbows, such as spirals or shells.
• Use ½ cup sharp cheddar, gruyère, or monterey jack cheese instead of parmesan, though this will raise the fat content.
• To increase your vegetable intake, add a grated carrot with the zucchini in step 2.
• Reduce macaroni to 3 ounces and add ¼ cup frozen baby peas to the pan for the last 5 minutes of cooking. Return the water to a boil after adding the peas.

1 Preheat the broiler to high. Bring a large saucepan of water to a boil. Add the macaroni, return to a boil, and stir. Reduce the heat, partly cover the pan, and boil for 12 minutes or according to package directions, until the macaroni is cooked.

2 Meanwhile, finely grate the zucchini and cut the peppers in half lengthwise, scraping out the seeds but leaving on the stems. Combine the cheese, grated zucchini, and chives. Reserve 1 tablespoon of parmesan, stir the remainder into the mixture, and set aside. Place the peppers on a broiler pan and broil, cut sides down, for 3 minutes, or until the skins begin to blister. Turn over and broil for another 3 minutes, brush with oil, and broil for a final 3 minutes, or until tender.

3 Drain the macaroni, return it to the pan, and stir in the cheese and zucchini mixture. Spoon the macaroni into the pepper shells and sprinkle with paprika and the reserved parmesan. Place the peppers back under the broiler for 5 minutes to warm through and brown them on top.

COOK'S TIPS
● During the final broiling, after brushing with a little oil, the peppers may bubble up inside, but they will shrink back when removed from the broiler. Watch them closely to avoid burning the skins and edges.
● Replace the cheese sauce with a white sauce made with low-fat (1%) milk, if desired.

SUPER FOOD

LOW-FAT DAIRY FOODS
Reduced-fat and low-fat dairy foods provide valuable protein, phosphorus, some B vitamins, zinc, vitamin A, and calcium, which is good for bone health. Three servings of low-fat dairy products per day—along with a diet rich in fiber, fruit, and vegetables—helps to reduce high blood pressure and lowers the risk of strokes.

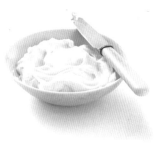

BELL PEPPERS

Cooked or raw, sweet bell peppers are packed with goodness. They are one of the best sources of vitamin C and are full of beneficial carotenes that may protect against lung cancer. Bell peppers are sold in many colors, depending upon variety and ripeness. Red, yellow, and green are the most common, with red bell peppers being the sweetest.

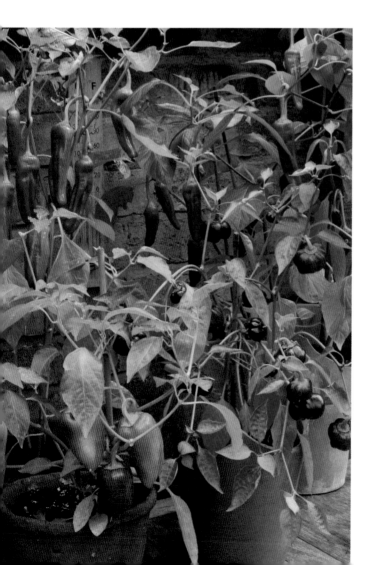

JUICY VEGETABLE KEBABS

Serves 4
Preparation 10 minutes Cooking 20 minutes

Each serving provides • 98 calories • 8 g fat
• 1 g saturated fat • 6 g carbohydrates • 1 g protein
• 2 g fiber

Preheat the broiler to high. Cut **2 red bell peppers** in half and put them on a broiler pan, skin side up. Brush them with **1 tablespoon olive oil** and broil for 15 minutes, turning occasionally, until softened and starting to blister. Reduce broiler setting to medium. Remove the peppers, cool slightly, and cut into bite-sized squares. Crush **2 medium cloves garlic** with a little salt and pepper and stir in **1 tablespoon olive oil, ½ finely chopped red chile**, and **1 teaspoon of balsamic vinegar**. Remove the stems from **12 small cremini mushrooms**. Use a pastry brush to coat the mushrooms with the flavored olive oil. Thread the mushrooms and peppers onto four metal or wooden skewers. Broil for 5 minutes, turning once, and basting with any remaining oil.

COOK'S TIPS

● Soak wooden skewers for 30 minutes in cold water before threading the vegetables to prevent the wood from burning under the hot broiler.
● Serve the kebabs as a appetizer on a bed of curly endive or other lettuce with crusty whole-grain bread.

RED PEPPER AND TOMATO SAUCE

Serves 4
Preparation 10 minutes Cooking 6 minutes

Each serving provides • 158 calories • 11 g fat
• 1 g saturated fat • 11 g carbohydrates • 4 g protein
• 3 g fiber

Heat **1 tablespoon olive oil** in a saucepan over medium heat. Add **1 finely chopped onion** and **2 diced red bell peppers** and cook for 5 minutes until softened. Stir in **2 crushed cloves garlic**. Cook for 1 minute, then add **1 cup tomato juice**. Transfer to a blender or use a stick blender, and purée until smooth. Stir in **¼ cup ground almonds** and blend for another 5 seconds. Gently reheat the sauce in the pan but don't boil. Season with salt and pepper to taste before serving.

● This sauce makes a colorful accompaniment to broiled tuna steaks or any robust white fish.

● The sweet flavor of the peppers and almonds also marries well with roast or broiled chicken.

● Reduce the tomato juice to 2 tablespoons for a rich dip with a light and refreshing taste. Serve with crudités, breadsticks, or baked cheese straws.

GOLDEN CHICKEN AND AVOCADO SALAD

Serves 4
Preparation 10 minutes Cooking 15 minutes

Each serving provides • 333 calories • 26 g fat • 5 g saturated fat • 7 g carbohydrates • 18 g protein • 4 g fiber

Preheat the broiler to medium-high. Cut **2 yellow bell peppers** lengthwise into ¼-inch-thick slices, halve the slices, and transfer them to a large bowl. Pour **3 tablespoons olive oil, juice of ½ lime** and **1 teaspoon honey** into a small bowl to make a dressing. Stir and season to taste and add to the the pepper slices. Broil **2 boneless, skinless chicken breasts** for 15 minutes, or until cooked through and lightly browned. Cool for 1–2 minutes then cut into four or five slices. Peel and slice **2 ripe avocados**. Arrange a layer of **mixed salad greens** on four plates. Layer the peppers, chicken, and avocado slices on top. Drizzle any remaining dressing on each portion and serve.

COOK'S TIP
● Serve the salad as a starter or double the quantity of chicken for a light lunch accompanied with minted new potatoes. Layer the pepper and avocado slices on top of the salad, then slice 4 broiled chicken breasts, adding one breast to each plate.

SESAME-FLAVORED PEPPERS AND BROCCOLI

Serves 4
Preparation 10 minutes Cooking 10 minutes

Each serving provides • 150 calories • 13 g fat • 2 g saturated fat • 5 g carbohydrates • 4 g protein • 3 g fiber

Heat **2 tablespoons sesame oil** in a frying pan. Thinly slice **1 large green and 1 large orange bell pepper** and add them to the pan with ¾ **cup broccoli florets**. Cook over medium-high heat for 8 minutes, or until the

pepper softens and browns, but the broccoli is still firm. Add **1 crushed clove garlic, 1 teaspoon finely chopped fresh ginger, 2 teaspoons light soy sauce** and **2 teaspoons sesame seeds**. Stir for 1 minute. Add salt and pepper to taste and transfer to four plates. Spoon any pan juices over the vegetables and drizzle with **2 teaspoons sesame oil** and an additional **2 teaspoons sesame seeds**.

COOK'S TIPS
● Serve as a healthy side dish with broiled turkey kebabs or a fish fillet. A baked potato or dollop of mashed potatoes makes a filling accompaniment.

● As an alternative to the broccoli, use ⅔ cup sugarsnap peas but omit the ginger and soy sauce.

FETA, CHILE, AND PEPPER SANDWICH SPREAD

Serves 4
Preparation 10 minutes Cooking 10 minutes

Each serving provides • 142 calories • 12 g fat • 6 g saturated fat • 3 g carbohydrates • 6 g protein • 1 g fiber

Heat **1 tablespoon olive oil** in a small frying pan. Add **1 chopped red or orange bell pepper**. Cook over medium-high heat for 8 minutes, or until softened. Add **1 finely chopped fresh jalapeño pepper** and cook for another 2 minutes before adding **a dash of chili sauce**. Crumble ⅔ **cup feta** into a bowl. Add the pepper mixture and mash with a fork to make a chunky spread.

COOK'S TIPS
● Use a jar of roasted peppers if fresh peppers are not available.

● Spread on chunks of crusty bread, use as a sandwich filling, or serve as a canapé on toast or crackers.

MALAYSIAN LAKSA WITH
SHRIMP AND VEGETABLES

This simple version of a classic Asian recipe is laden with vegetables in a broth just bursting with aromatic spices. Reduced-fat coconut milk provides the authentic traditional flavor.

Serves 4
Preparation 15 minutes
Cooking 10 minutes

1 onion
1 red chile
⅓ cup grated fresh ginger
1⅓ cups shredded napa cabbage
1 small cucumber
1 scallion
1 cup bean sprouts
2 tablespoons olive oil or canola oil
2 cloves garlic, crushed
1 teaspoon ground turmeric
4 cups hot fish stock
1 can (**14** ounces) light coconut milk
1⅔ cups fine rice noodles
⅔ pound large peeled cooked shrimp
8 chopped fresh mint leaves

Each serving provides
• 663 calories • 21 g fat • 10 g saturated fat • 94 g carbohydrates • 24 g protein • 3 g fiber

ALTERNATIVE INGREDIENTS
• Use bok choy or choy sum (mustard greens) instead of napa cabbage. Add any frozen mixed stir-fry vegetables instead of fresh ones.
• For a touch of lemony sharpness, crush 1 piece of lemongrass and add it to the onion mixture in step 1. Remove before serving.

1 Thinly slice the onion, finely chop the chile, cut the cucumber into thin strips, and finely slice the scallion. Thoroughly wash the bean sprouts. Heat the oil in a large saucepan over high heat. Add the garlic, onion, and chile, reduce heat to medium, and cook for 2 minutes.

2 Stir in the ginger, turmeric, hot fish stock, and coconut milk and bring to a boil. Reduce the heat, cover, and simmer for 5 minutes. Stir in the rice noodles, cabbage, and bean sprouts and simmer for another minute before adding the shrimp.

3 Continue to cook for 30 seconds to warm the shrimp, but don't let the liquid boil or the shrimp will be tough. Ladle into bowls and sprinkle with cucumber, scallion, and mint before serving.

COOK'S TIP
● Frozen grated ginger is a great ingredient to have on hand. Buy good-quality fresh ginger—look for large, plump, smooth, thin-skinned roots. Peel, chop in a food processor, or grate using a metal grater, then spread the ginger on a plastic tray covered with plastic wrap and freeze. Once frozen, drop the block of ginger into a freezer bag, seal, and tap against a work surface to break it into pieces. You can use the ginger frozen.

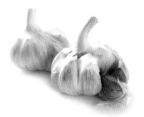

SUPER FOOD

GARLIC
A member of the onion family, garlic is rich in allyl sulphur compounds, a group of antioxidants believed to play a role in reducing the risk of cancer by stimulating enzymes that help the body to get rid of harmful chemicals.

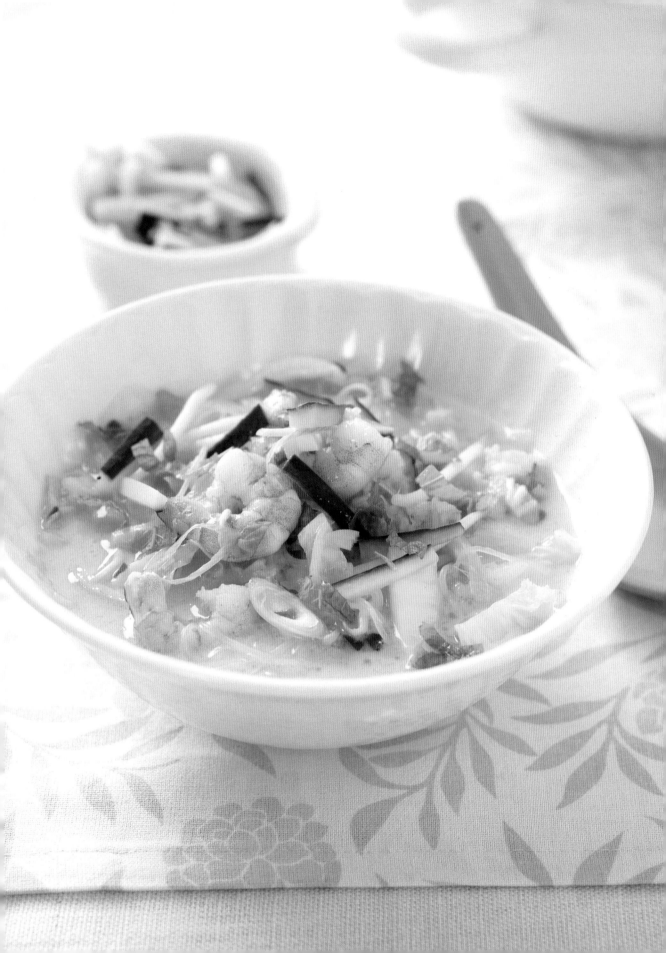

THAI **NOODLES** WITH **CASHEWS** AND STIR-FRIED **VEGETABLES**

Take a wonderfully simple recipe for Thai stir-fry and experiment with store-bought curry paste, sweet cashew nuts, and creamy soybeans for a quick, super-healthy meal any day of the week.

Serves 4
Preparation 10 minutes
Cooking 10 minutes

1 onion
⅓ cup mushrooms
1 red bell pepper
½ pound bok choy
⅔ cup bean sprouts
2 tablespoons olive oil or canola oil
2 cloves garlic, crushed
⅓ cup unsalted cashew nuts
½ cup frozen soybeans
1 tablespoon Thai green curry paste
14 ounces fresh egg noodles

Each serving provides
• 649 calories • 28 g fat • 5 g saturated fat • 82 g carbohydrates • 22 g protein • 8 g fiber

ALTERNATIVE INGREDIENTS
• If time is short, cook the garlic and onion and add 2 cups mixed stir-fry vegetables in step 3 instead of the mushrooms, pepper, bok choy, and bean sprouts.
• Try unsalted peanuts as a change from cashew nuts.
• Stir-fry strips of raw chicken or pork with the onion in step 1 and omit the soybeans. The meat strips should be cooked through and lightly browned before adding the curry paste.

1 Finely slice the onion and mushrooms and dice the pepper. Wash and shred the bok choy and thoroughly wash the bean sprouts. Heat the oil in a large frying pan or wok over high heat. Add the garlic, onion, mushrooms, and pepper.

2 Stir-fry the vegetables for 2 minutes, then add the cashew nuts and continue to cook for another 3 minutes. Add the frozen soybeans and Thai green curry paste. Stir in the noodles, breaking them up with a spoon, then add the bok choy.

3 Stir-fry the mixture for 2 minutes, adding 1–2 tablespoons of cold water if it becomes too dry and the bok choy doesn't wilt. Add the bean sprouts and cook for a final minute before serving.

COOK'S TIPS
● A broad selection of red and green Thai curry paste is available in food stores and oriental markets. They vary in their spice mix and chile heat, so try a few to find your favorite.
● Frozen soybeans are bright green, creamy in flavor, and firm. They are a good freezer standby for adding nutrition, great texture, and flavor to meat-free meals.

SUPER FOOD

SOYBEANS
Soybeans are rich in vitamins and protein, and packed with nutrients that offer antioxidant-boosting and cholesterol-lowering benefits. They are a good source of fiber, vitamin C, iron, and B vitamins thiamin and folate, which help to maintain a healthy heart.

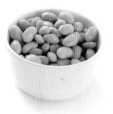

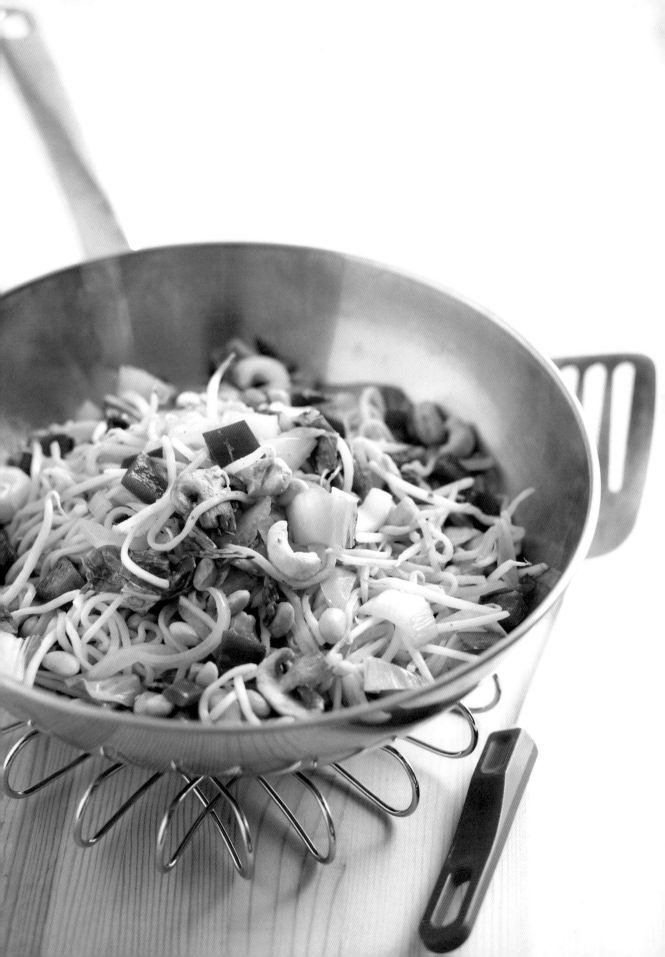

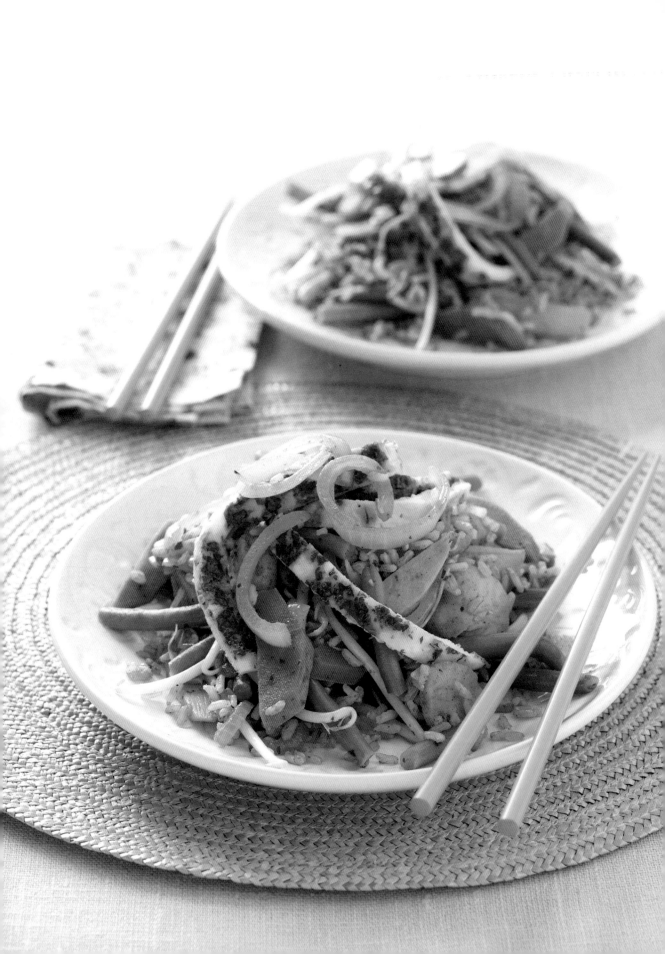

INDONESIAN FRIED **RICE** WITH **EGG** AND **VEGETABLES**

Known as *nasi goreng*, this dish of egg-topped fried rice is a traditional way of using leftovers. Crunchy water chestnuts, bamboo shoots, and bean sprouts complement the soft rice perfectly.

Serves 4
Preparation 15 minutes
Cooking 28 minutes

1 cup brown rice
2½ cups hot vegetable stock
2 onions
2 small carrots
1 can (8 ounces) water chestnuts
1 can (8 ounces) sliced bamboo shoots
⅓ cup bean sprouts
3 tablespoons olive oil or canola oil
1 teaspoon sesame oil
3 cloves garlic, crushed
½ cup frozen green beans, thawed
½ tablespoon medium curry powder
1 scallion
3 eggs
3 tablespoons chopped fresh cilantro

Each serving provides
• 432 calories • 20 g fat • 3 g saturated fat • 54 g carbohydrates • 13 g protein • 5 g fiber

ALTERNATIVE INGREDIENTS
• Use jasmine rice instead of brown rice and reduce the cooking time to 15 minutes, or according to the package directions.
• Use a 18-ounce package of fresh mixed stir-fry vegetables instead of the carrots, green beans, and bean sprouts.

1 Add the rice to a large saucepan with the hot stock. Cover, bring to a boil, and stir once. Reduce heat and simmer for 25 minutes, or according to package directions, until the rice is tender and the stock has been absorbed. Slice the onions. Thinly slice the carrots at an angle, drain and slice the water chestnuts, drain the bamboo shoots, and wash the bean sprouts.

2 Halfway through cooking the rice, heat 1 tablespoon olive oil or canola oil in a frying pan over high heat. Add the onions, reduce heat to medium, and cook for 7 minutes, or until browned. Set aside and keep warm. When the rice is almost done, heat 1 tablespoon of the olive oil or canola oil in the frying pan. Add the sesame oil, garlic, carrots, water chestnuts, bamboo shoots, green beans, and curry powder. Stir-fry for 2 minutes, or until the vegetables are tender. Add the bean sprouts and stir-fry for 1 minute, or until piping hot. Toss vegetables together with the rice and season to taste.

3 Slice the scallion. Beat the eggs with the scallion and cilantro. Add the remaining tablespoon of oil to the frying pan over high heat. Add the egg and cook for 1 minute on each side, or until set. Cut the omelet into thin strips. Divide the rice among four bowls and top with the fried onions and omelet strips.

COOK'S TIP
● Boil the rice uncovered for a few seconds if there is any excess liquid left at the end of cooking in step 1.

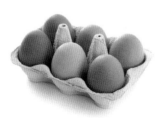

SUPER FOOD

EGGS
Egg yolks are one of the few foods that contain vitamin D, which helps reduce the risks of some cancers and heart disease, boosts the immune system, and fights diabetes. Eggs are also a complete protein; they contain all nine of the essential amino acids that cannot be made by the body.

BUTTERNUT SQUASH CASSEROLE WITH PAPAYA

Succulent butternut squash, delicate papaya, and firm borlotti beans make a satisfying one-pot meal that helps keep blood glucose levels steady. Serve with a side salad of mixed greens.

Serves 4
Preparation 15 minutes
Cooking 10 minutes

½ butternut squash, about
   1¼ pounds
1 medium papaya
1 red onion
1 tablespoon olive oil or canola oil
4–6 large fresh sage leaves
1 teaspoon ground cinnamon
juice of 1 large orange, about ½ cup
1 can (14 ounces) borlotti beans,
   drained

Each serving provides
• 179 calories • 4 g fat • 1 g saturated fat • 29 g carbohydrates
• 7 g protein • 9 g fiber

ALTERNATIVE INGREDIENTS
• Try other types of squash if butternut is not available.
• Mango goes well with squash. Select a ripe but firm mango, peel and slice it off the pit, and cut the flesh into chunks. While papaya mellows the flavor of the orange juice, mango accentuates its tanginess.
• Substitute chickpeas or cannellini beans for the borlotti beans.
• For a meaty version of this dish, broil and slice four good-quality sausages and gently add them to the mixture before serving.

1 Peel and seed the butternut squash and dice the flesh into ¾-inch chunks. Seed and peel the papaya (see Cook's Tips below), slice it, and set aside. Thinly slice the onion.

2 Heat the oil in a large covered frying pan. Add the onion and squash and cook over high heat, stirring occasionally, for 1 minute. Reduce heat to medium or medium-low, cover the pan, and cook for 2 minutes.

3 Shred the sage leaves and stir them into the pan with the cinnamon and orange juice. Bring to a boil, reduce heat to low, and cover. Simmer for 5 minutes, stirring once, until squash is tender but not soft.

4 Stir in the beans, cover the pan, and heat gently for 2 minutes. Top with the papaya and serve immediately.

COOK'S TIPS
● To prepare papaya, cut the fruit in half and scoop out the round black seeds with a spoon. Peel the thin skin from the fruit with a knife.
● Cut onions in half before slicing them so the cut side can be placed flat on a cutting board to prevent the onion from slipping.

SUPER FOOD

BEANS
A good, low-fat source of protein, beans also have a low glycemic index (GI), which means they provide a steady energy release without causing spikes in blood glucose levels. The borlotti beans in this recipe are rich in lysine, an essential protein-building amino acid that is often lacking in plant proteins.

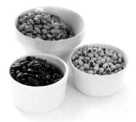

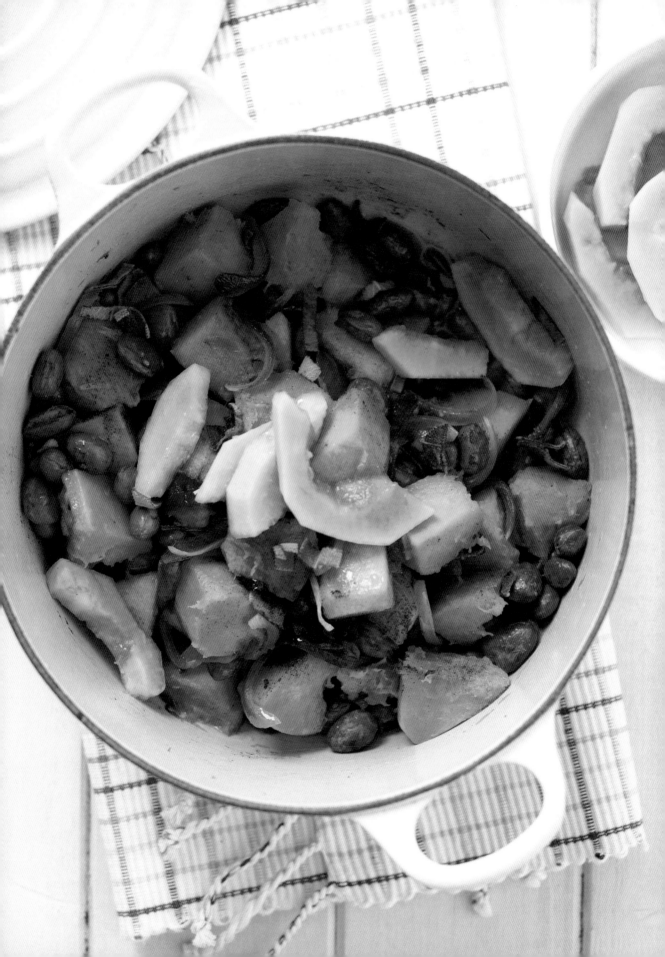

MINTED MIXED GRAIN SALAD

Fresh summery salad ingredients, plump grains, plus plenty of aromatic parsley, mint, and lemon, combine to make this zesty lunchtime treat both refreshing and surprisingly filling.

Serves 4
Preparation 10 minutes,
plus 15 minutes cooling
Cooking 15 minutes

⅓ cup bulgur
⅓ cup quinoa
1 small cucumber
2 large tomatoes
1 large green bell pepper
2 scallions
1 teaspoon sugar
grated zest and juice of 1 lemon
3 teaspoons olive oil
5 chopped large mint sprigs
¼ cup chopped fresh parsley
1 head romaine lettuce, to serve

Each serving provides
• 267 calories • 13 g fat • 2 g saturated fat • 32 g carbohydrates
• 7 g protein • 3 g fiber

ALTERNATIVE INGREDIENTS
• Use young zucchini instead of cucumber and add a crushed clove of garlic in step 2.
• Try the vegetable and herb mixture with rice as a change from bulgur and quinoa. Cook jasmine rice for an aromatic salad or sushi rice for a delicious, slightly sticky dish.

1 Place the bulgur and quinoa in a saucepan with 4 cups of boiling water. Return to a boil, reduce heat, cover and simmer for 15 minutes, or until the bulgur and quinoa are tender. Drain any water that was not absorbed. Finely dice the cucumber, tomatoes, and pepper, and thinly slice the scallions.

2 Mix the sugar, lemon zest, and juice in a large bowl, stirring until the sugar dissolves. Whisk in the oil and add the cucumber, tomatoes, pepper, and scallions. Stir in the cooked bulgur and quinoa, cover, and let cool for 15 minutes.

3 Stir the mint and parsley into the salad and season to taste just before serving. Divide the salad among four bowls and serve with a selection of lettuce leaves for wrapping and scooping.

COOK'S TIPS
● To finely dice a cucumber, slice it lengthwise, stack the slices together, cut them into strips, and cut across the strips to dice.
● The easiest way to 'chop' herbs is to hold the large leaves in a bunch and shred them finely with scissors.

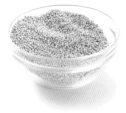

SUPER FOOD

QUINOA
Perfect in salads, quinoa provides whole-grain, high-fiber goodness to a meal. Quinoa has the highest protein content of all grains and contains all nine essential amino acids, making it a great choice for vegetarians.

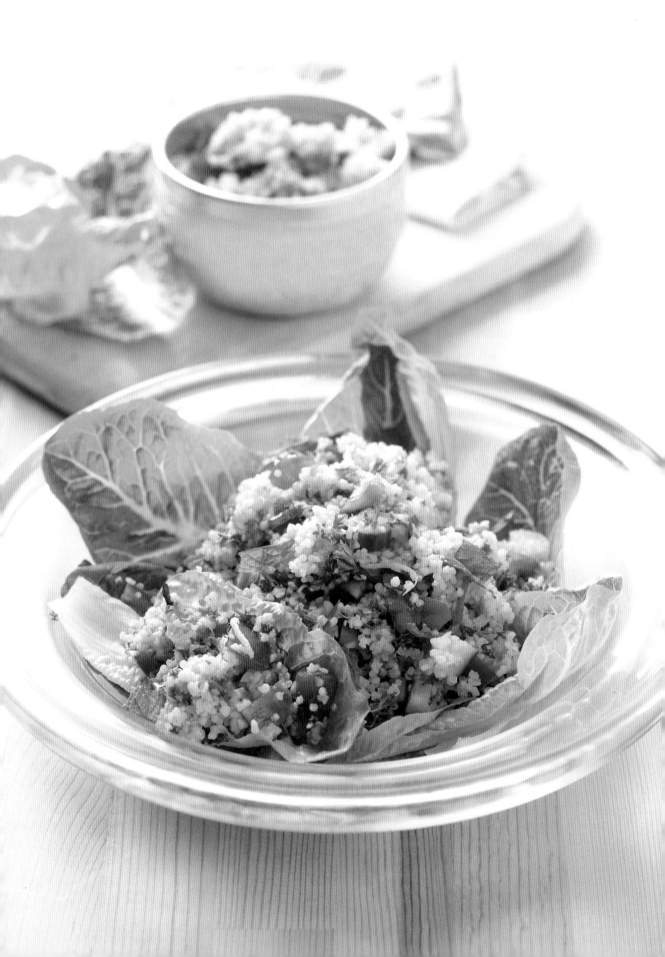

SEAFOOD AND VEGETABLE RICE

Vegetables and seafood pair perfectly with savory rice for a quick alternative to paella. With a healthy variety of ingredients, this dish also provides a real nutrition boost.

Serves 4
Preparation 15 minutes
Cooking 35 minutes

2 onions
2 large bell peppers (1 yellow, 1 red)
1 tablespoon olive oil or canola oil
2 large cloves garlic, crushed
2 bay leaves
1 cup brown rice
2½ cups hot vegetable stock
1 cup frozen peas
1 cup frozen green beans
¾ pound frozen cooked
   mixed seafood
lemon wedges and chopped
   fresh parsley, to garnish

Each serving provides
• 397 calories • 9 g fat • 2 g
saturated fat • 59 g carbohydrates
• 24 g protein • 11 g fiber

ALTERNATIVE INGREDIENTS
• Frozen diced bell peppers are a good ingredient to have on hand. Add them with the rice at step 2 instead of cooking them with the onions. Frozen mixed vegetables can also be used instead of the peas and beans.
• For a tomato-based version, reduce the stock to 1¼ cups in step 2, and add a 14½-ounce can of chopped tomatoes.
• If you don't like mixed seafood, use 1 pound cooked large shrimp.

1 Thinly slice the onions and peppers. Heat the oil in a large frying pan and add the onions, garlic, and bay leaves. Add the peppers and cook, stirring over high heat for 2 minutes, or until the vegetables soften.

2 Stir in the rice and add the stock. Return to a boil and stir the ingredients. Reduce heat to low so the liquid simmers. Cover and cook for 20 minutes, or until the liquid has almost evaporated.

3 Use a fork to gently add the frozen peas and beans. Return to a boil, reduce heat, and cover the pan. Simmer gently for another 5 minutes.

4 Add the frozen cooked seafood to the rice. Cover the pan and cook for a final 5 minutes until the rice is tender, the seafood is hot, and most of the liquid has evaporated. Garnish with lemon wedges and chopped parsley. Season with ground black pepper before serving.

COOK'S TIPS
• Garnish with mussels in their shells. Rinse and scrub the shells clean, and steam the mussels with 4 tablespoons white wine in a covered pan for 5–7 minutes, or until the shells open. Discard any mussels that do not open.
• Serve with a salad of lettuce and cherry tomatoes.

SUPER FOOD

SEAFOOD
Full of goodness, seafood contributes many nutrients to a balanced diet. It contains immune-boosting zinc and the antioxidant selenium, which helps to protect against heart disease. It's also a rich source of iodine, needed for a healthy metabolism.

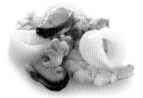

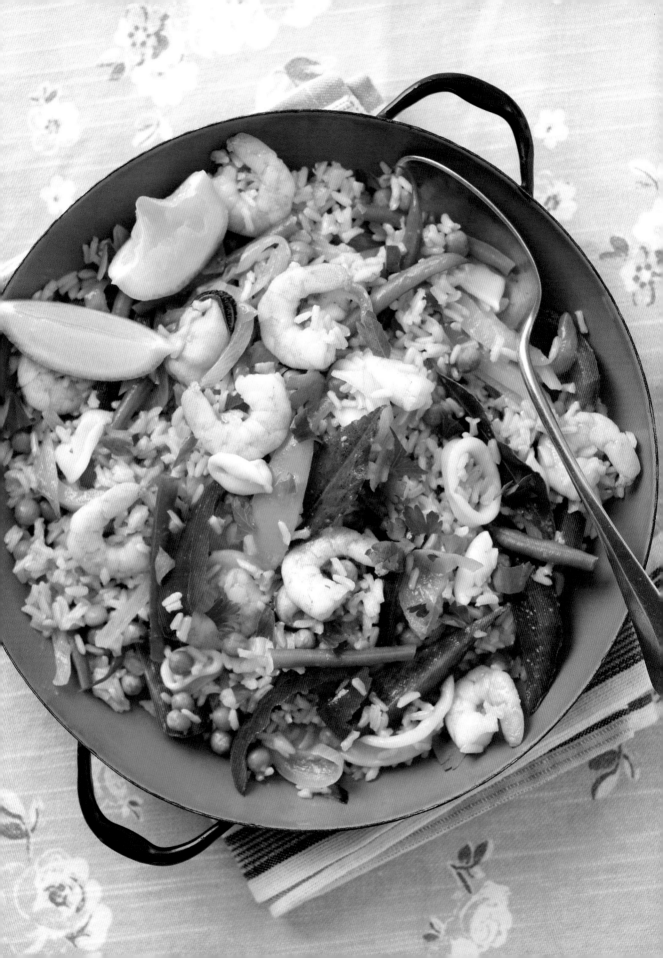

CURRIED SMOKED FISH WITH
SWEET CORN AND BROCCOLI

In an updated classic, the full-bodied flavor of smoky fish is balanced by refreshing vegetables. The golden hue of this dish comes from the turmeric-colored rice, the sweet corn, and the yolks of boiled eggs.

Serves 4
Preparation 15 minutes, plus
5 minutes standing
Cooking 25 minutes

1 large onion
⅔ pound skinless smoked cod
  or haddock fillet
2 tablespoons olive oil or canola oil
1 cup basmati rice
1½ teaspoons cumin seeds
1½ teaspoons turmeric
4 cups hot fish stock
1 cup frozen sweet corn
4 eggs
1 cup small broccoli florets
grated zest of 1 lemon
2 tablespoons chopped fresh parsley

Each serving provides
• 537 calories • 17 g fat • 3 g saturated fat • 68 g carbohydrates • 31 g protein • 4 g fiber

ALTERNATIVE INGREDIENTS
• Chunks of fresh salmon are fine in place of smoked fish.
• Omit the uncooked fish in step 2 and serve the rice topped with shredded smoked salmon, allowing ½ pound per person, or use smoked mackerel, allowing ⅔ pound per person.
• For a vegetarian kedgeree, add ⅓ cup red lentils to the rice and omit the smoked haddock. Use vegetable stock in step 1 and increase the amount to 5¼ cups.

1 Finely chop the onion and cut the smoked fish into ¾-inch pieces. Heat the oil in a large saucepan over high heat. Add the onion and cook for 2 minutes. Reduce heat and stir in the rice, cumin seeds, and turmeric. Add the hot stock, return to a boil, and reduce heat to low. Cover and simmer for 5 minutes.

2 Add the frozen corn and return to a boil. Add the fish, reduce the heat, cover, and simmer for 15 minutes, or until all the stock has been absorbed. Meanwhile, cook the eggs for 8 minutes in a pan of boiling water. Remove the rice from the heat and let it stand, covered, for 5 minutes.

3 Drain the boiled eggs, rinse them under cold water, and shell and quarter them. Place the broccoli in a saucepan, add boiling water to cover, and return to a boil. Reduce the heat, simmer for 3 minutes, and drain. Add the broccoli and lemon zest to the kedgeree. Top with the eggs and parsley and season with black pepper.

COOK'S TIPS
● Smoked fish is available dyed yellow or undyed. Where you can, opt for the natural version.
● Running hard-boiled eggs under cold water stops the cooking process and prevents a gray-green ring from forming around the yolk.

SUPER FOOD

SWEET CORN
In addition to the naturally occurring phytochemical lutein, good for eye health, corn is also a useful source of fiber, folate, and antioxidants. All three of these are associated with a lower risk of cancer.

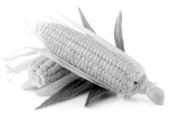

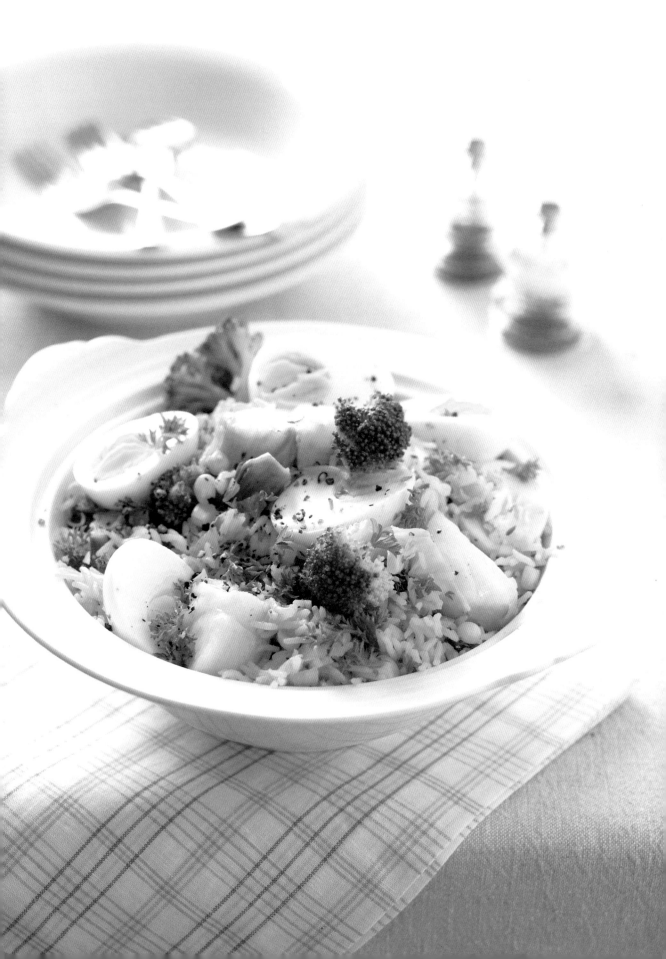

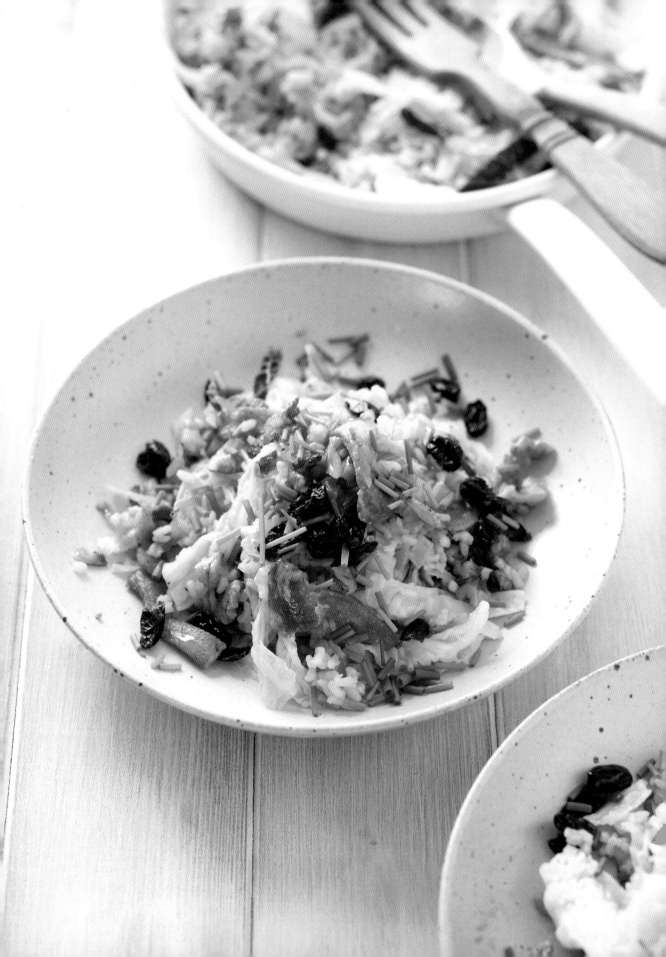

BACON PILAF WITH BERRIES AND NUTS

The brown rice in this pilaf lends a lovely nutty taste and wholesome goodness to the dish. The flavors of walnuts, cranberries, and bacon combine to make a palate-pleasing plateful.

Serves 4
Preparation 15 minutes
Cooking 45 minutes

¼ pound lean bacon
1 onion
2 celery stalks
¾ pound head of cabbage
⅓ cup coarsely chopped walnuts
1 tablespoon olive oil
1⅓ cups brown rice
4 cups hot chicken stock
¼ cup dried cranberries
4 tablespoons snipped fresh chives

Each serving provides
• 565 calories • 26 g fat • 3 g saturated fat • 71 g carbohydrates • 16 g protein • 8 g fiber

ALTERNATIVE INGREDIENTS
• Use thin slices of pepperoni or chorizo instead of bacon.
• For vegetarian pilaf, omit the bacon and heat ⅓ cup pine nuts or roughly chopped macadamia nuts in a dry frying pan until lightly browned. Set aside and add with the walnuts in step 4. Use vegetable stock in place of the chicken stock.
• Use chopped dried apricots or peaches instead of cranberries.

1. Cut the bacon into thin strips. Finely chop the onion and celery, and shred the cabbage. Add the bacon to a large dry frying pan over medium-high heat and fry for 5 minutes until browned. Add the walnuts, cooking them with the bacon for 1 minute. Remove the bacon and walnuts and set aside.

2. Add the oil, onion, and celery to the pan and cook over high heat for 2 minutes, or until the onion softens. Add the rice and continue to cook for 2 minutes, stirring frequently, until the rice grains are opaque.

3. Add 2 cups chicken stock, bring to a boil, reduce heat to medium, cover, and simmer for 5 minutes. Add the remaining stock, return to a boil and cook for another 10 minutes.

4. Pile the cabbage on top of the rice, cover, and cook over low heat for 20 minutes, or until the rice is tender and the cabbage is cooked. Add the fried bacon and walnuts plus the cranberries for the last minute of cooking and warm through. Season to taste and divide the pilaf among four plates. Sprinkle with chives and serve.

COOK'S TIPS
● Savoy cabbage or any green cabbage works well in this recipe. Collard greens or curly kale are also good choices.
● Take care adding the first batch of stock to the hot pan. It will sizzle and steam as the liquid hits the bottom of the pan.

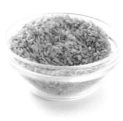

SUPER FOOD

BROWN RICE
Research shows that the risk of both heart disease and type 2 diabetes may be up to 30 percent lower in people who regularly eat whole grains such as brown rice as part of a low-fat diet and healthy lifestyle. It is the combination of health-promoting nutrients working together in brown rice that offers protection against these life-threatening disorders.

GREEK SALAD WITH **CHICKPEAS**

Food doesn't get much healthier than this salad low in fat, high in fiber, and full of antioxidants. This dish conjures visions of lazy days in the sun, and delivers on taste with every mouthful.

Serves 4
Preparation 10 minutes

1 can (15 ounces) chickpeas
1 small onion
1 green bell pepper
1 small cucumber
1 cup cherry tomatoes
2 tablespoons olive oil
1 clove garlic, crushed
20 pitted black olives
4 tablespoons chopped fresh parsley
1 cup crumbled feta
8 ounces mixed salad greens
lemon wedges, to garnish

Each serving provides
• 258 calories • 14 g fat • 7 g saturated fat • 19 g carbohydrates • 15 g protein • 3 g fiber

ALTERNATIVE INGREDIENTS
• Try adding baby new potatoes, instead of or in addition to the chickpeas. Use ½ pound potatoes, cook them in boiling water for 10 minutes until tender, and toss with the oil and garlic dressing while still hot.
• Feta is traditional in Greek salad, but try diced mozzarella for a lighter flavor.

1 Drain the chickpeas and thinly slice the onion. Coarsely dice the pepper and cucumber. Cut the cherry tomatoes in half.

2 Mix the oil, garlic, olives, chickpeas, onion, pepper, and cucumber together in a large bowl. Stir in the tomatoes and parsley. Add the feta and gently toss together.

3 Divide the mixed salad greens among four plates or bowls. Spoon the Greek salad over the greens and garnish with lemon wedges.

COOK'S TIPS
● Most of this salad can be prepared ahead, except for adding the tomatoes, parsley, and feta. It can be covered and set aside for several hours. Once complete, the salad is best served within 2–3 hours.
● If you don't like raw garlic, use the old-fashioned French method of rubbing a cut clove around the serving bowl to impart a mild garlic flavor before adding the salad. Another option is to cook the garlic in a little oil over low heat for 1–2 minutes to mellow its flavor. Cool, then add to the salad in step 1.

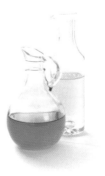

SUPER FOOD

OLIVE OIL
For decades, olive oil has been linked to good health. Recent research shows that people who follow a Mediterranean diet (olive oil, fruit, vegetables, whole grains, nuts, and fish) do indeed enjoy better health and live longer than people who follow a more traditional meat-based diet.

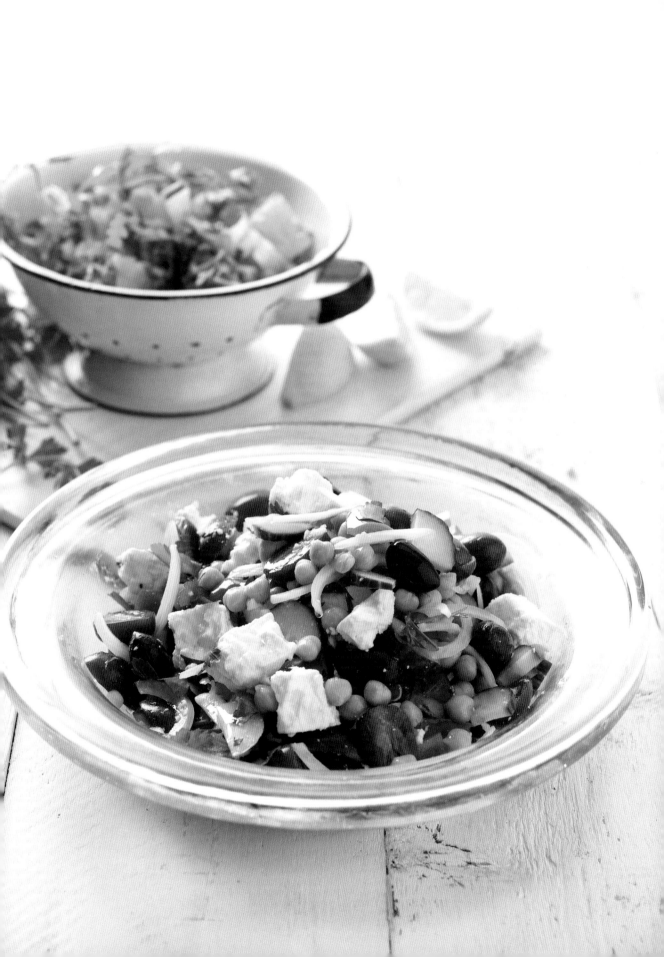

THREE BEAN SALAD WITH LEMON AND WALNUT DRESSING

A tart dressing transforms a plate of mixed beans into a richly satisfying dish, served either as a main meal or as a side dish. Crisp croutons and lively lemon zest also add texture.

Serves 4
Preparation 10 minutes
Cooking 7 minutes

8 thick baguette slices
2 tablespoons olive oil
grated zest of 2 lemons and juice
  of 1 lemon
3 tablespoons honey
1 clove garlic, crushed
3 tablespoons walnut oil
1 cup green beans
1 can (**14** ounces) red kidney beans
1 can (**14** ounces) butter beans

Each serving provides
• 483 calories • 21 g fat • 2 g saturated fat • 62 g carbohydrates • 16 g protein • 12 g fiber

ALTERNATIVE INGREDIENTS
• Try soybeans or chickpeas instead of kidney beans and butter beans.
• Use hazelnut oil as a change from walnut oil.
• A rustic light rye bread or Italian ciabatta also make good croutons.

1 Preheat the broiler to high. Place the slices of baguette on a broiler pan and brush lightly with 1 tablespoon of the olive oil. Toast for about 2 minutes, or until crisp and golden. Turn the slices, brush with the remaining 1 tablespoon olive oil and toast for another 2 minutes. Cut into chunky croutons and set aside to cool.

2 To make the lemon and walnut dressing, whisk together the lemon zest and juice, honey, garlic, and walnut oil in a large bowl. Trim the green beans and drain the kidney beans and butter beans.

3 Place the green beans in a saucepan. Add boiling water to cover and return to a boil. Reduce heat slightly and simmer for 3 minutes, or until lightly cooked but still crunchy. Drain the beans, shaking off the cooking water, and toss them with the dressing.

4 Add the kidney beans and butter beans to the dressing. Mix well and divide the salad among four bowls, spooning any remaining dressing in the bowl over each portion. Top with croutons and serve.

COOK'S TIP
● Canned butter beans are widely available in major supermarkets. You can also soak and cook your own dried butter beans, following package directions. Drain cooked beans and add to ziplock bags or containers while hot, then chill and freeze. Thaw at room temperature before use.

SUPER FOOD

BUTTER BEANS
These large beans (which are mature lima beans) are a good source of protein and iron, which play an important role in physical well-being. Just 3 tablespoons count as one of your seven-a-day. Butter beans are also virtually fat-free and packed with fiber to promote digestive health.

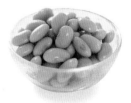

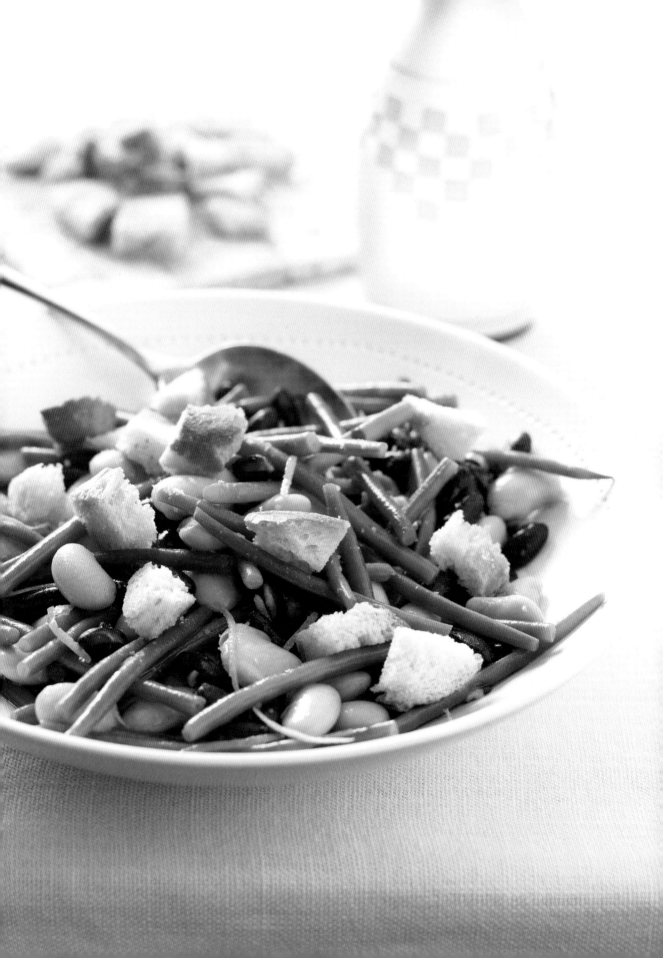

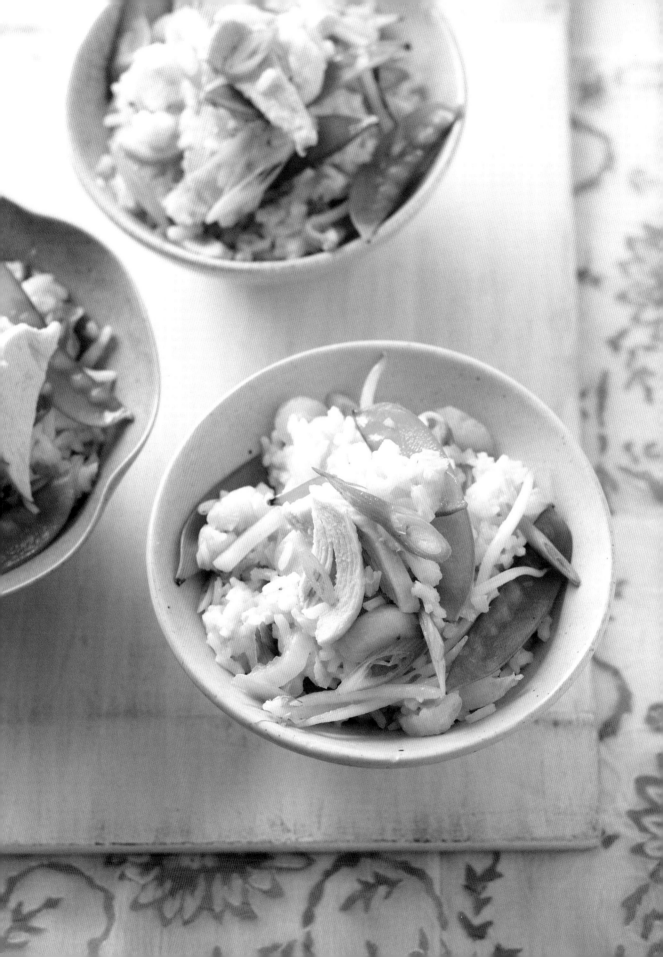

CHICKEN AND GINGER FRIED RICE

Take a little cooked chicken breast, add some delightfully crunchy vegetables and warming fresh ginger, combine with rice, and you have a simple dinner that is really hard to beat.

Serves 4
Preparation 10 minutes
Cooking 25 minutes

¾ pound cooked boneless, skinless
  chicken breast
1 can (8 ounces) water chestnuts
1 cup bean sprouts
4 scallions
2 tablespoons olive oil or canola oil
¼ cup peeled, grated fresh ginger
2 cloves garlic, crushed
1⅓ cups long-grain rice
1 teaspoon sesame oil
4 cups hot low-sodium chicken stock
1 cup finely shredded napa cabbage
1 cup snow peas

Each serving provides
• 595 calories • 18 g fat • 3 g
saturated fat • 72 g carbohydrates
• 35 g protein • 5 g fiber

ALTERNATIVE INGREDIENTS
• Brown rice works well in this recipe,
but allow an additional cup of stock
and cook for an extra 10 minutes
in step 2.
• Instead of adding the cooked chicken
in step 3, add ¾ pound peeled, cooked
shrimp in step 4, heating them briefly
before serving.
• Add a diced red or green bell pepper
with the snow peas in step 4.
• Try sugarsnap peas instead of snow
peas, or add frozen peas or green
beans in step 3.
• For vegetarian fried rice, replace the
chicken stock with vegetable stock
and add 12 ounces of tofu or tempeh
instead of the chicken.

1 Slice the chicken into small strips. Drain and slice the water chestnuts. Wash the bean sprouts and slice the scallions.

2 Heat the olive oil or canola oil in a large saucepan over high heat. Add the ginger, garlic, and rice and cook, stirring, for 3 minutes, or until the rice becomes opaque.

3 Pour in the sesame oil and hot stock. Return to a boil, reduce heat to low, cover, and simmer for 10 minutes. Add the chicken, water chestnuts, and cabbage, but don't stir. Make sure the stock is simmering and cover the pan. Cook gently for another 7 minutes.

4 Add the snow peas, bean sprouts, and scallions to the pan. Cover and cook for 2 minutes, or until the bean sprouts are piping hot. Toss the ingredients gently with the rice and serve.

COOK'S TIP
● This is a good recipe for using leftover roast chicken. Remove all the meat from the bones and cut into bite-sized pieces, checking for any bone fragments. Store cooked chicken in a sealed container in the fridge for up to 3 days.

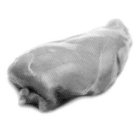

SUPER FOOD

CHICKEN
Boneless, skinless, chicken breast contains 30 percent high-quality protein and is low in fat—great for weight control. Chicken also contains some B vitamins, especially niacin, and when eaten with carbohydrates, such as rice and pasta, it can help to fight fatigue and improve mood.

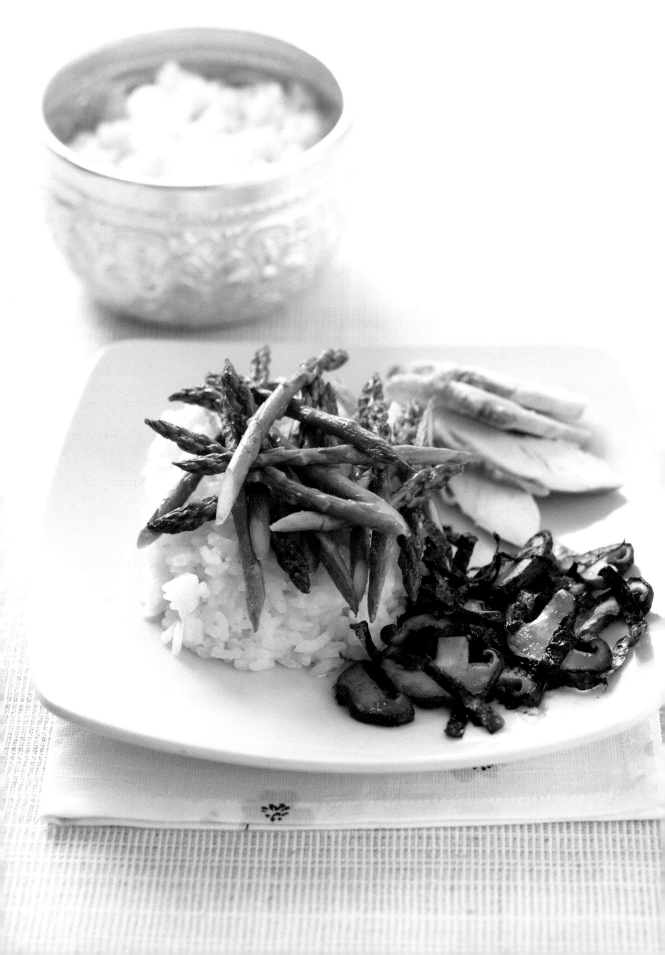

ASPARAGUS AND MUSHROOM RICE

Sticky sushi rice is a perfect base for tender Japanese-style vegetables, topped with fiber-packed, mineral-rich seaweed. Serve with sliced chicken.

Serves 4
Preparation 10 minutes, plus
5 minutes standing
Cooking 20 minutes

1 cup sushi rice
4 sheets roasted nori
2 tablespoons Japanese rice vinegar
¼ teaspoon salt
1 tablespoon sugar
3 tablespoons olive oil or canola oil
1 cup asparagus tips
⅓ cup thinly sliced shiitake mushrooms
2 tablespoons sake or dry sherry
1 tablespoon soy sauce

Each serving provides
- 338 calories • 12 g fat • 1 g saturated fat• 46 g carbohydrates
- 7 g protein • 2 g fiber

ALTERNATIVE INGREDIENTS
- Add 1 cup shredded smoked chicken or ham, or ⅓ pound diced smoked salmon, to the rice instead of or in addition to the asparagus tips.
- Sauté 1 pound raw large peeled shrimp instead of the asparagus tips. Cook for 2–4 minutes, or until they turn pink. Add them to the rice.
- You can substitute 2 tablespoons vegetable stock for the sake or sherry if you prefer.

1 Add the rice to a large saucepan with 1¼ cups of boiling water. Return to a boil, stirring once, reduce heat to low, cover, and simmer for 15 minutes, or until the water has been absorbed.

2 Cut each sheet of nori into four strips, then across into fine shreds and set aside. Mix the vinegar, salt, and sugar and add to the cooked rice. Cover the pan and set aside to infuse for 5 minutes.

3 Meanwhile, heat 1 tablespoon of the oil in a large frying pan over high heat. Add the asparagus tips and cook for 3 minutes, or until tender. Heat the remaining oil in another pan, add the mushrooms, and cook over high heat for 2 minutes. Add the sake or sherry and soy sauce to the mushrooms and boil for a few seconds, stirring the mushrooms in the liquid.

4 Divide the sushi rice among four plates, forming each portion into a neat oblong shape, and top with the asparagus tips. Transfer the mushrooms to the plates and top them with nori strips before serving.

COOK'S TIP
● Nori is an edible seaweed. Sheets of toasted nori are available in the international section of most large supermarkets or in Asian markets. Once opened, store the packet of nori in a ziplock bag for 1–2 days, though it is best eaten on the first day.

SUPER FOOD

NORI
Rich in fiber, nori is good for aiding digestive health. In addition, it's a good source of protein, iron, vitamin B_{12}, potassium, and iodine, which together help prevent anemia and regulate blood pressure. Rich in carotenoids, nori has powerful antioxidant properties, too.

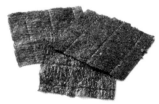

PEPPER **TABOULEH** WITH **CRANBERRIES**

Marjoram, nutmeg, and chile bring a hint of warmth, and dried cranberries add eye-catching color to this lighter version of a classic Middle Eastern salad. Serve with crisp lettuce leaves and soft tortillas.

Serves 4
Preparation 10 minutes,
plus 30 minutes soaking

1 cup bulgur
1 large red bell pepper
1 medium-hot red chile
½ red onion
¼ cup dried cranberries
1 tablespoon red wine vinegar
2 tablespoons olive oil
4 sprigs fresh marjoram, chopped
pinch of grated nutmeg

Each serving provides
• 309 calories • 9 g fat • 1 g saturated fat • 53 g carbohydrates • 6 g protein • 2 g fiber

ALTERNATIVE INGREDIENTS
• For a color change, use an orange bell pepper instead of a red one.
• Use walnut oil as an alternative to olive oil for a nuttier tabouleh.
• Dried blueberries are just as tasty as cranberries in this dish. Currants or raisins—golden or regular—work well.
• Try fresh thyme instead of marjoram or use a mix of herbs such as parsley and fennel for an aromatic twist.
• For a tangy tabouleh, add the grated zest and juice of 1 orange in step 2.

1 Place the bulgur in a heatproof bowl and add boiling water to cover. A ratio of one part bulgur to two parts water works well. Cover the bowl with plastic wrap and let it soak for 30 minutes, or until the bulgur has doubled in volume.

2 Meanwhile, finely dice the pepper and chile, and finely chop the onion. In a large bowl, mix the pepper, chile, onion, cranberries, vinegar, oil, marjoram, and nutmeg. Cover and set aside until the bulgur is ready.

3 Drain the bulgur in a sieve to remove any excess water and add it to the pepper mixture. Season to taste and serve.

COOK'S TIPS
● The flavor of the tabouleh is enhanced by letting the flavors develop for 2 hours or more before eating. If you have time, prepare and cover the tabouleh, and store it in the fridge until needed. It will stay fresh for up to 2 days when chilled.
● Tabouleh goes well with barbecued food, either as a first course or a side dish. It is also great packed in lunches or for picnics.

SUPER FOOD

CRANBERRIES
Similar to other red berries such as raspberries and strawberries, cranberries are rich in a phytochemical called ellagic acid. Some studies have shown that ellagic acid can help to prevent the growth of cancerous cells. Fiber-rich cranberries also help support a healthy digestive system.

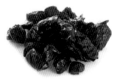

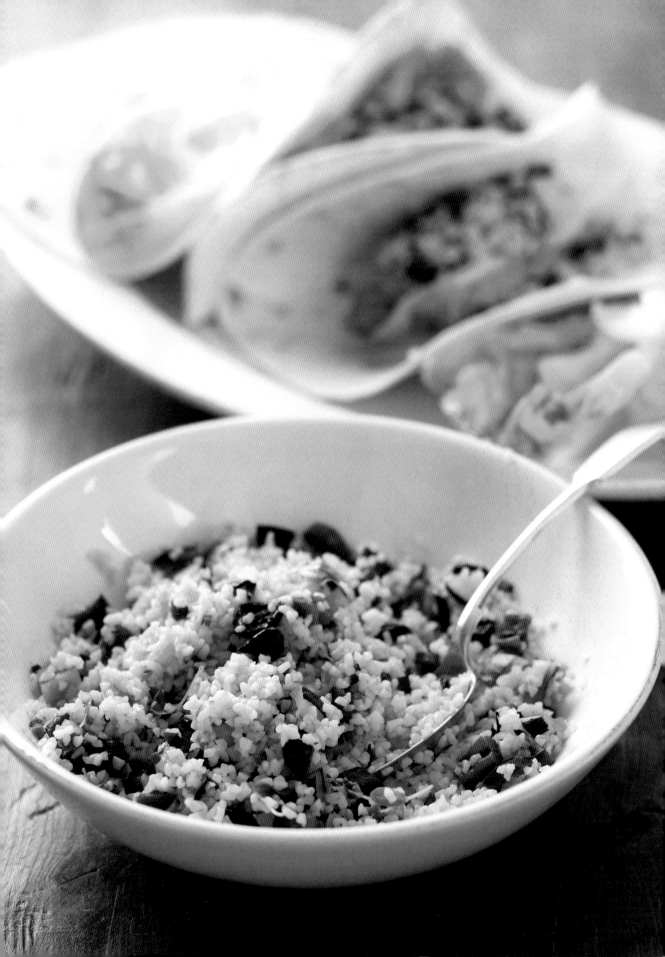

QUINOA WITH SUMMER VEGETABLES

The creamy, slightly crunchy texture and nutty taste of quinoa make it a great partner for sweet beans and juicy tomatoes. Top with a mild gouda cheese and serve with salad greens.

Serves 4
Preparation 5 minutes
Cooking 18 minutes

1 cup quinoa
1¾ cups hot chicken stock
1 cup baby lima beans, thawed
   if frozen
4 scallions
1⅔ cups halved cherry tomatoes
2 tablespoons olive oil
6 fresh basil sprigs
⅓ cup gouda cheese shavings

Each serving provides
• 333 calories • 16 g fat • 5 g saturated fat • 35 g carbohydrates • 15 g protein • 5 g fiber

ALTERNATIVE INGREDIENTS
• Use pearl barley if quinoa is not available. Cook barley in boiling water for 30 minutes, allowing 2½ cups water to 1 cup of barley.
• Use frozen soybeans instead of lima beans, adding them still frozen to the quinoa and increasing the cooking time by 2 minutes.
• Use a firm-textured aged gouda, or try manchego, gruyère, or a sharp cheddar. For a completely different flavor, use a smoked gouda or add crumbled feta.

1 Add the quinoa to a large saucepan with the hot stock. Cover, bring to a boil, reduce heat to medium, and simmer for 10 minutes. Add the baby lima beans to the pan. Cover, return to a boil, and simmer for another 5 minutes.

2 Increase the heat and boil the mixture, uncovered, for 1 minute to evaporate excess stock. If any remains in the pan after this time, drain the quinoa through a fine-meshed sieve.

3 Thinly slice the scallions. Pour the oil into a serving bowl and add the scallions and tomatoes. Shred the basil leaves on top, transfer the cooked quinoa and beans to the mixture, and stir to combine. Season to taste, divide among four bowls, and top with the gouda cheese shavings.

COOK'S TIPS
● Quinoa is cooked when the grains burst open and you can see that the germ inside the grain has formed an opaque curl. The grains should be tender but not mushy. Quinoa is gluten-free, so this recipe is suitable for people with celiac disease or gluten sensitivity.
● Baby lima beans can be eaten with their skins, but you can squeeze them off to reveal the delicate bright-green legumes, if you prefer. Larger lima beans benefit from this, as their skins can be tough.

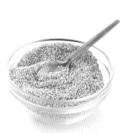

SUPER FOOD

QUINOA
Pronounced 'keen-wah,' quinoa is a whole grain with a low glycemic index (GI) that produces a slow rise in blood glucose levels and may help protect against type 2 diabetes. It's also a source of magnesium, needed for healthy bones, muscle, and nerve functions, and high in protein—good news for vegetarians.

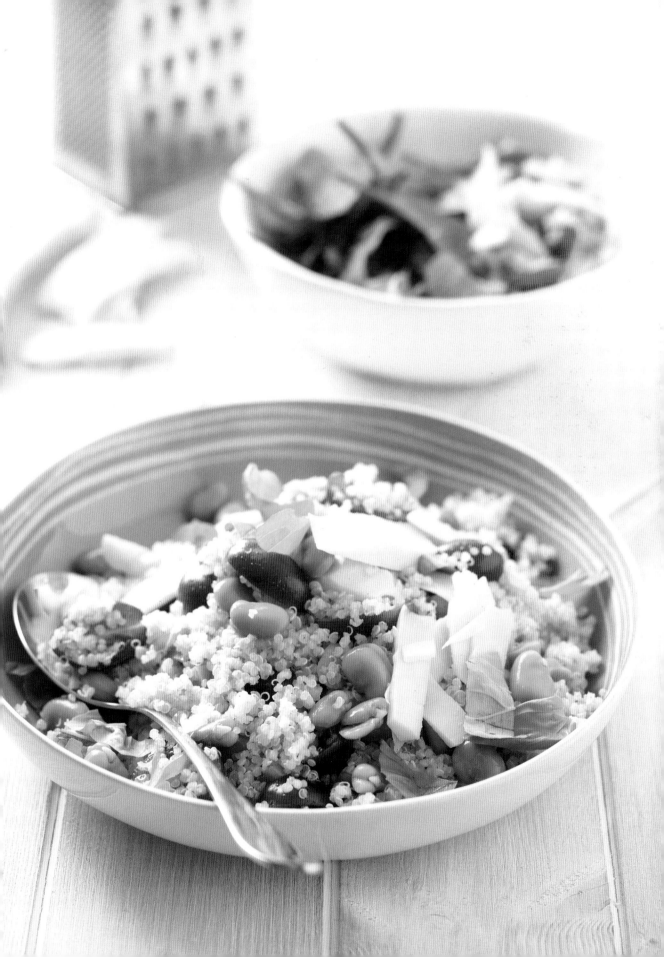

PEARL BARLEY PILAF WITH GREEN VEGETABLES

Whole-grain pearl barley is tossed with blueberries and pine nuts for an unusual combination that really works. With fresh green vegetables, it is as easy on the eye as it is on the palate.

Serves 4
Preparation 10 minutes
Cooking 25 minutes

1 cup pearl barley
1 bay leaf
2 large leeks
3 celery stalks
3 tablespoons olive oil
8 ounces spinach
1 clove garlic, crushed
¼ cup pine nuts
⅓ cup dried blueberries

Each serving provides
• 59 calories • 22 g fat • 3 g saturated fat • 79 g carbohydrates
• 16 g protein • 6 g fiber

ALTERNATIVE INGREDIENTS
• For a change, use a mix of brown rice and pearl barley, which have similar cooking times. Other types of rice that make a good pilaf include red rice and wild rice.
• Try raisins or golden raisins instead of dried blueberries, and sunflower seeds instead of pine nuts.
• Baby turnips make a tasty alternative to the spinach. Thinly slice 1 pound of baby turnips and cook them in the olive oil in step 3 with the pine nuts and garlic.

1 Add the pearl barley to a large saucepan with the bay leaf and 2½ cups of boiling water. Return to a boil, stir once, reduce heat, partly cover the pan, and cook for 25 minutes, or until the water has been absorbed and the barley is tender.

2 Meanwhile, thinly slice the leeks and celery. Heat 2 tablespoons of the oil in a frying pan over high heat. Add the leeks and celery and cook, stirring frequently, for 5 minutes, or until the vegetables are tender. Add the vegetables to the cooked barley and season to taste.

3 Add the remaining tablespoon of oil to the pan. Add the spinach and cook over medium heat for 3 minutes, or until wilted. Add the garlic, pine nuts, and dried blueberries and cook for 1 minute. Remove the bay leaf and divide the barley among four plates. Top with spinach, blueberries, and pine nuts and serve.

COOK'S TIP
● If you don't have a garlic press, peel the garlic, flatten the clove on a cutting board with the side of a large knife blade, and chop it. Whether garlic is crushed, chopped, or sliced influences its flavor in the finished dish. Crushed garlic gives the most intense result.

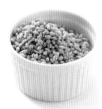

SUPER FOOD

PEARL BARLEY
A member of the grain family, pearl barley contains many nutrients, including B vitamins and folate, which help produce healthy red blood cells and prevent a type of anemia known as macrocytic anemia. Pearl barley also contains soluble dietary fiber that's effective in lowering cholesterol.

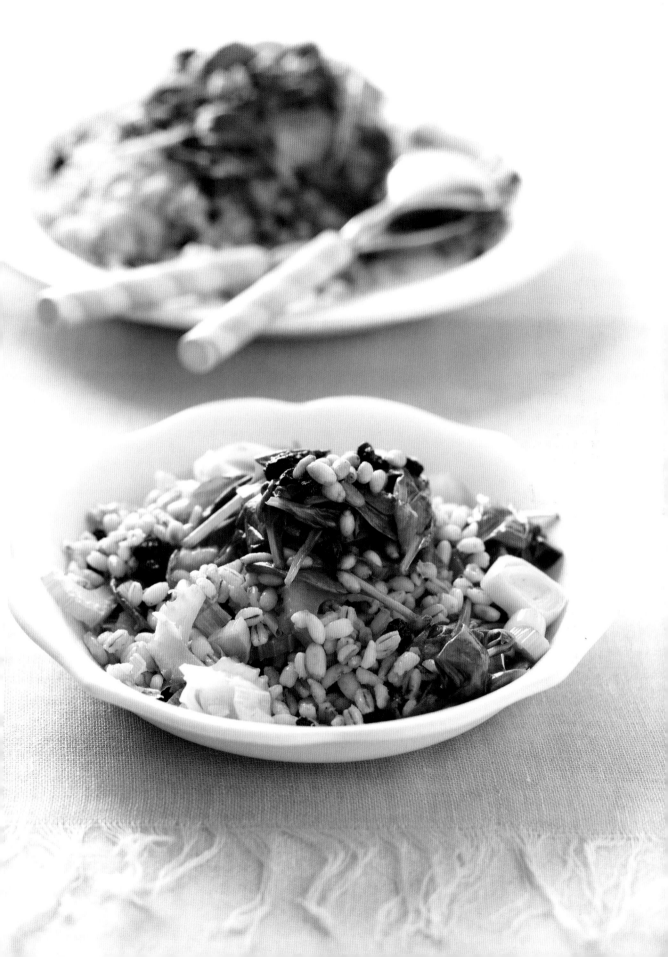

SPINACH

Dark leafy greens, especially spinach, have a rich supply of carotenoids, a group of plant compounds with strong antioxidant properties. When eaten regularly, vegetables containing carotenoids help build the body's resistance to disease. Spinach is also a good source of heart-healthy folate.

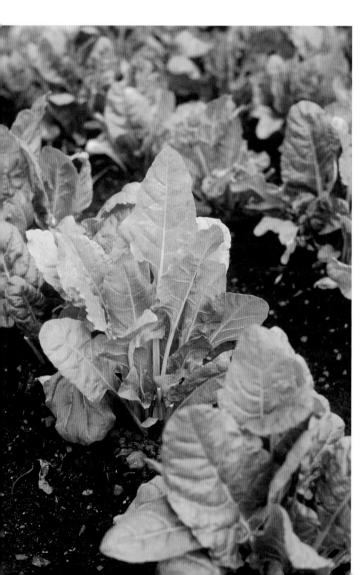

BUTTERNUT SQUASH, SPINACH, AND HAZELNUT GRATIN

Serves 4
Preparation 15 minutes Cooking 35 minutes

Each serving provides • 250 calories • 11 g fat • 5 g saturated fat • 24 g carbohydrates • 14 g protein • 6 g fiber

Preheat the oven to 375°F. Peel **1 small butternut squash**, halve lengthwise, remove the seeds, and cut into ½-inch slices. Cut **⅔ pound potatoes** into small cubes. Steam the squash and potatoes together for 8 minutes, or until just tender. Season with ground black pepper. Meanwhile, wilt **18 ounces fresh spinach** with a tablespoon of water in a large saucepan over medium-high heat, stirring, for 5 minutes. Remove from heat when the spinach leaves have turned dark green but not broken up. Drain any liquid, stir in **1 teaspoon grated fresh nutmeg (or 2 teaspoons ground nutmeg)**, and set aside. Spoon half of the squash and potato mixture into a shallow, greased baking dish and top with half the spinach. Sprinkle with **2 tablespoons chopped hazelnuts**. Continue layering the dish and top with a creamy sauce made by with **⅔ cup Greek yogurt, 1 beaten egg, 2 tablespoons grated parmesan** and **¼ cup crumbled feta**. Sprinkle **2 tablespoons whole-grain breadcrumbs** over the top and bake for 25 minutes, or until golden.

COOK'S TIPS

● Try sweet potatoes instead of white potatoes.
● If you don't have a steamer, place the butternut squash and potatoes in a colander set over a large pan of boiling water. Cover with a lid and steam as above. Or boil them for 5 minutes then drain, but be sure not to overcook them or the gratin will be mushy.

EGGS FLORENTINE

Serves 4
Preparation 15 minutes Cooking 15 minutes

Each serving provides • 311 calories • 22 g fat • 11 g saturated fat • 11 g carbohydrates • 19 g protein • 4 g fiber

Preheat the broiler to high. Make a cheese sauce by melting **¾ ounce butter** in a nonstick pan with **1 ounce all-purpose flour**. Stir over a medium heat for 2 minutes then gradually beat in **1⅓ cups low-fat (1%) milk** until it forms a smooth sauce. Add **¼ cup grated cheddar** and **1 teaspoon dijon mustard**. Wilt **20 ounces baby spinach**

leaves with 1 tablespoon of water in a large pan over medium-high heat for 5 minutes. Drain thoroughly and whisk in **1 tablespoon butter**. Divide among four individual ovenproof dishes or gratin dishes, and make a hollow in the center of each portion. Poach **4 eggs** in a pan of simmering water until the whites are cooked, remove the eggs using a slotted spoon, drain on paper towels, and place one in each spinach hollow. Pour the sauce over the spinach and egg, sprinkle each portion with **1 tablespoon grated cheddar** and broil for 2 minutes, or until golden.

COOK'S TIP

● This dish makes a hearty appetizer or serve it as a light supper with crusty bread.

SAVORY SPINACH WITH PEAS

Serves 4
Preparation 5 minutes Cooking 8 minutes

Each serving provides • 122 calories • 9 g fat
• 1 g saturated fat • 5 g carbohydrates • 6 g protein
• 8 g fiber

Cook ⅔ **cup baby peas** for 3 minutes in a small pan of boiling water. Drain and set aside. Meanwhile, heat **1 tablespoon olive oil** in a large pan. Add **8 chopped scallions** and cook over medium heat for about 5 minutes, or until softened. Add **18 ounces fresh spinach** and an extra **1 tablespoon olive oil**, stirring until wilted. Stir in the peas and the **juice of ½ lemon** and serve.

COOK'S TIP

● As an alternative to baby peas, use fresh shelled peas. They must be sweet and small—large peas contain more starch and and are not as tasty.

SPINACH-FILLED PHYLLO TARTS

Serves 4
Preparation 15 minutes Cooking 20 minutes

Each serving provides • 213 calories • 11 g fat
• 5 g saturated fat • 14 g carbohydrates • 13 g protein
• 3 g fiber

Preheat the oven to 375°F. Wash **18 ounces baby spinach leaves** in a colander, shake dry, and cook in a large saucepan for 5 minutes over medium heat, with just the water clinging to the leaves. Drain the spinach,

if necessary, and transfer it to a large bowl with **1 cup ricotta, 2 egg yolks**, and **1 crushed clove garlic**. Mix well, season with ground black pepper, and set aside. Chop **2 slices prosciutto** into ½-inch strips. Cut **4 phyllo pastry sheets** into four squares each and lightly brush with a little **olive oil**. Layer four squares of pastry into four individual metal tart pans and fill with the spinach mixture. Top each tart with a few slices of prosciutto and sprinkle **1 tablespoon grated parmesan** over each. Bake for 15 minutes, or until the pastry is golden and the filling has set.

COOK'S TIP

● Serve the tarts warm or cold with a mixed greens salad or a tomato and onion salad.

SPINACH AND MUSHROOM PASTA

Serves 4
Preparation 5 minutes Cooking 12 minutes

Each serving provides • 558 calories • 29 g fat
• 4 g saturated fat • 61 g carbohydrates • 17 g protein
• 6 g fiber

Cook **10 ounces penne** in a saucepan of boiling water for 10 minutes, or according to package directions, until the pasta is tender but still firm to the bite. Drain. Meanwhile, heat **2 tablespoons olive oil** in a large frying pan and add **2 finely chopped shallots**, **1 cup sliced mushrooms**, and **2 crushed cloves garlic**. Stir over a medium heat until softened. Add **14 ounces baby spinach leaves** and **1 teaspoon grated nutmeg**. Stir until the spinach has wilted and add an additional **1 tablespoon olive oil**. Toss the vegetables with the hot pasta and season to taste. Divide among four plates and sprinkle each portion with **½ tablespoon grated parmesan** and **½ tablespoon pine nuts**.

COOK'S TIP

● For a creamy dish, add ⅓ cup low-fat sour cream or low-fat cream cheese instead of the last tablespoon of olive oil.

SUMMER **CHICKEN** RISOTTO WITH GREEN **PEAS**

The creaminess of Italian arborio rice develops with the slow cooking of this mouthwatering and simple dish. The sweetness of fresh green peas adds the taste of a summer garden.

Serves 4
Preparation 20 minutes, plus
5 minutes standing
Cooking 28 minutes

1 onion
1 pound boneless, skinless
   chicken breasts
1¾ cups fresh peas or
   1 cup frozen baby peas
2 tablespoons olive oil
1 cup arborio rice
3¾ cups hot chicken stock

Each serving provides
• 460 calories • 11 g fat • 2 g
saturated fat • 60 g carbohydrates
• 32 g protein • 3 g fiber

ALTERNATIVE INGREDIENTS
• For a richer risotto, try a combination of wine and stock. Add 1¼ cups dry white wine in step 2 and reduce the chicken stock to 2½ cups. Top each portion of risotto with parmesan shavings before serving.
• Asparagus works well instead of peas. Trim off any woody ends from 8 asparagus spears, slice, and add to the pan in step 2 before adding the stock.

1 Finely chop the onion and cut the chicken into ¾-inch chunks. Shell the fresh peas, if using. Heat the oil in a large saucepan over high heat. Add the onion, reduce heat to medium, and cook for 1 minute. Add the chicken and cook, stirring, for 5 minutes, or until the chicken is firm and no pink color remains.

2 Add the rice and cook for 1 minute, stirring to coat the rice with the oil. Add 2 cups of hot stock to the pan and bring to a boil, stirring once or twice. Reduce heat to medium or low so the stock simmers, and cook for 10 minutes.

3 Add the fresh peas, if using, and stir in the remaining 1¾ cups stock. Return to a boil, reduce heat to medium or low, and simmer for 10 minutes. If using frozen peas, add them for the final 5 minutes of cooking time. Stir once or twice so the rice cooks evenly. At the end of the cook time, most of stock should be absorbed with a little remaining.

4 Season to taste, cover, and remove the pan from the heat. Let the risotto stand for 5 minutes—the rice will finish cooking and absorb the excess liquid, leaving it moist and creamy.

COOK'S TIP
● Simmer the stock gently for an authentic, creamy risotto. Don't let it boil or the stock will evaporate rather than being absorbed by the rice.

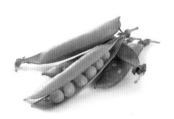

SUPER FOOD

PEAS
These little green wonders are bursting with antioxidants, including lutein, which can protect your eyesight by lowering the risk of developing age-related cataracts. Peas are also starchy and high in fiber—good for promoting a healthy heart and digestive system.

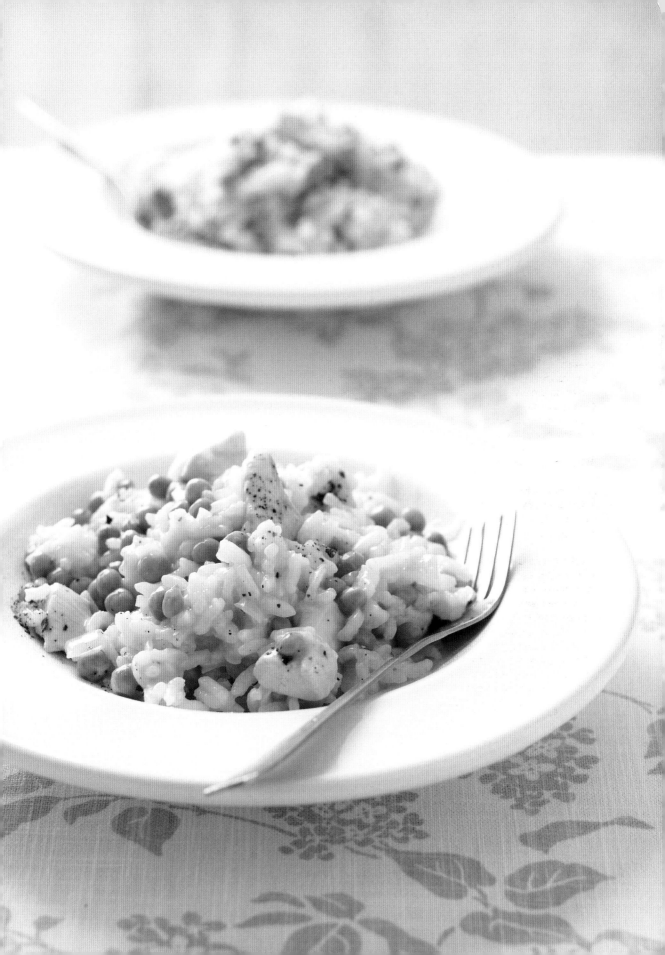

HERBED **BULGUR** WITH **CHORIZO**

Moist, chewy bulgur, flavored with herbs, peppers, and cucumber is a welcome change from everyday salad. Spicy chorizo adds plenty of punch, with some cooling yogurt served on the side.

Serves 4
Preparation 10 minutes,
plus 30 minutes soaking

1 cup bulgur
1¾ cups hot chicken stock
½ cucumber
2 red bell peppers
¼ pound cooked chorizo,
   thinly sliced
4 tablespoons snipped fresh chives
2 tablespoons chopped fresh dill
8 large sprigs fresh mint,
   leaves chopped
½ cup plain yogurt

Each serving provides
• 343 calories • 12 g fat • 5 g
saturated fat • 47 g carbohydrates
• 8 g sugars • 2 g fiber

ALTERNATIVE INGREDIENTS
• Use a variety of cooked meats—
spicy or full-flavored varieties work
best—such as pastrami, garlic
sausage,
or salami.
• Mixed grains, such as spelt, barley,
and buckwheat, make an ideal change
from bulgur. Follow the package
directions for individual soaking and
cooking times.
• For a meat-free alternative, top the
yogurt with chopped hard-boiled egg,
allowing one egg per portion and omit
the chorizo and mint. Replace the
chicken stock with vegetable stock.

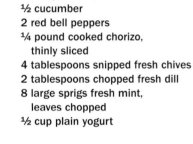

1 Place the bulgur in a heatproof bowl and add the hot stock. Cover with plastic wrap and let soak for 30 minutes, or until the bulgur is tender and doubled in volume.

2 Meanwhile, dice the cucumber and peppers and shred the chorizo. Remove any excess liquid from the bulgur by draining it through a sieve. Return it to the bowl and stir in the cucumber, pepper, chives, dill, and mint and season to taste.

3 Divide the bulgur among four bowls. Top each serving with the chorizo. Add some of the yogurt or serve it on the side.

COOK'S TIPS
● Use kitchen scissors to cut the chorizo into thin strips.
● If you need to measure yogurt, it is helpful to know that ½ cup of yogurt equals 4 ounces.

SUPER FOOD

RED BELL PEPPERS
As a fiber source, red bell peppers are good for promoting a healthy digestive system, and contain potassium to help regulate blood pressure. They are also packed with powerful antioxidant carotenes, which help protect the body against some cancers.

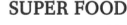

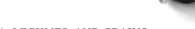

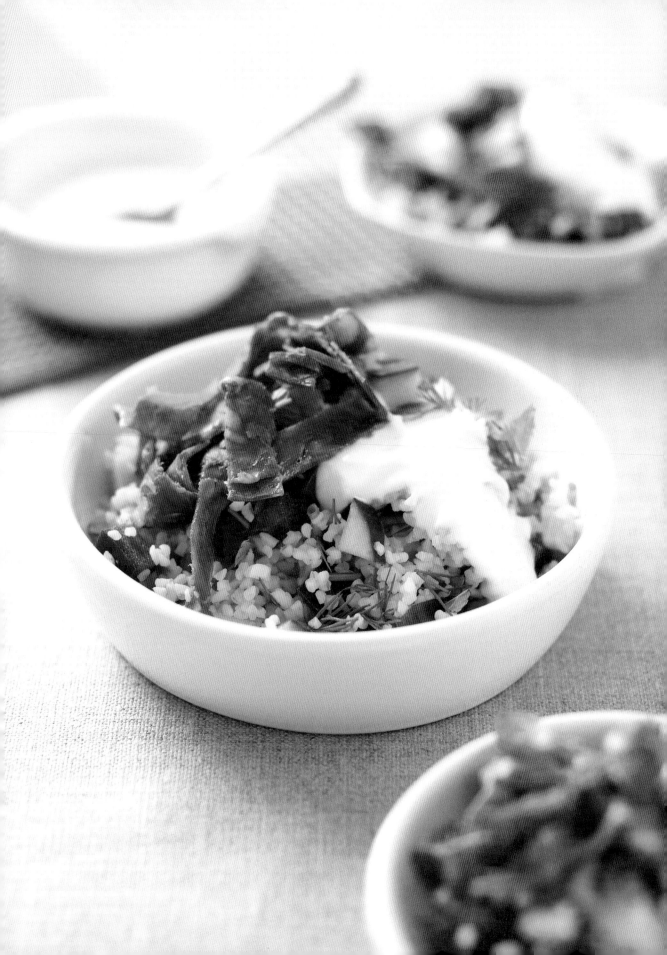

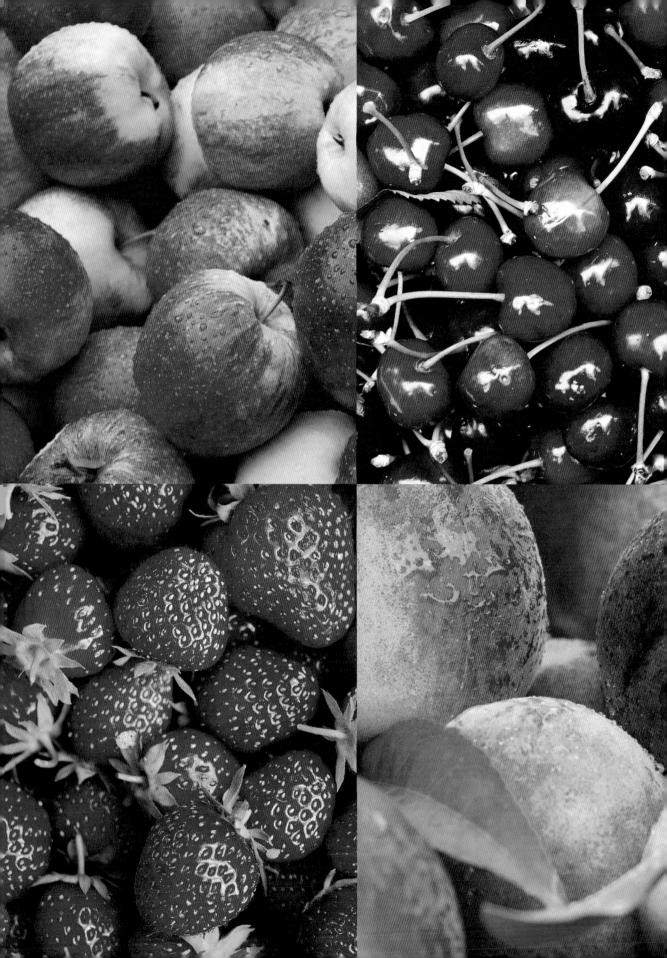

DESSERTS

RASPBERRY CREAMS WITH MANGO AND HONEY SAUCE

Everyone will love this lusciously smooth yet quick and healthy dessert. What's more, its bright jewel-like colors would look great on any dinner-party table.

Serves 4
Preparation 10 minutes

1 cup low-fat Greek yogurt
　or low-fat cream cheese
2 tablespoons confectioners' sugar
1 large ripe mango
1 tablespoon honey
1 cup raspberries

Each serving provides
• 170 calories • 2 g fat • 1 g
saturated fat • 30 g carbohydrates
• 6 g protein • 4 g fiber

ALTERNATIVE INGREDIENTS
• Use a variety of fruit instead of raspberries—sliced strawberries, whole blueberries, pitted cherries, halved black or green grapes, kiwifruit, pineapple chunks, or sliced bananas.
• Swap the yogurt or cream cheese for ricotta, beating it thoroughly with the confectioners' sugar in step 1 until it's smooth and creamy.
• As a change from mango, use 1½ cups of fruit such as peaches, nectarines, or plums to make a tasty purée to complement the raspberries.

1 Mix the yogurt or cream cheese with the confectioners' sugar. Cut the mango flesh from the pit, chop it into small chunks, and purée in a blender or food processor. Stir the honey into the mango purée.

2 Set aside 8 raspberries and reserve 4 teaspoons of the sweetened yogurt or cream cheese. Divide the remainder of the raspberries among four glass dishes and top with the yogurt mixture, smoothing the surface with a knife or the back of a spoon.

3 Spoon the mango purée over the yogurt to cover. Top each portion with a teaspoon of the reserved sweetened yogurt and decorate with 2 raspberries.

COOK'S TIP
● To measure honey, dip a metal spoon into boiling water, dry off the water, and scoop up the honey—it will easily slide off the hot spoon. For creamed honey, use a round-blade knife to fill the bowl of a measuring spoon, then scrape the honey into the mango purée.

SUPER FOOD

RASPBERRIES
Like other berries, raspberries are rich in anthocyanins and ellagic acid, powerful antioxidants that protect against cancer and heart disease. Raspberries also have a low glycemic index (GI), which means their natural sugars are released slowly into the bloodstream, helping keep blood glucose levels steady.

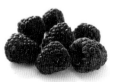

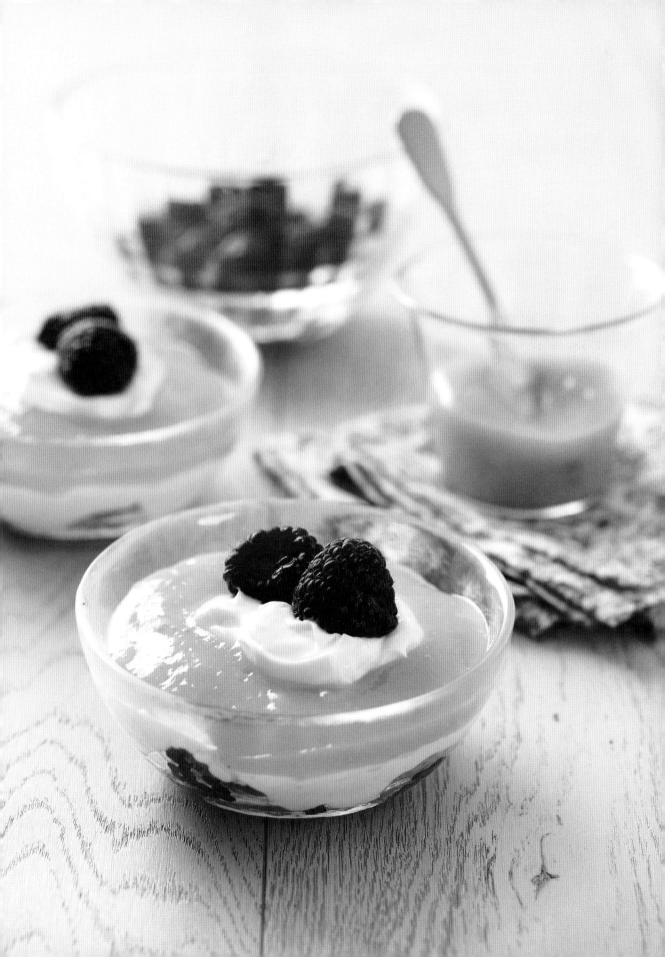

WARM SPICED **PLUMS** WITH **HAZELNUT** YOGURT

Speedy cooking brings out the best in firm plums, especially when they are sprinkled with a little cinnamon. Toasted hazelnuts, mixed with yogurt, add a burst of fiber and vitamin E goodness.

Serves 4
Preparation 10 minutes
Cooking 5 minutes

⅓ cup chopped toasted hazelnuts
1¾ cups low-fat Greek yogurt
2 tablespoons honey
1 tablespoon sugar
½ teaspoon cinnamon
1 pound firm ripe plums

Each serving provides
• 374 calories • 18 g fat • 3 g saturated fat • 39 g carbohydrates
• 12 g protein • 5 g fiber

ALTERNATIVE INGREDIENTS
• Use chopped pecans and maple syrup rather than hazelnuts and honey.
• Broil 8 ripe pear halves instead of of plums. Halve 1 pear per portion, remove the cores and place, cut sides up, in the dish. Use a little grated nutmeg instead of the cinnamon, which is too strong a flavor for pears. Sprinkle pear halves with the juice of ½ lemon and the spiced sugar before broiling in step 2.
• For a weekend breakfast, serve the plums on heated waffles or pancakes and top with the hazelnut yogurt.

1 Preheat the broiler to high. Reserve 4 tablespoons of hazelnuts and mix the remaining hazelnuts with the yogurt. Drizzle in the honey, mix gently, cover, and set aside in the fridge while preparing the plums.

2 Mix the sugar and cinnamon. Halve and pit the plums (see Cook's Tips), cutting the halves in quarters if they are large. Place the plums in an ovenproof dish and sprinkle with cinnamon sugar. Broil for 5 minutes, or until the sugar has dissolved and the plums begin to brown. Cooking time will depend on the ripeness of the fruit.

3 Divide the plums among four serving plates and spoon any cooking juices on each portion. Add a spoonful of hazelnut yogurt and sprinkle with the reserved hazelnuts.

COOK'S TIPS
● To pit plums, cut the fruit in half from the top, following the natural dimple. Twist the halves and they will separate easily, leaving the pit in one half. Use a small pointed knife or your fingers to remove the pit.
● To toast hazelnuts, place the nuts on a baking sheet and roast in the oven for 5 minutes at 425°F, or until browned, checking regularly to be sure they don't burn.
● Prepare the hazelnut yogurt in advance so it's handy for an easy weekend breakfast treat.

SUPER FOOD

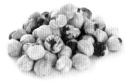

HAZELNUTS
Highly nutritious, hazelnuts are rich in heart-healthy fats. They are also a good source of B vitamins, especially thiamine (B_1) and B_6. Full of fiber, nuts help to maintain digestive health and a handful will provide your daily dose of vitamin E.

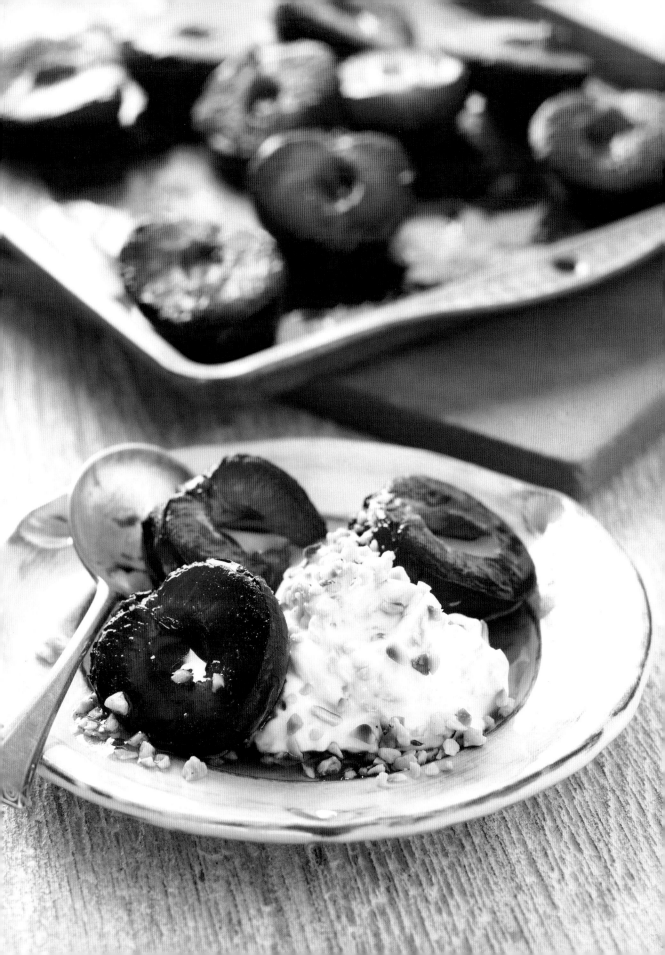

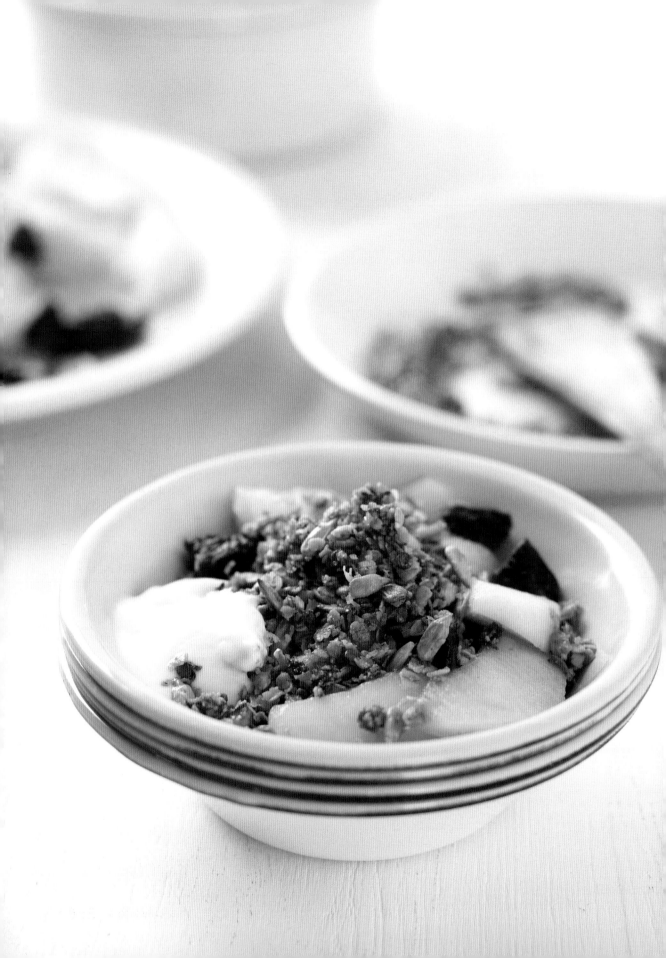

JUICY **APPLES** WITH **OAT** AND **SEED** CRUNCH

A fresh and fiber-rich take on the classic crumble, these lightly stewed apples and prunes with a golden oat topping are a special treat with a spoonful of yogurt or vanilla pudding.

Serves 4
Preparation 5 minutes
Cooking 8 minutes

1 pound cooking apples
½ cup apple juice
½ cup quartered pitted prunes
2 tablespoons butter
½ cup whole rolled oats
2 tablespons sunflower seeds
2 tablespoons raw sugar
¼ cup plain yogurt

Each serving provides
• 273 calories • 11 g fat • 4 g saturated fat • 41 g carbohydrates • 6 g protein • 5 g fiber

ALTERNATIVE INGREDIENTS
• Almost any dried fruit can be used to sweeten the apples instead of prunes: peaches, pears, apricots, golden or regular raisins, cranberries, or any mixed dried fruit.
• Add ¼ cup chopped walnuts with the sugar in step 3.
• Try mixed seeds, such as sesame, sunflower, and pumpkin, or use a combination of chopped mixed nuts and seeds.

1 Peel, core, and cut the apples into ½-inch slices. Place in a saucepan and add the juice. Bring to a boil, reduce the heat, and cover. Simmer for about 5 minutes, stirring occasionally, until soft but not mushy. Add the pieces of prunes and gently toss them into the pan. Cover and set aside off the heat.

2 Melt the butter in a frying pan over medium heat. Add the oats and sunflower seeds, increase heat to medium-high, and cook, stirring, for about 2 minutes, or until the oats and seeds are browned.

3 Add the sugar and stir until it melts and coats the mixture. Remove pan from the heat. Divide the apple among four dishes and top with the oat mixture. Spoon a tablespoon of yogurt onto each portion and serve hot or warm.

COOK'S TIP
● Make double the quantity and freeze in individual portions. You can also do this if you have leftover stewed apples. The crunchy topping can be frozen separately and sprinkled over ice cream or yogurt.

SUPER FOOD

APPLES
Apples have been called nature's toothbrush. While they don't actually cleanse the teeth, biting and chewing an apple stimulates the gums, and the sweetness of the apple prompts an increased flow of saliva, which reduces tooth decay by lowering the levels of bacteria in the mouth.

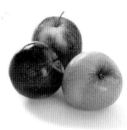

CHOCOLATEY **ORANGE** AND **BLUEBERRY** SOUFFLÉS

A gooey soufflé, with its tempting deep cocoa color, is baked over a vitamin-filled blueberry base, proving that even such an irresistible dessert can be good for you.

Serves 4
Preparation 10 minutes
Cooking 12 minutes

1 cup blueberries
2 eggs
4 tablespoons superfine sugar
3 tablespoons all-purpose flour
2 tablespoons unsweetened
   cocoa powder
grated zest and juice of 1 orange
½ teaspoon confectioners' sugar,
   for dusting

Each serving provides
• 208 calories • 5 g fat • 2 g
saturated fat • 35 g carbohydrates
• 7 g protein • 3 g fiber

ALTERNATIVE INGREDIENTS
• When fresh blueberries are not
available, use frozen ones or use
frozen mixed berries.

1 Preheat the oven to 425°F. Place four 1-cup (4-inch diameter) ramekins on a baking sheet and divide the blueberries among them.

2 Separate the eggs, putting the whites in a thoroughly clean bowl and the yolks in a separate bowl. Add the sugar, flour, cocoa powder, orange zest, and juice to the egg yolks and beat to form a smooth batter. Beat the egg whites with a whisk until they stand in stiff peaks. Use a large metal spoon to fold the egg whites into the batter.

3 Spoon the batter over the blueberries, leveling each surface, and bake for 12 minutes, or until the soufflés rise and are set. Dust with confectioners' sugar and serve immediately.

COOK'S TIPS

● When whisking egg whites, the bowl and beaters must be totally clean and grease-free or the whites will not stiffen.
● If you are preparing this dessert ahead of time, mix the chocolate batter a couple of hours in advance, cover, and set it aside until needed. Put the egg whites in a separate bowl and whisk just before folding them into the chocolate batter.

SUPER FOOD

BLUEBERRIES
Acclaimed as one of the ultimate super foods, blueberries are packed full of phytochemicals, especially anthocyanins, which are thought to have anti-inflammatory effects in the body. Researchers believe that the berries may help to protect against some cancers and heart disease.

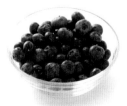

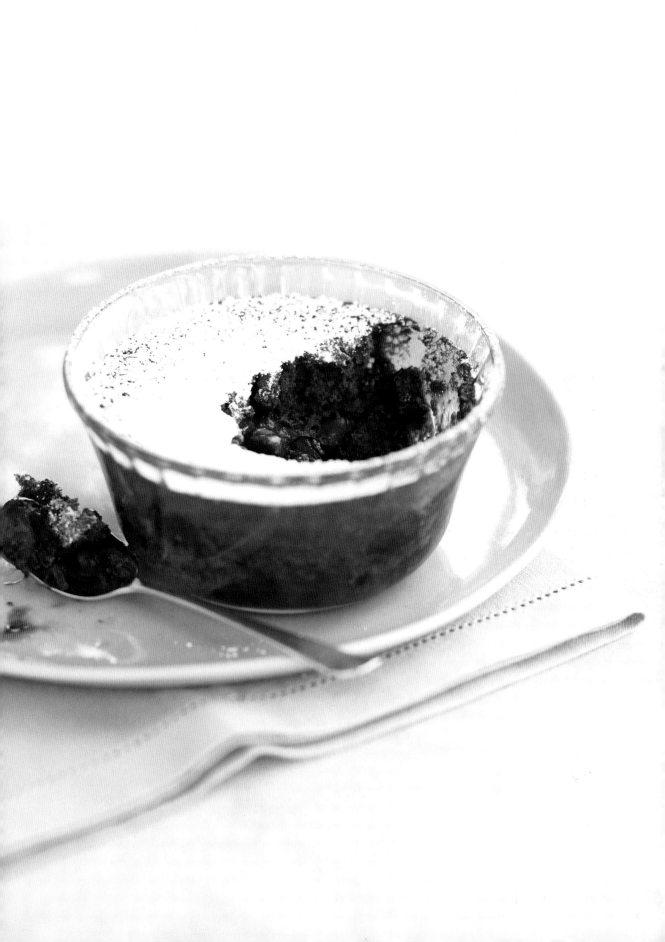

ORANGE AND BANANA MEDLEY

Cinnamon and orange are a perfect match for banana in a quick, refreshing, and filling dessert full of flavor, essential vitamins, and minerals. Serve with a dollop of low-fat vanilla ice cream.

Serves 4
Preparation 10 minutes
Marinating 10–15 minutes
Cooking 2 minutes

4 large seedless oranges
¼ cup raisins or golden raisins
1 stick cinnamon
2 large or 4 small bananas

Each serving provides
• 180 calories • 1 g fat • 0 g saturated fat • 43 g carbohydrates • 4 g protein • 6 g fiber

ALTERNATIVE INGREDIENTS
• Use dried cranberries (often sold as 'craisins') or cherries instead of raisins or golden raisins.
• Try strawberries as a change from bananas, leaving the strawberries whole or halving large ones.
• Spiced pineapple is a refreshing alternative to banana and orange. Use 1 peeled ripe pineapple, 1 star anise and ¼ teaspoon ground cinnamon.

1 Use a zester to remove the zest of 1 orange, halve the orange, and squeeze the juice. Add water, if necessary, to make 5 ounces of juice. Pour the juice into a saucepan. Add the zest, raisins or golden raisins, and the cinnamon stick (or half a stick if you prefer). Bring to a boil, remove from the heat, cover, and set aside.

2 Slice the ends off the remaining 3 oranges, and cut away the peel in wide strips, working down the fruit to remove all the pith. Slice the oranges, discarding any seeds.

3 Place the sliced oranges in a serving dish, adding any juice that came from preparation. Pour the juice mixture over the fruit. Cover and set aside for 10–15 minutes.

4 Peel and slice the bananas and add them to the oranges just before serving, mixing to coat the slices in the orange juice mixture so that they don't discolor.

COOK'S TIPS
● The banana and orange medley can also be served warm, especially when using a good-quality fresh cinnamon stick, which will provide plenty of flavor. Prepare the recipe as above but don't set the syrup or fruit aside in either step 1 or step 3.
● Oranges can be prepared, cooled, and chilled overnight in an airtight container.

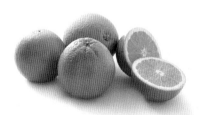

SUPER FOOD

ORANGES
Oranges are renowned for their high content of vitamin C, which, as well as being a powerful antioxidant, is good for eye health and the immune system.

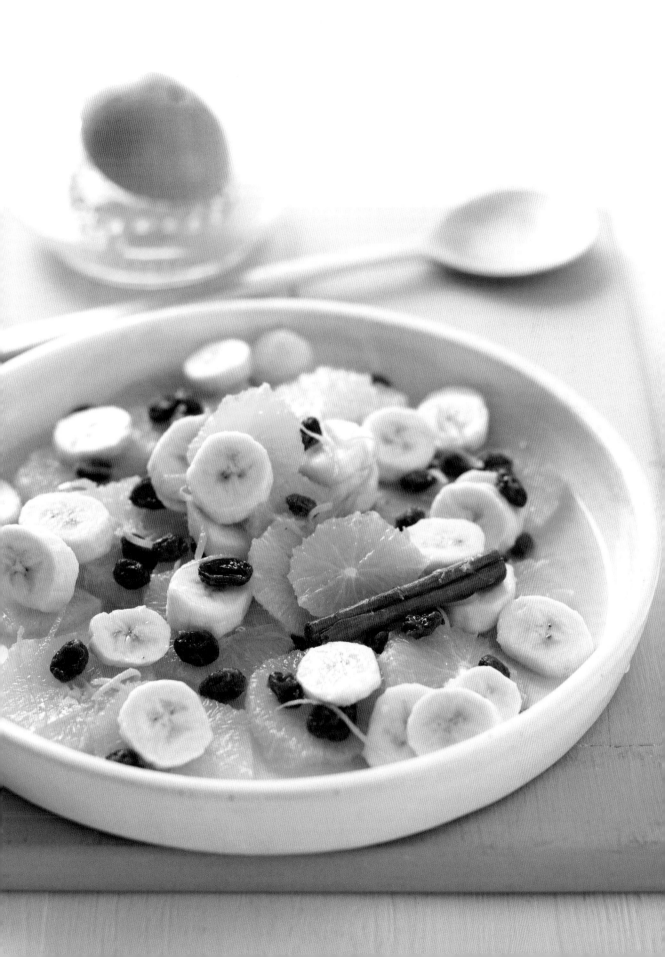

BANANAS

The fiber in bananas, both soluble and insoluble, helps to protect the body against bowel cancer, stabilize blood glucose levels, and lower harmful blood cholesterol. Bananas also contain vitamin B_6, important for making red blood cells and breaking down protein and fats.

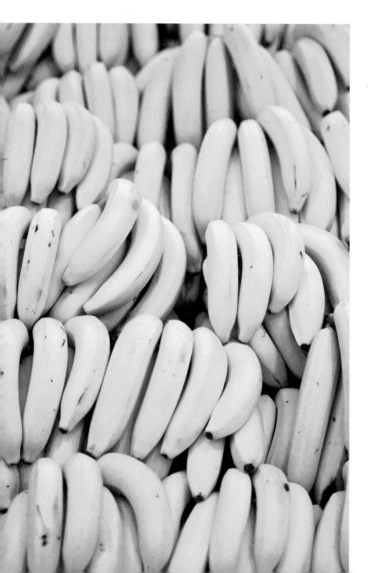

FRUITY QUICK BREAD

Makes 8 slices
Preparation 10 minutes Cooking 40 minutes

Each serving provides • 275 calories • 14 g fat • 2 g saturated fat • 31 g carbohydrates • 8 g protein • 3 g fiber

Preheat the oven to 350°F. Grease a 9x5x3-inch loaf pan and line it with parchment paper. In a bowl, combine **⅔ cup self-rising flour, ½ cup whole-wheat self-rising flour, ⅔ cup ground almonds, ½ teaspoon baking powder** and **½ teaspoon ground ginger**. In another bowl, combine **3 mashed very ripe bananas, 2 eggs, ¼ cup honey** and **⅓ cup low-fat (1%) milk**. Stir the dry ingredients into the wet ingredients, then fold in **⅓ cup chopped pecans**. Pour the mixture into the prepared loaf pan and bake for 40 minutes, or until golden and a skewer comes out clean when inserted in the center of the bread. Cool completely before slicing.

COOK'S TIP

● This yummy bread is a healthy alternative for breakfast, picnics, and lunchboxes. If desired, spread with butter or low-fat all-fruit preserves before serving.

APRICOT AND BANANA CRUMBLE

Serves 4
Preparation 10 minutes Cooking 35 minutes

Each serving provides • 342 calories • 12 g fat • 4 g saturated fat • 54 g carbohydrates • 7 g protein • 6 g fiber

Preheat the oven to 350°F. Simmer **⅔ cup dried apricots** in water to cover for 15 minutes, or until tender. Meanwhile, peel and slice **3 bananas** and place in an ovenproof dish. Add the juice of **1 lemon**. Drain the apricots, reserving the cooking liquid, chop into quarters and spoon them over the sliced bananas. Pour in 4 tablespoons of the reserved cooking liquid. In a bowl, combine **¾ cup rolled oats** with **¼ cup chopped mixed nuts** and **1 tablespoon sunflower seeds**. In a small saucepan, add **1 tablespoon honey, 2 tablespoons butter,** and **1 tablespoon soft brown sugar**. Warm over medium heat until the sugar has dissolved. Mix together and add to the dry ingredients, stirring to combine. Spoon the oaty topping over the fruit and bake for 20 minutes, or until the crumble topping is cooked and golden.

● When melting the sugar with the honey and butter, do not place the pan over high heat or the sugar may burn and make the crumble topping bitter. Stir the mixture regularly.

BANANA SPLIT WITH FROZEN YOGURT

Serves 4
Preparation 10 minutes, plus 30 minutes cooling
Cooking 5 minutes Freezing 5 hours

Each serving provides • 410 calories • 6 g fat • 3 g saturated fat • 81 g carbohydrates • 13 g protein • 4 g fiber

To make the iced yogurt, dissolve **⅓ cup superfine sugar** in **3 tablespoons hot water** in a saucepan for 5 minutes over low heat. Remove from heat and cool for 30 minutes. Combine this syrup with **2¾ cups full-fat plain yogurt** and **½ teaspoon vanilla extract**. Freeze in an ice-cream maker following manufacturer's directions, or transfer to a covered plastic container and freeze for at least 5 hours, removing every hour and beating to prevent ice crystals from forming. In a blender or food processor, blend **1⅓ cups fresh raspberries** with **¼ cup superfine sugar** and the **juice of 1 lemon**. Strain the purée through a fine-meshed sieve to remove seeds, stirring in 1 tablespoon of water to thin slightly, if necessary. Peel **4 ripe bananas,** halve them lengthwise and arrange in four dishes. Top each banana with a scoop of frozen yogurt, **⅓ cup fresh raspberries, 1 tablespoon chopped almonds** and 2 tablespoons of the purée.

COOK'S TIPS

● If short on time, use prepared raspberry coulis and store-bought frozen yogurt or ice cream.
● For a big vanilla boost, try vanilla bean paste instead of vanilla extract.

BANANA SMOOTHIE

Serves 4
Preparation 5 minutes Chilling 30 minutes

Each serving provides • 136 calories • 1 g fat • 0 g saturated fat • 30 g carbohydrates • 4 g protein • 1 g fiber

Add **2 ripe bananas** to a blender with **2 tablespoons honey, ½ teaspoon ground cinnamon** and **1 heaping tablespoon wheat germ**. Blend for 10 seconds, then add **1 cup low-fat plain yogurt, 1¼ cups orange juice** and the **juice of ½ lemon**. Blend again until smooth. Chill for 30 minutes in the fridge before pouring into four tall glasses.

COOK'S TIPS

● Wheat germ is a tiny part of the wheat kernel that is high in protein, vitamin E, and potassium. You will find it in the cereal aisle in the supermarket or in health food stores.
● This smoothie is best drunk within an hour of making because it will thicken as the wheat germ absorbs liquid and the vitamin C content will begin to deteriorate.

PAN-FRIED BANANAS IN A SWEET CITRUS SAUCE

Serves 4
Preparation 5 minutes Cooking 5 minutes

Each serving provides • 163 calories • 6 g fat • 2 g saturated fat • 28 g carbohydrates • 1 g protein • 1 g fiber

Cut **4 just-ripe bananas** into bite-sized diagonal chunks. Heat **1 tablespoon butter** in a large frying pan with **2 teaspoons sunflower oil**. Add the banana chunks to the pan and cook for 3 minutes over medium heat until golden, then add the **juice of 1 orange, 1 tablespoon soft dark brown sugar** and a **dash of orange liqueur (optional)**. Stir for 2 minutes until bubbling then transfer to four plates, spoon the pan juices onto each plate and serve.

COOK'S TIPS

● For an oven-baked dessert, add 4 whole bananas to an ovenproof dish with the flavorings and bake at 350°F for 20 minutes, basting once or twice. Remove from the oven and sprinkle with 1 teaspoon dried coconut per portion.
● A spoonful of crème fraîche would make a tasty addition to the bananas.

KIWIFRUIT CHEESECAKE WITH LIME HONEY

Sinfully yummy—but not sinfully high in calories—this healthy take on traditional cheesecake blends low-fat yogurt or cream cheese with toasted muesli and a fruity combo bursting with vitamin C.

Serves 4
Preparation 10 minutes
Cooking 2 minutes

½ cup muesli
1 cup low-fat **Greek yogurt** or low-fat cream cheese
1 teaspoon **confectioners' sugar**
grated zest of **2 limes** and juice of 1 lime
2 tablespoons **honey**
4 ripe **kiwifruit**

Each serving provides
- 246 calories • 3 g fat • 1 g saturated fat • 47 g carbohydrates
- 8 g protein • 5 g fiber

ALTERNATIVE INGREDIENTS
- Try 3 crushed chocolate-chip cookies per portion instead of muesli.
- To make a red berry cheesecake, use a handful of raspberries or ripe strawberries per portion and leave out the kiwifruit.
- For a more substantial dessert, coarsely mash 2 bananas and mix them with the yogurt or cream cheese in step 1.

1 Preheat the broiler to high. Cover the broiler pan with foil and sprinkle the muesli evenly over it. Toast the muesli under the broiler for 2 minutes, stirring once or twice to prevent it from burning. Mix the yogurt or cream cheese with the confectioners' sugar and zest of 1 lime. Stir the lime juice into the honey. Peel and slice the kiwis.

2 Divide half of the toasted muesli among four dessert plates or bowls, spooning the cereal into small mounds. Top with the yogurt or cream cheese and sprinkle with the rest of the muesli. Flatten each portion into a 'cake' using a knife or the back of a spoon.

3 Arrange the kiwi slices on top of each cheesecake and sprinkle with the remaining lime zest. Drizzle with the lime and honey mixture just before serving.

COOK'S TIPS
● The exact weight of the muesli may vary slightly depending on the brand and its ingredients. As a guide, each cheesecake uses roughly 2 tablespoons of muesli.
● Instead of mounding the cheesecakes on plates, layer the muesli, cheese, and fruit into 3-inch cooking rings to form a tidy shape. Remove the rings just before serving.

SUPER FOOD

LIMES
Like all citrus fruit, limes are packed with vitamin C, which is essential for healthy skin, muscles, and bones and a booster for the body's immune system. Vitamin C also offers protection from some cancers and heart disease, and helps the body absorb essential iron.

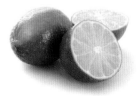

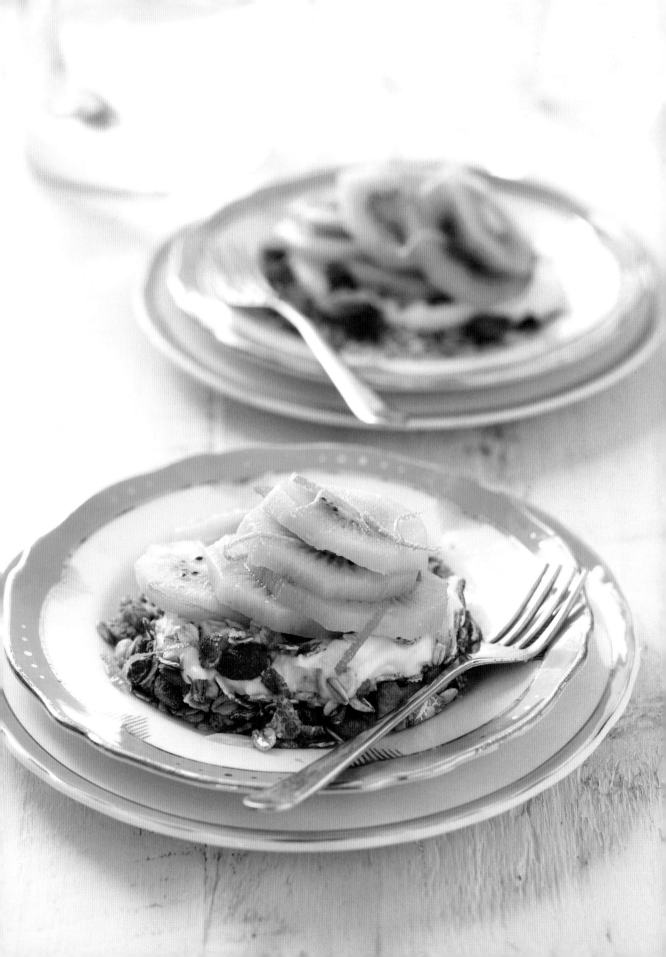

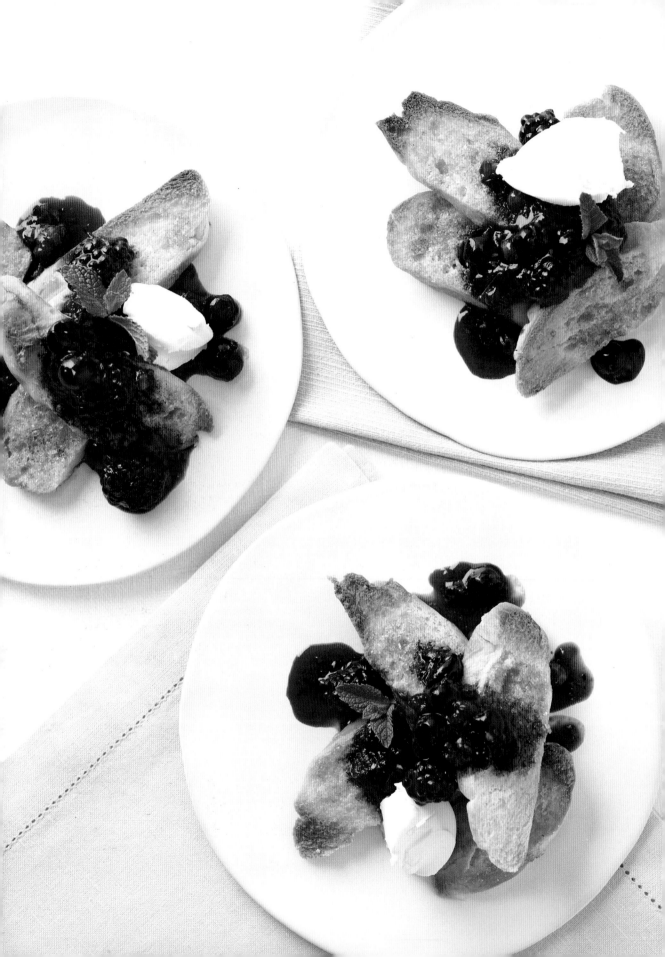

WARM **BERRIES** ON TOASTED **BRIOCHE**

A vibrant fruit mix, served over buttery brioche with a creamy mascarpone topping makes a flavor-drenched dessert. Even better, it's bursting with vitamins and fiber for your good health.

Serves 4
Preparation 5 minutes
Cooking 4 minutes

¼ cup raw sugar
3 tablespoons butter
4 brioche rolls
1 cup mixed berries, thawed
   if frozen
2 large fresh mint leaves, chopped
½ cup mascarpone
4 sprigs mint, to garnish

Each serving provides
• 257 calories • 12 g fat • 8 g saturated fat • 37 g carbohydrates • 4 g protein • 4 g fiber

ALTERNATIVE INGREDIENTS
• When berries are in season, this recipe can be made using fresh fruit. Choose from black currants, black cherries, raspberries, red currants, and strawberries.
• Greek yogurt makes a good alternative to mascarpone.

1 Preheat the broiler to high. Beat half of the sugar into the butter. Trim the rounded ends off the brioche rolls, then cut each one at a slant into four slices. Toast the slices under the broiler on one side.

2 Place the fruit in a small saucepan. Add 2 tablespoons of water and the remaining sugar, and bring to a boil over medium heat, stirring frequently. Cook for 1–2 minutes, or until the sugar dissolves and the fruit releases its juices. Remove the pan from the heat and add the chopped mint.

3 Spread the untoasted sides of the brioche with the sweetened butter. Toast under the broiler for 1 minute, or until the sugar melts and the edges of the slices are crisp and browned.

4 Transfer the brioche to four plates and spoon the hot mixed fruit over each portion. Top with a large spoonful of mascarpone and garnish with a sprig of mint before serving.

COOK'S TIPS
● Cook the mixed fruit over medium rather than high heat to avoid boiling the juices rapidly, which will toughen the skins. Remove the pan from the heat as soon as the juice boils.
● Currants and berries freeze well and can be cooked from frozen. Allow an extra 3–5 minutes cooking time in step 2 if using frozen fruit. If you grow your own raspberries, strawberries, or currants, rinse and freeze them as soon as possible after picking.

SUPER FOOD

MIXED BERRIES
Vividly colored berries contain valuable antioxidants that can slow down brain aging and enhance memory. They may also prevent and even repair skin damaged by the sun. Berries are also rich in pectin, a form of soluble fiber that can lower total cholesterol levels.

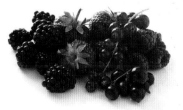

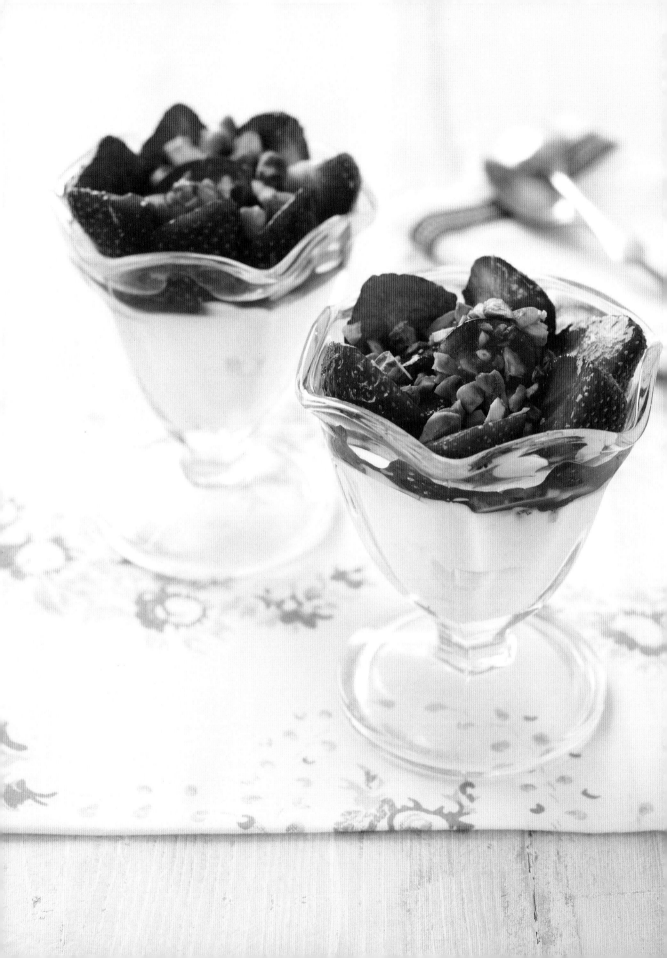

STRAWBERRY, GRAPE, AND PISTACHIO FLOWERS

What a tempting dessert! Simply arrange fresh strawberry 'petals' around a rosewater and cinnamon-infused grape center for an enticing bouquet of summertime treats.

Serves 4
Preparation 10 minutes

¼ teaspoon ground cinnamon
1 teaspoon rosewater
2 tablespoons honey
¾ cup seedless black grapes
1 tablespoon confectioners' sugar
½ teaspoon vanilla extract
1 cup low-fat Greek yogurt
1 cup low-fat cream cheese
1⅓ cups strawberries
2 tablespoons chopped pistachios

Each serving provides
• 273 calories • 7 g fat • 4 g saturated fat • 36 g carbohydrates • 15 g protein • 2 g fiber

ALTERNATIVE INGREDIENTS
• Use all Greek yogurt instead of half yogurt and half low-fat cream cheese for a more tangy flavor.
• Try sliced and quartered oranges instead of grapes, removing the bitter pith before mixing them with the cinnamon, rosewater, and honey.
• Sliced dried peaches or pears make great alternatives to the grapes. Allow two pieces of dried fruit per portion.

1 Mix the cinnamon, rosewater, and honey in a large bowl. Cut the grapes in half and toss them with the honey mixture.

2 In another bowl, lightly beat the confectioners' sugar and vanilla extract with the yogurt and softened cream cheese until smooth. Divide among four ice-cream dishes or tall dessert dishes. Level the surface of the mixture with the back of a spoon or a round-blade knife.

3 Hull the strawberries and cut them in half, slicing any large ones into smaller pieces. Arrange the strawberries around the edge of each dish to look like the petals of a flower. Spoon the grape mixture into the center of each portion and sprinkle with pistachios.

COOK'S TIPS
● Rosewater contributes a flowery flavor that goes perfectly with honey. It is usually found in the baking aisle of the supermarket.
● If you can't buy chopped pistachios, buy whole nuts and process them in a food processor for 10 seconds, or until finely chopped.

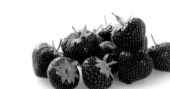

SUPER FOOD

STRAWBERRIES
A summer favorite, strawberries are rich in vitamin C, helping to boost the body's immune system and protect against aging. Strawberries also contain ellagic acid, an antioxidant found in berries and thought to have anti-cancer properties.

PINEAPPLE AND KIWIFRUIT WITH GINGERSNAP CREAM

Mint and preserved ginger are the surprise ingredients in a refreshing exotic fruit dessert. The kiwifruit and pineapple pieces are sweetly sharp, while a crunchy, gingersnap cream cheese adds just a hint of indulgence.

Serves 4
Preparation 20 minutes

½ pineapple
4 kiwifruit
4 pieces preserved ginger stem
6 large fresh mint leaves
4 gingersnaps
1 cup low-fat cream cheese, softened
4 sprigs fresh mint, to garnish

Each serving provides
• 217 calories • 5 g fat • 2 g saturated fat • 33 g carbohydrates • 9 g protein • 4 g fiber

ALTERNATIVE INGREDIENTS
• Instead of kiwifruit, use 1 cup seedless green grapes, cutting them in half first.
• Try ginger or chocolate shortbread cookies as a change from gingersnaps, or use almond macaroons if you want a softer texture.
• Crystallized ginger is more economical than preserved stem ginger. Use 1 heaping teaspoon chopped crystallized ginger per portion.

1 Peel, core, and slice the pineapple into wedges (see Cook's Tip). Peel, thickly slice the kiwifruit, and cut each slice in half. Thinly slice the preserved stem ginger. Shred the mint leaves and toss with the pineapple and kiwifruit.

2 In a plastic bag, crush the gingersnaps with a rolling pin to make fine crumbs. Stir the gingersnap crumbs into the cream cheese.

3 Arrange the pineapple and kiwifruit on four plates with a large spoonful of gingersnap cream cheese on the side. Top the cream cheese with sliced ginger and garnish each portion with a mint sprig.

COOK'S TIP
● To prepare a whole pineapple, cut off the leafy top and stem end. Slice off the skin with a sharp knife, working down the fruit to remove any eyes and spines. Divide the pineapple in half lengthwise and remove the tough core from both halves. Slice into semicircles and cut into wedges.

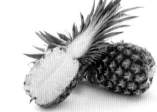

SUPER FOOD

PINEAPPLE
Like all fruit, pineapple is a low-calorie, health-promoting food. It contains fiber and potassium to help to regulate the body's blood pressure and fluid balance. With a glycemic index (GI) that is relatively high for fruit, pineapple is best eaten in combination with a low-GI food such as low-fat yogurt.

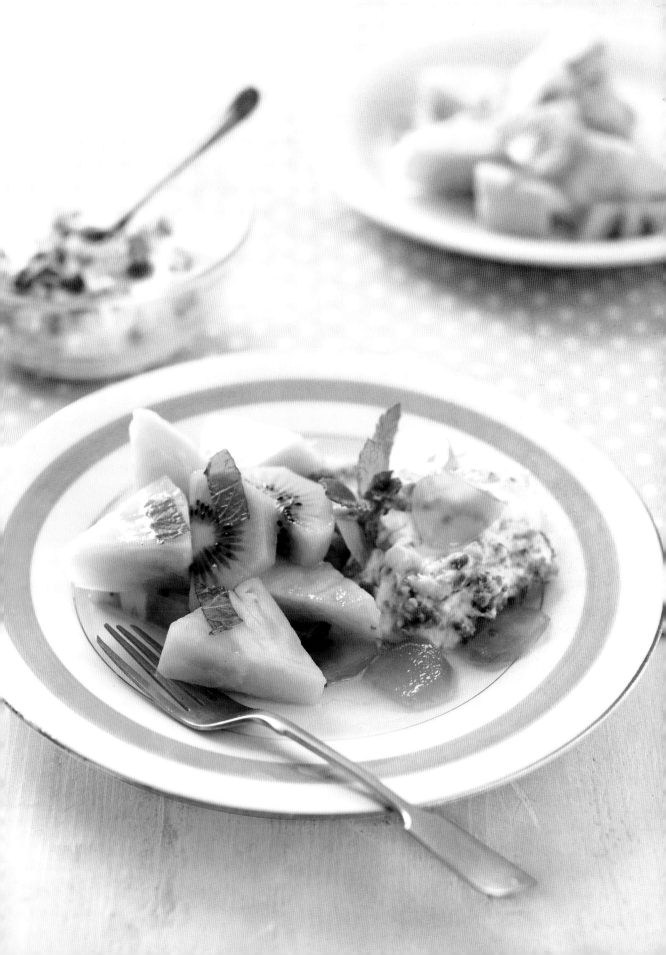

RED BERRY PANCAKES

Warm fruity pancakes make a feast for any meal, be it brunch or weekday family desserts. Use plenty of rich red berries, and finish with a little Greek yogurt.

Serves 4
Preparation 15 minutes
Cooking 8 minutes

⅔ cup self-rising flour
1 teaspoon sugar
1 egg
⅓ cup low-fat (1%) milk
½ cup red currants
12 strawberries
2 tablespoons unsalted butter
2–3 teaspoons superfine sugar
½ cup low-fat Greek yogurt

Each serving provides
• 265 calories • 8 g fat • 5 g saturated fat • 39 g carbohydrates
• 9 g protein • 3 g fiber

ALTERNATIVE INGREDIENTS
• Try fresh or frozen black currants, gooseberries, raspberries, or blueberries instead of red currants.
• Seasonal raspberries, blackberries, or pitted cherries make very tasty alternatives to strawberries.
• For a lactose-free dessert, make the batter with ⅓ cup unsweetened fruit juice, such as cranberry, apple, or orange juice, instead of milk.

1 Sift the flour into a bowl and stir in the sugar. Beat in the egg and a little of the milk to form a thick paste. Gradually add the rest of the milk, beating to remove any lumps until it forms a smooth, thick batter. Pull the stems off the red currants, if necessary, and stir the berries into the batter. Hull and halve the strawberries.

2 Heat a large frying pan over medium heat and melt half the butter. Use shaped molds (see Cook's Tips) to make the pancakes or cook four heaping teaspoonfuls of batter, spaced well apart, for 2 minutes, or until they are firm, set, and golden underneath.

3 Flip and cook for another minute, turning the heat down if the pancakes begin to burn. Transfer the pancakes to a dish and keep warm. Carefully wipe any berry juice from the pan with a paper towel, add the remaining butter, and cook four more pancakes using the rest of the batter. Transfer the pancakes to the dish and keep warm.

4 Add the strawberries to the hot pan for 30 seconds to warm through. Transfer the pancakes to four plates, top with the strawberries, some of the superfine sugar, and serve with Greek yogurt.

COOK'S TIPS
● To create shaped pancakes, place four heatproof molds in the frying pan, carefully spoon the batter into each mold, and let cook until firm. Carefully remove the molds and flip the pancakes to cook the other side.
● Currants are small, tart berries that can be sold fresh, frozen, or dried. Dried currants resemble small raisins, and won't work well in this recipe. If you can't find fresh or frozen currants, substitute other small fresh or frozen berries such as gooseberries, raspberries, or blueberries.

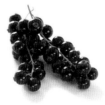

SUPER FOOD

RED CURRANTS
This versatile fruit, often used to make jelly, is rich in nutrients and high in health-promoting fiber. Red currants also contain potassium, which helps to regulate blood pressure, and vitamin C for healthy bones, teeth, and gums.

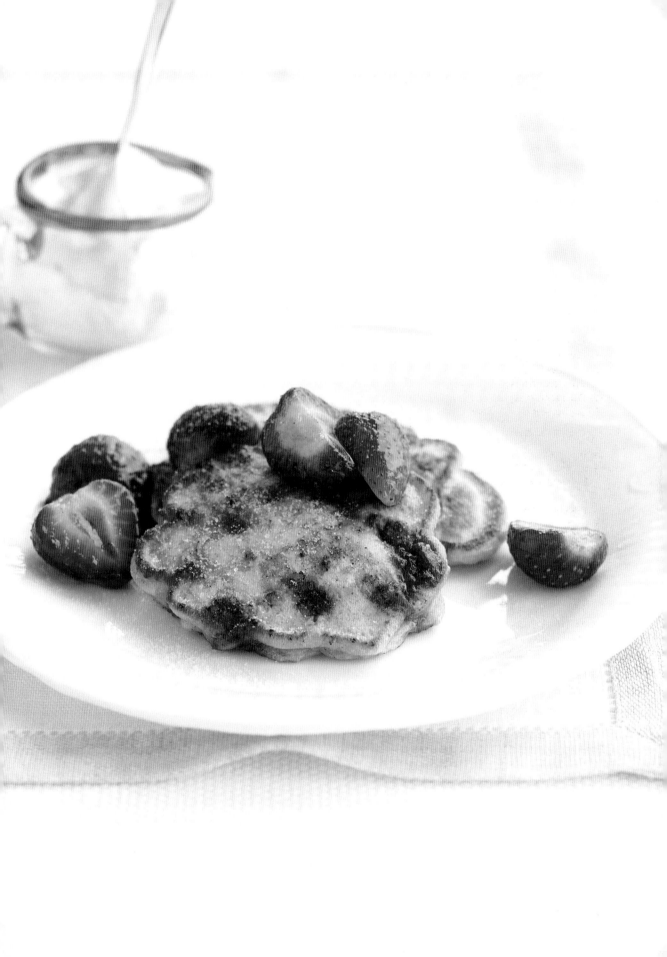

QUICK MIXED **BERRY** AND **ALMOND** DELIGHTS

A nutty but light topping of fiber-rich almonds and oats transforms a package of frozen mixed berries into a supercharged dessert that combines comfort food eating with healthy treating.

Serves 4
Preparation 10 minutes
Cooking 20 minutes

1¾ cups frozen mixed berries
⅓ cup ground almonds
¼ cup rolled oats
2 eggs
2 tablespoons honey
⅓ cup low-fat (1%) milk
½ teaspoon almond extract

Each serving provides
• 325 calories • 19 g fat • 2 g saturated fat • 29 g carbohydrates • 12 g protein • 6 g fiber

ALTERNATIVE INGREDIENTS
• Add some frozen cherries to the mixed berries. As they are larger, cherries will need an extra 5 minutes to cook.
• For a lactose-free dish, use apple juice instead of milk.

1 Preheat the oven to 400°F. Divide the frozen berries among four one-cup (4-inch-diameter) ramekins.

2 Mix the ground almonds and oats in a bowl and make a well in the center. Separate the eggs, adding the yolks with the almond mixture and the whites in a separate, clean bowl. Pour the honey, milk, and almond extract into the well in the oat mixture and beat the ingredients together to form a soft, dropping consistency (see Cook's Tip).

3 Whisk the egg whites until stiff and beat one-third of them into the oat mixture. Use a metal spoon to fold in the remaining egg whites. Spoon the pudding mixture over the frozen berries, levelling the top.

4 Place the ramekins on a baking sheet and bake for 20 minutes, or until the mixture browns, rises, and is slightly cracked and firm to the touch. Serve hot.

COOK'S TIP
● A dropping consistency is achieved when the mixture drops easily off your spoon when tapped against the side of the bowl. The mixture should be firm and not sloppy.

SUPER FOOD

ALMONDS
There is good evidence that a handful of nuts, especially almonds, eaten daily, can lower harmful cholesterol. Almonds contain 7 g fiber per ⅓ cup, good news because high-fiber foods may protect against bowel cancer.

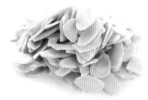

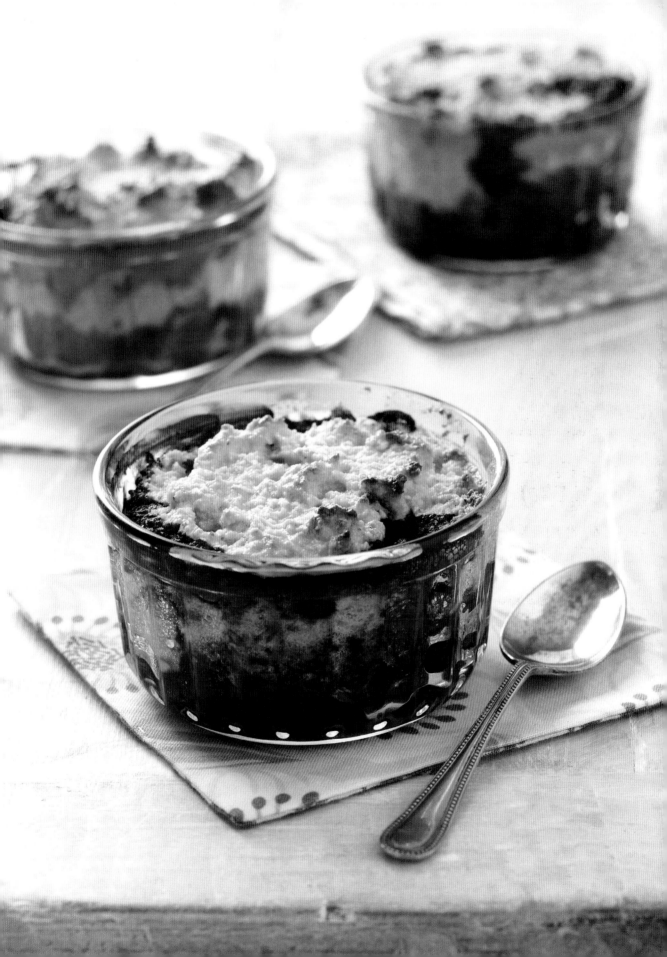

SPICED **RHUBARB** AND **BLUEBERRY** COMPOTE

Ginger delivers a delicious spike to this versatile compote that can be served warm or chilled, for breakfast or dessert—perfect with a scoop of ice cream or yogurt. The fruit provides a mouthwatering cocktail of vitamins.

Serves 4
Preparation 5 minutes
Cooking 10 minutes
Chilling 30 minutes (optional)

1¼ pounds rhubarb
3 tablespoons sugar
3 tablespoons crystallized ginger
½ cup blueberries

Each serving provides
• 83 calories • 0 g fat • 0 g saturated fat • 20 g carbohydrates
• 1 g protein • 3 g fiber

ALTERNATIVE INGREDIENTS
• Frozen blueberries can be used in place of fresh ones, but the rhubarb must be fresh, not canned.
• Strawberries are a traditional partner with rhubarb.
• Serve the rhubarb and blueberry compote with muesli and yogurt for a nutritious breakfast.
• Pit ½ to ¾ pounds of cherries and add them to the rhubarb, omitting the blueberries and ginger and adding an extra tablespoonful of sugar.
• Serve as a healthy topping for pancakes or waffles.

1 Cut rhubarb into ¾- to 1¼-inch lengths and place in a large saucepan. Sprinkle sugar over the fruit and add 1 tablespoon water. Cook over high heat for 30 seconds, or until sugar begins to dissolve.

2 Reduce heat to medium or medium-low, so the fruit simmers. Cover and simmer for 5–8 minutes, stirring once, until the rhubarb is tender but still firm.

3 Cut the crystallized ginger into ⅛-inch slices. Remove pan from the heat and add the ginger and blueberries. Stir gently and divide among four bowls. Serve immediately or chill for 30 minutes.

COOK'S TIPS
● Small, fresh rhubarb stalks are usually tender and only need the ends of the trimmed and the poisonous leaves discarded. Larger or older stalks should be thinly peeled to remove the skin, which can be stringy.
● Make the stewed rhubarb and keep it in a covered container in the fridge for up to 3 days. Add the blueberries and ginger just before serving.

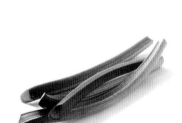

SUPER FOOD

RHUBARB
A low sugar content, and therefore a low glycemic index (GI), means that rhubarb can help steady blood glucose levels, which is great for weight control and keeping hunger at bay. With fiber and potassium as extra nutritional benefits, rhubarb helps to maintain a healthy digestive system.

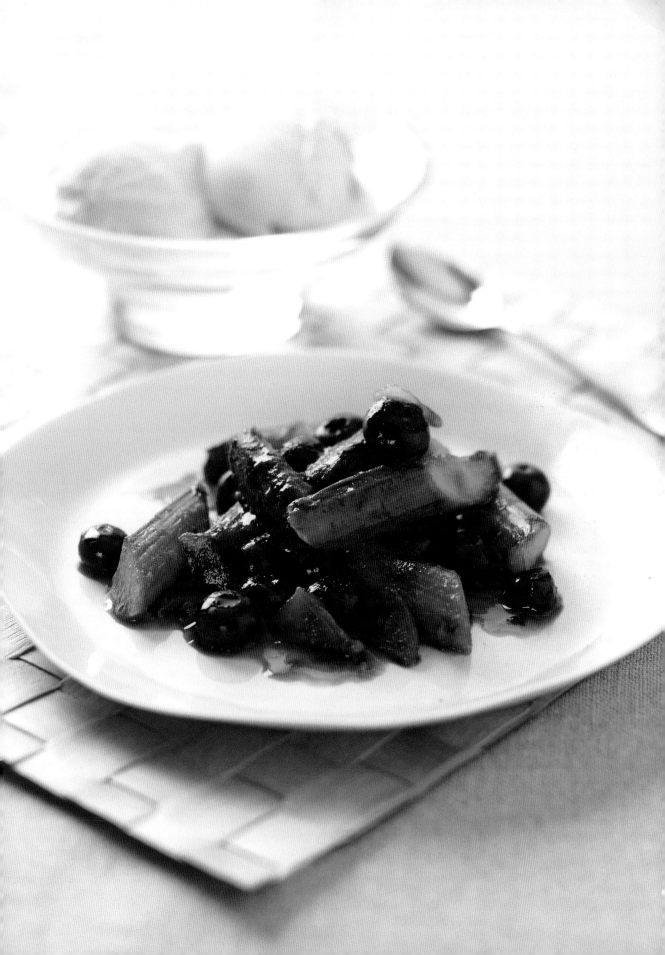

BLUEBERRIES

A nutritional supernova, blueberries are bursting with antioxidants that can offer protection against long-term health problems such as some cancers and heart disease. As fiber providers, blueberries also do their part in supporting a healthy digestive system.

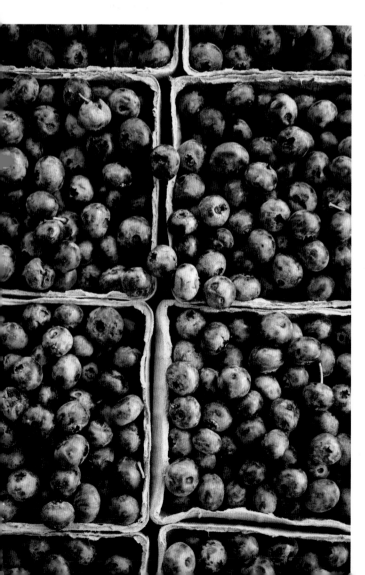

INDIVIDUAL SUMMER PUDDINGS

Serves 4
Preparation 5 minutes Cooking 5 minutes
Chilling 1½ hours

Each serving provides • 175 calories • 3 g fat • 1 g saturated fat • 35 g carbohydrates • 5 g protein • 5 g fiber

Poach **1 cup blueberries** and **1 cup raspberries** in a saucepan with 3 tablespoons of water, **3 tablespoons superfine sugar** and the **juice of 1 lemon** for 5 minutes, or until the juices are released. Line four dariole molds or large popover cups with plastic wrap. Remove the crusts from **5 thin brown bread slices**, cut each slice into four squares, use them to line the molds, placing one square on the bottom and four around the sides. Spoon the fruit and juice into the lined molds, wrap in plastic wrap, and chill in the fridge for 1½ hours. Lift the puddings out of the molds using the plastic wrap and transfer to four plates. Top each pudding with **1 tablespoon reduced-fat crème fraîche** and serve.

COOK'S TIP

● When pouring the fruit juice into the molds, make sure that it covers as much of the bread as possible.
● Dariole molds are small metal cylindrical cups that are often used for making small pastries. Popover cups have deep, steep-sided wells that are designed to make popovers. If you don't have either, you can use regular small cups or glasses.

BERRY FROZEN YOGURT

Serves 4
Preparation 5 minutes Cooking 15 minutes
Freezing 5 hours

Each serving provides • 309 calories • 6 g fat • 2 g saturated fat • 56 g carbohydrates • 11 g protein • 3 g fiber

Place **1¾ cups blueberries** in a small saucepan with **2 tablespoons superfine sugar** and 2 tablespoons of cold water. Bring to a boil over high heat, lower heat, and simmer the fruit for 5 minutes. Let cool. Whisk **2 egg yolks** in a bowl with **⅓ cup superfine sugar** and **1 cup low-fat Greek yogurt**. Transfer to a small saucepan and warm gently over low heat, stirring continuously, for 10 minutes, or until the mixture thickens slightly. Remove from the heat. Mash **1 ripe banana** with **¼ teaspoon ground cinnamon, juice of ½ lemon** and **1 cup low-fat plain yogurt**. Stir this mixture into the pan. Add the blueberries with any juice and stir again. Freeze in an ice-cream maker following the manufacturer's directions, or transfer to a covered plastic container and freeze for at least 5 hours, removing from the freezer every hour and beating to remove any ice crystals. When ready to serve, leave the frozen yogurt at room temperature for 15 minutes to thaw slightly and scoop into bowls.

COOK'S TIP
● Serve two scoops of frozen yogurt in a bowl with one crunchy cookie or wafer per person.

BLUEBERRY CRÈME BRÛLÉE

Serves 4
Preparation 5 minutes Cooking 12 minutes
Chilling 1 hour

Each serving provides • 185 calories • 13 g fat
• 8 g saturated fat • 16 g carbohydrates • 2 g protein
• 1 g fiber

Preheat the broiler to high. Put **½ cup blueberries**, 1 tablespoon of water, and **2 teaspoons superfine sugar** in a saucepan over a medium-high heat and simmer for 2 minutes. Spoon the blueberries, and any juice, into four 1 cup (4-inch diameter) ramekins. Put **2 graham crackers** in a plastic bag and crush them with a rolling pin. Gently beat **1¼ cups low-fat crème fraîche** with **1 teaspoon vanilla extract** in a bowl and stir in the cookie crumbs. Spoon the mixture over the blueberries and level the surface. Sprinkle **1 level tablespoon brown sugar** evenly over each ramekin and broil for 10 minutes, or until the sugar caramelizes. Cool slightly before transferring to the fridge to chill for 1 hour, or until the tops harden.

COOK'S TIP
● For a nutty crème brûlée, replace the graham crackers with 2 tablespoons chopped blanched almonds.

BLUEBERRY AND BUTTERMILK MUFFINS

Makes 6
Preparation 20 minutes, plus 15 minutes cooling
Cooking 25 minutes

Each serving provides • 287 calories • 6 g fat
• 1 g saturated fat • 52 g carbohydrates • 9 g protein
• 4 g fiber

Preheat the oven to 350°F. In a large bowl, combine **⅔ cup self-rising flour** with **⅔ cup whole-wheat**

self-rising flour, **1 teaspoon baking powder**, **zest of ½ lemon** and **¼ cup soft light brown sugar**. In another bowl, beat **1 egg** and stir in **⅔ cup cup buttermilk** and **1 tablespoon sunflower oil**. Using a large metal spoon, gently stir the wet ingredients into the dry ingredients. Add **½ cup blueberries**. Spoon the mixture into a six-muffin pan lined with paper liners and bake for 25 minutes, or until golden. Cool in the pan for 15 minutes and transfer to a wire rack.

COOK'S TIPS
● Use half low-fat (1%) milk and half low-fat plain yogurt if you can't get buttermilk.
● The muffins will keep fresh for 48 hours in an airtight container but are best eaten right after baking.

FRUIT EXPLOSION MUESLI

Serves 4
Preparation 10 minutes, plus 15 minutes standing

Each serving provides • 295 calories • 12 g fat
• 1 g saturated fat • 41 g carbohydrates • 8 g protein
• 6 g fiber

Place **⅓ cup rolled oats** in a large bowl and stir in **1 tablespoon sunflower seeds**, **1 tablespoon pumpkin seeds**, **2 tablespoons chopped hazelnuts**, **2 tablespoons chopped almonds** and **1 tablespoon finely chopped dried apricots**. Add **2 grated apples** with the skins on and **½ cup blueberries**. Pour in **1 cup orange juice**, stir and let soak for 15 minutes. When ready to serve, divide the muesli among four bowls, add **½ teaspoon brown sugar**, and **1 heaping tablespoon plain yogurt** to each bowl.

COOK'S TIPS
● For variety, include a mixture of whole grains, such as wheat germ or rye flakes, in addition to rolled oats.
● For muesli with added crunch, roughly chop the apricots and leave the almonds whole.

POACHED **PEACHES** AND **PEARS** IN A **BLUEBERRY** JUS

Few things are more mouthwatering than a juicy peach and a ripe pear, and poaching is a great way to make them extra delectable. Using nothing but the goodness of fresh fruit and juice guarantees a sweet but healthy dessert.

Serves 4
Preparation 5 minutes
Cooking 30 minutes

4 cups blueberry juice drink
2 large firm peaches
2 large pears
½ cup blueberries

Each serving provides
• 194 calories • 0 g fat • 0 g saturated fat • 48 g carbohydrates • 1 g protein • 5 g fiber

ALTERNATIVE INGREDIENTS
• A smart way to combine the first pears of the season with late-season raspberries is to use raspberry juice drink instead of blueberry juice drink and top the peaches and pears with ½ cup raspberries in place of blueberries.
• If you can't find blueberry or raspberry juice drink, red grape juice will also work.
• Try dried peaches or mango slices instead of fresh peaches. Use 2 dried peach halves per portion or 3 mango slices. Poach the dried fruit with the pears for 5 minutes.

1 Pour the blueberry juice drink into a large saucepan. Halve and pit the peaches, leaving the skins on, and add them to the pan as they are prepared. Peel, halve, and core the pears and add them to the pan.

2 Bring the blueberry juice drink to a boil over high heat, reduce heat to medium so the juice is simmering, and poach the fruit for 10 minutes, or until tender, testing the fruit with the tip of a knife. Use a slotted spoon to transfer the fruit to a bowl, then set aside.

3 Increase heat to high and boil the blueberry juice drink for 20 minutes, or until it is reduced to a thick glaze. Watch it carefully after 10 minutes so it doesn't boil over. Divide the fruit among four bowls and spoon a little glaze over each portion. Top with fresh blueberries and serve.

COOK'S TIPS

● Firm peaches do not shed their skins when cooked but become tender and juicy. They also retain heat better than peeled fruit and remain warm while the juice drink is being reduced.
● For a healthy breakfast treat, prepare the glazed fruit the day before, cool, cover, and store in the fridge overnight.

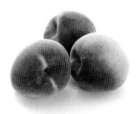

SUPER FOOD

PEACHES
Low in calories, peaches make a perfect healthy snack or dessert, with vitamin C to fortify the body's immune system. Peaches also contain beta-carotene, which the body converts to vitamin A for healthy skin and eyes.

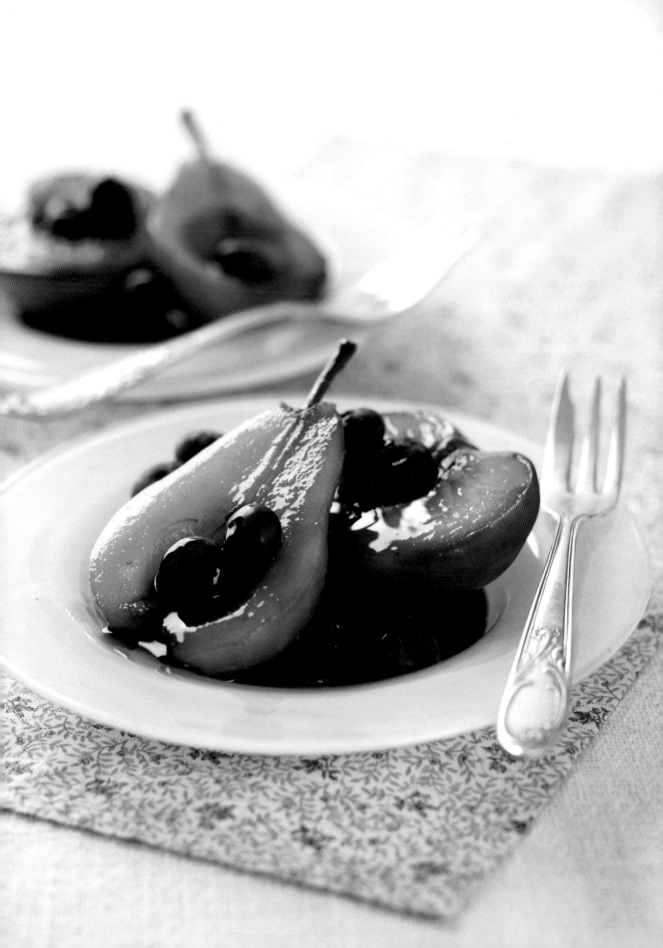

CHOCOLATE AND PECAN DIP WITH FRUIT

Rich dark chocolate, crunchy nuts, and sweet honey combine for a tempting dip that is actually chock-full of healthy fruit. A little goes a long way, so take it easy and you'll be more saint than sinner.

Serves 4
Preparation 10 minutes
Cooking 5 minutes

4 ounces dark chocolate
4 teaspoons honey
¼ cup finely chopped pecans
½ cup low-fat cream cheese, softened
Fresh fruit, such as bananas, pineapple chunks, mandarin orange segments, strawberries, pitted cherries (about ¾ cup per person)

Each serving provides
• 370 calories • 23 g fat • 9 g saturated fat • 32 g carbohydrates • 9 g protein • 5 g fiber

1 Break the chocolate into 1-inch pieces and place them in a small heatproof bowl. Drizzle in the honey and put the bowl over a saucepan of simmering water set over low heat for 5 minutes, stirring occasionally, or until the chocolate has melted.

2 Remove the bowl from the pan and cool slightly. Stir in 2 tablespoons of the cream cheese and the pecans. Gradually stir in the remaining cream cheese and transfer the dipping sauce to a large serving bowl or four individual bowls.

3 Prepare a selection of fresh fruit for serving with the chocolate and nut dipping sauce. Cut the fruit into bite-sized pieces and arrange them on a serving dish. Serve the sauce warm with the fresh fruit to dip.

COOK'S TIP
● To prevent chocolate from separating when it is being melted, use a small pan that fits neatly under the bowl. It is essential to avoid getting water or steam in the chocolate because this will make the fat separate from the chocolate solids, causing the chocolate to become stiff and grainy. Do not overheat chocolate, as it burns easily.

SUPER FOOD

PECANS
Rich in beneficial cholesterol-lowering unsaturated fats, pecans are good for the heart. In addition, they are high in fiber, omega-3s, B vitamins, and vitamin E for healthy skin. Pecans also contain flavonoids, potent plant-based antioxidants that may help to protect against cancer.

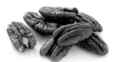

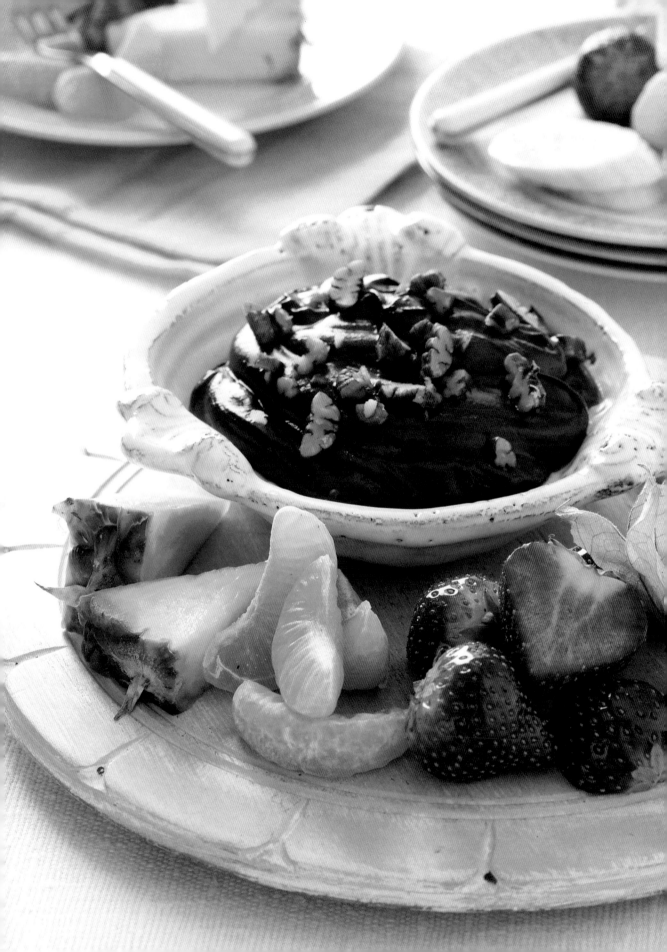

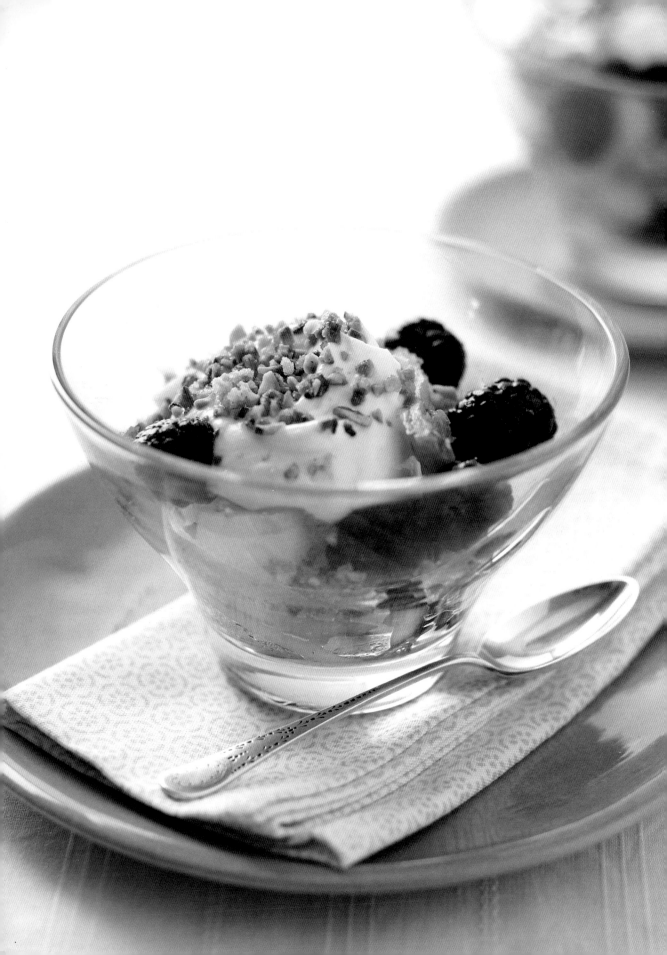

HOT **FRUIT PUDDINGS** TOPPED WITH **HAZELNUT PRALINE**

Succulent dried pears, tart apples, and luscious raspberries are topped with a layer of creamy yogurt and sprinkled with a crunchy nut praline. Each mouthful promises plenty of vitamins and calcium.

Serves 4
Preparation 5 minutes, plus
2 minutes standing
Cooking 10 minutes
Chilling 30 minutes

¾ pound tart apples, such as
　Granny Smith
⅓ cup dried pears, cut in
　½-inch wedges
1 cup raspberries
2 cups low-fat Greek yogurt
⅓ cup roasted chopped hazelnuts
¼ cup sugar

Each serving provides
• 459 calories • 20 g fat • 3 g
saturated fat • 57 g carbohydrates
• 15 g protein • 9 g fiber

ALTERNATIVE INGREDIENTS
• Pitted cherries make a succulent
replacement for raspberries.
• Sliced almonds are a good
alternative to hazelnuts. Buy them
already toasted or broil for a minute
under medium-hot heat before adding
the sugar.

1 Peel, core, and slice the apples into ½-inch wedges and place in a large saucepan. Add 4 tablespoons boiling water and return to a boil over high heat. Cover, reduce heat, and simmer for 4 minutes, stirring once.

2 Add the pears to the apples and remove the pan from the heat. Mix in the raspberries and divide the fruit among four bowls. Spoon the yogurt over the fruit. Cover, let cool, and chill in the fridge for 30 minutes, ready for finishing with the nut topping.

3 To make the praline, mix the hazelnuts and sugar in a heavy frying pan. Cook over high heat for 1–2 minutes, or until the sugar begins to melt. Shake the pan and continue to cook, stirring frequently, for another 1–2 minutes, or until the sugar turns golden brown.

4 Working quickly so the sugar doesn't burn in the hot pan, spoon the praline on top of each desserts. Let stand for 1–2 minutes so the praline can cool slightly before being served.

COOK'S TIPS
● Praline is a crunchy sweet made by boiling nuts in sugar. If serving the desserts in glass dishes, spread the praline out on a lightly oiled baking sheet to cool slightly, otherwise the heat might crack the glass.
● The praline topping can be made, cooled, and stored in an airtight jar. It will keep for several months, ready for sprinkling over fruit compotes or yogurt.

SUPER FOOD

YOGURT
One small dish of yogurt a day provides nearly one-third of your daily calcium needs. Probiotic yogurt contains lactobacillus and bifido bacteria, which, if eaten regularly, can boost 'friendly' bacteria in the bowel and colon, helping to maintain and promote healthy digestion.

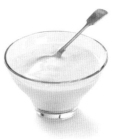

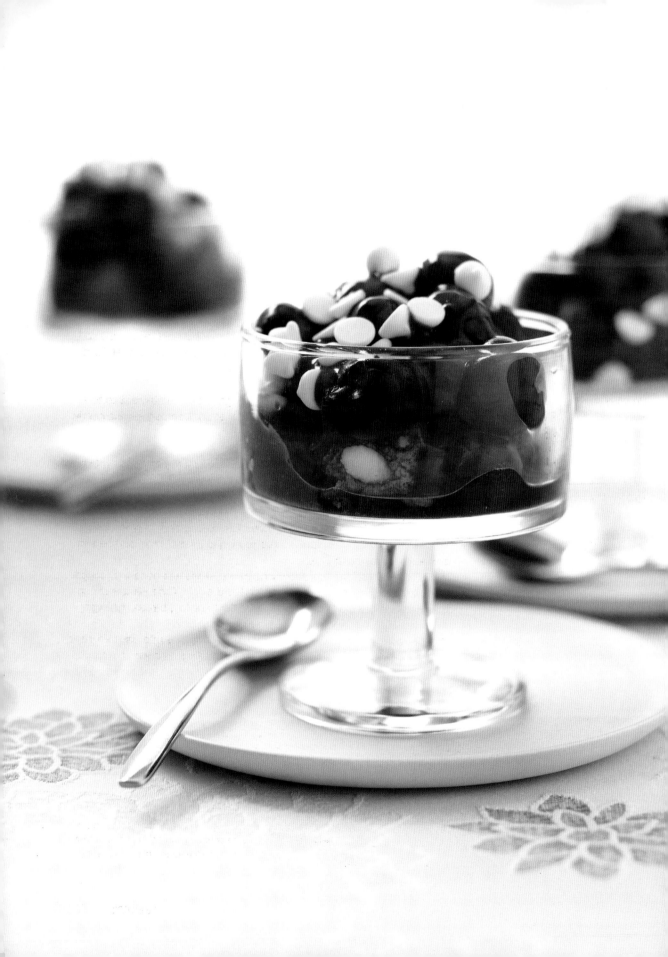

WARM **CHERRY** AND **CHOCOLATE** TRIFLE

Biscotti make a crunchy base for a medley of cherries and blueberries, coated in a smooth chocolate sauce. The fruit bursts with potassium, which helps to keep blood pressure under control.

Serves 4
Preparation 10 minutes
Cooking 5 minutes

6 biscotti, about 6 ounces
1 can (15 ounces) pitted cherries
   in juice or syrup
⅔ cup blueberries
2 tablespoons cornstarch
2 tablespoons cocoa powder
1⅓ cups low-fat (1%) milk
1 teaspoon vanilla extract
2 tablespoons sugar
¼ cup white chocolate chips

Each serving provides
• 479 calories • 11 g fat • 6 g saturated fat • 89 g carbohydrates • 9 g protein • 2 g fiber

ALTERNATIVE INGREDIENTS
• Use amaretti cookies or almond macaroons instead of biscotti.

1 Break the biscotti in half and divide them among four dishes, 3 halves per dish. Drain the cherries over a bowl to catch the juice. Spoon the juice over the biscotti and let them soak for 5 minutes before topping with the cherries and blueberries.

2 Whisk the cornstarch and cocoa powder with a little milk in a small saucepan. Gradually whisk in the remaining milk. Use a spatula to scrape up any cornstarch from the bottom of the pan.

3 In the pan over medium to medium-high heat, bring the sauce to a boil, whisking continuously. Reduce heat and simmer, stirring gently, for 2 minutes. Whisk in the vanilla extract and sugar.

4 Pour the sauce over the fruit. Sprinkle with chocolate chips and use the tip of a knife to swirl the chocolate around as it melts.

COOK'S TIPS
● Try flavored biscotti, such as almond, chocolate, or pistachio.
● Be sure cherries are pitted before you buy them as some bottled and canned cherries contain pits.
● Adding sugar to the milk and cocoa sauce at the end of cooking helps to prevent it from browning and sticking to the pan. The milk and cocoa sauce may seem too thick before the sugar is added, but as the sugar melts, your sauce will thin to the proper consistency.
● Instead of chocolate chips, break a bar of chocolate into squares, drop them into a strong plastic bag, and use a rolling pin to crush into pieces.

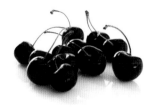

SUPER FOOD

CHERRIES
High in fiber, cherries are good for digestive health. They are rich in health-protecting anthocyanins, and also contain plenty of potassium that can help to regulate blood pressure.

INDEX

Super foods are shown in **bold**.
Page numbers in *italic* indicate where super food nutritional information can be found.

Reader's digest

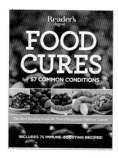

Discover how highly nutritional foods can be used to treat common ailments naturally, safely, and deliciously. Includes 75 recipes formulated to help you live pain free, disease free, and worry free.

ISBN 978-0-76210-797-1
$17.99 paperback
352 pages/75 recipes/7¾ x 10
Over 200 photos & illustrations

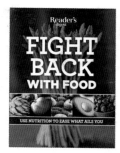

An authoritative, easy-to-use reference arranged in an A-to-Z format, revealing 50 superstar foods to help fight 50 common ailments. Includes over 100 recipes for treating and fighting disease.

ISBN 978-0-76210-840-4
$17.99 paperback
352 pages/100+ recipes/8 x 10¼
Over 200 photos & illustrations

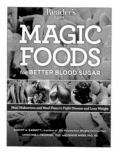

Discover 57 magic foods that can change your life, with 100 appetizing recipes designed to rein in insulin resistance, offload dangerous belly fat, guard against diabetes, and leave you ready to embrace life.

ISBN 978-0-76210-895-4
$17.99 paperback
304 pages/100+ recipes/7¾ x 10
Over 100 photos & illustrations

Reader's Digest books can be purchased through retail and online bookstores.